Posttraumatic Stress Disorder

Diagnosis, Management, and Treatment

Second Edition

Edited by

David J Nutt, PhD, MA, DM, FRCP, FRCPsych, FMedSci
Department of Neuropsychopharmacology and Molecular Imaging
Imperial College London
Hammersmith Hospital
London
United Kingdom

Murray B Stein, MD, FRCPC, MPH
Department of Psychiatry
University of California at San Diego
La Jolla, California
United States of America

and

Joseph Zohar, MD
Division of Psychiatry
Chaim Sheba Medical School
Tel Hashomer
and Sackler School of Medicine
Tel Aviv University
Tel Aviv
Israel

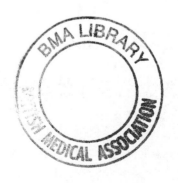
informa
healthcare

First published in 2009 by Informa Healthcare, Telephone House, 69-77 Paul Street, London EC2A 4LQ. Informa Healthcare is a trading division of Informa UK Ltd. Registered Office: 37/41 Mortimer Street, London W1T 3JH. Registered in England and Wales number 1072954.

A CIP record for this book is available from the British Library.
Library of Congress Cataloging-in-Publication Data

Data available on application

ISBN-13: 9780415395717

Distributed in North and South America by

Taylor & Francis
6000 Broken Sound Parkway, NW (Suite 300)
Boca Raton, FL 33487, USA

Within Continental USA

Tel: 1 (800) 272 7737; Fax: 1 (800) 374 3401

Outside Continental USA

Tel: 1-859-727-5000
Fax: 1-859-647-4028
E-mail: orders@taylorandfrancis.com

Orders in the rest of the world

Informa Healthcare
Sheepen Place
Colchester
Essex CO3 3LP
UK

Telephone: +44 (0)20 7017 5540
Email: CSDhealthcarebooks@informa.com

Typeset byC&M Digitals (P) Ltd, Chennai, India
Printed and bound in Great Britain by MPG Books Ltd, Bodmin, Cornwall, UK

Contents

List of contributors   **v**

Foreword   **vii**
Simon Wessely

1   Posttraumatic stress disorder: Diagnosis, history, and longitudinal course   1
Arieh Y Shalev

2   Epidemiology of traumatic events and posttraumatic stress disorder   12
Tracie O Afifi, Gordon JG Asmundson, and Jitender Sareen

3   Diagnostic dilemmas in assessing posttraumatic stress disorder   25
Berthold PR Gersons and Miranda Olff

4   Neuroimaging and posttraumatic stress disorder   36
Sarah N Garfinkel and Israel Liberzon

5   Brain circuits in posttraumatic stress disorder   51
Eric Vermetten and Ruth Lanius

6   The genetics of posttraumatic stress disorder   70
Eduard Maron and Jakov Shlik

7   Setting apart the affected: A novel animal model for posttraumatic stress disorder and its translational perspective   88
Joseph Zohar, Michael Matar, and Hagit Cohen

8   Psychosocial treatments of posttraumatic stress disorder   99
Kerry J Ressler and Barbara O Rothbaum

9   Pharmacotherapy of posttraumatic stress disorder   116
Lakshmi N Ravindran and Murray B Stein

10   Early interventions following traumatic events   127
Jonathan I Bisson, Arieh Y Shalev, and Joseph Zohar

11   Traumatic stress disorders in children   147
Soraya Seedat

12   Ethnocultural issues   163
Alexander McFarlane and Devon Hinton

13   Posttraumatic stress disorder after disasters   176
Andrea R Maxwell and Sandro Galea

14   Symptom exaggeration in posttraumatic stress disorder   187
Alzbeta Juven-Wetzler, Rachel Sonnino, Danit Bar-Ziv, and Joseph Zohar

15   Future directions   195
Joseph Zohar, Murray B Stein, and David Nutt

Index   201

List of contributors

Tracie O Afifi
Anxiety and Illness Behaviors Laboratory
University of Regina
Regina, Saskatchewan, Canada

Gordon JG Asmundson
Anxiety and Illness Behaviors
    Laboratory
Department of Psychology
University of Regina
Regina, Saskatchewan, Canada

Danit Bar-Ziv
Chaim Sheba Medical Center
Tel Hashomer, Israel

Jonathan I Bisson
School of Medicine
Cardiff University
Cardiff, UK

Hagit Cohen
Israel Ministry of Health Mental Health
    Center
and
Anxiety and Stress Research Unit
Faculty of Health Sciences
Ben-Gurion University of the Negev
Beer-Sheva, Israel

Sandro Galea
Medical School
School of Public Health
Institute for Social Research
University of Michigan
Ann Arbor, Michigan, USA

Sarah N Garfinkel
Department of Psychiatry
University of Michigan
Ann Arbor, Michigan, USA

Berthold PR Gersons
Department of Psychiatry
Amsterdam Medical Center
Amsterdam, The Netherlands

Devon Hinton
Harvard Medical School
Boston, Massachusetts, USA

Alzbeta Juven-Wetzler
Chaim Sheba Medical Center
Tel Hashomer, Israel

Ruth Lanius
Department of Psychiatry
University of Western Ontario
London, Ontario, Canada

Israel Liberzon
Department of Psychiatry
University of Michigan
and Ann Arbor VA Medical Center
Ann Arbor, Michigan, USA

Eduard Maron
Department of Mental Health
The North Estonian Regional Hospital
    Psychiatry Clinic
Tallinn, Estonia
and Department of Psychiatry
University of Tartu
Tartu, Estonia

Michael Matar
Israel Ministry of Health Mental Health
    Center
and Anxiety and Stress Research Unit
Faculty of Health Sciences
Ben-Gurion University of the Negev
Beer-Sheva, Israel

Andrea R Maxwell
Department of Epidemiology
University of Michigan School of Public
    Health
Ann Arbor, Michigan, USA

Alexander McFarlane
The Centre for Military and Veterans' Health
The University of Adelaide,
Adelaide, Australia

David J Nutt
Department of Neuropsychopharmacology
    and Molecular Imaging
Imperial College London
Hammersmith Hospital
London, UK

Miranda Olff
Center for Psychological Trauma
Department of Psychiatry
Academic Medical Center
University of Amsterdam
Amsterdam, The Netherlands

Lakshmi N Ravindran
Mood and Anxiety Program
Centre for Addiction and Mental Health
Toronto, ON, Canada

Kerry Ressler
Department of Psychiatry and Behavioral
    Sciences
Yerkes Research Center
Emory University
Atlanta, Georgia, USA

Barbara O Rothbaum,
Trauma and Anxiety Recovery Program
Department of Psychiatry
Emory University School of Medicine
Atlanta, Georgia, USA

Jitender Sareen
Department of Psychiatry
and
Department of Community Health Sciences
University of Manitoba
Winnipeg, Manitoba, Canada

Soraya Seedat
Department of Psychiatry
University of Stellenbosch
Cape Town, South Africa

Arieh Y Shalev
Department of Psychiatry
Hadassah University Hospital
Jerusalem, Israel

Jakov Shlik
Department of Psychiatry
University of Ottawa
and
Anxiety Disorders Program
Royal Ottawa Mental Health Centre
Ottawa, Ontario, Canada

Rachel Sonnino
Chaim Sheba Medical Center
Tel Hashomer, Israel

Murray B Stein
Department of Psychiatry
University of California at San Diego
La Jolla, California, USA

Eric Vermetten
Military Mental Health Center
and
Rudolf Magnus Institute of Neurosciences
University Medical Center
Utrecht, The Netherlands

Simon Wessely
King's Centre for Military Health Research
Institute of Psychiatry
King's College London
London, UK

Joseph Zohar
Chaim Sheba Medical Center
Tel Hashomer
Sackler School of Medicine
Tel Aviv University
Tel Aviv, Israel

Foreword

When writing an introduction to an already established text the easiest option is to turn to the first edition and see what has changed over the years. And so never one to turn down the easy route, that is what I have done.

Many things remain much the same, which is reassuring, as one sign of a maturing field is stability. Some problems have not been solved. Diagnostic dilemmas remain, both as a chapter, and as a problem. Neuroscience was the great prospect in 2000, and remains a great prospect today. The sense of optimism conveyed in the final chapters in 2000 is undiminished, and indeed some progress has been made. Neuroimaging has delivered at least some goods, although the hope that this would translate into treatment advances expressed ten years ago remains a hope today. Nevertheless, Vermetten is able to highlight for example a study in which long-term treatment of PTSD with paroxetine increased hippocampal volume, suggesting some neurogenerating actions of 5HT, which if replicated represents a genuine advance. Likewise, using the tryptophan depletion paradigm Professor Nutt's team have elegantly shown that 5HT might be critical to restraining the expression of anxiety in PTSD when treated with SSRIs, although this in turn also takes us back to the issue of comorbidity and whether PTSD is just another shuffling of the anxiety disorder cards, rather than a unique diagnostic and biological entity.

A new and impressive addition is an authoritative chapter on genetics. The concept that hereditary factors might play a role in the etiology of PTSD was a baby thrown out with the 1980 bathwater when they sat down to redraft the DSM and turned their backs on the previous half century of thinking on predisposition, so it is good to see it back in there.

And what about treatment? The chapter on debriefing has gone, now incorporated into a general discussion of early interventions. The reawakening of interest into the older literature that suggested that ordinary people are and remain fairly resilient is starting to influence our approaches and reminds us that sometimes in this area we go round and round, and not always forwards. We have rediscovered what was known a generation ago—that the best immediate mental health interventions in the hours and days after a disaster concern issues such as shelter, safety, information, and communication. It is not necessary to immediately ask, "How was it for you?" while the smoke and dust are literally and metaphorically still settling—because the answers might be curt and unprintable. There are also signs of a more sensible public mental health approach gaining ground—not wasting money on immediate treatments of large numbers of people who are going to get better anyway (and who, as study after study shows, vote with their feet in rejecting formal mental health interventions at that stage), but instead concentrating a few weeks later on the smaller numbers who are still in trouble—the policy of "watchful waiting" followed by "screen and treat" advocated in the UK NICE Guidelines and used to good effect in the aftermath of the London bombs.(1)

So how should we be treating the smaller numbers of those who are still in trouble perhaps some months after the event? The book reflects the fact that differences of opinion still exist here. The final chapter, in which the editors use their prerogative to give their own views, have not changed much over the decade. In 2000 SSRIs are the first-line treatment, and remain so in 2009. But in the equally scholarly psychological treatment chapter Ressler and Rothbaum draw attention to the recent statements from the respected US Institute of Medicine that exposure-based psychotherapy remains the best validated treatment, and just like our own NICE Guidelines, are less taken with the evidence for medications.

In truth most people don't get very much anyway. In our studies of UK veterans with mental health problems the majority never get near a doctor, and when they do they tend to get given antidepressants, followed by counseling.(2) Only a very few will receive the NICE- or IOM-approved "best practice" of trauma-focused therapy. Getting any decent treatment is the challenge.

Perhaps the most challenging chapter comes from Professor McFarlane, writing alone in 2000 but now joined by Devon Hinton, who brings his experience of working in Cambodia to the table. I thoroughly commend this chapter to the reader because it is a thoughtful and wide-ranging contribution that does not duck some difficult questions. For example, the authors use Robert Hughes's "Culture of Complaint," one of my favorite books (3) to suggest that how society conceptualizes personal responsibility is dramatically influenced by the adversarial tradition. But Hughes also goes on to reflect about the cultural role of the victim, of a person defined not by what he or she does, but by what was done to him or her, and identifies the growth of what he called "victim culture" as a source of concern. Hughes is not alone in having these concerns—influential sociologist Frank Furedi, for example, goes even further.(4) As a specialty we have perhaps had a tendency to ignore views that run counter to our own narrative, so it is refreshing for McFarlane and Hinton to be joining in this debate, as well as reminding us of the need to take a broader historical perspective on what we have done and are doing.

If I have a personal hobby horse (and of course I do), it is to take issue with the view that in the field of posttraumatic stress disorder, we are following an upward trajectory, always moving along the path of knowledge in a Whiggish progress from ignorance to enlightenment. My reading of the historical literature suggests that while this is partly true, it is also true that we have also moved in a more circular trajectory during the past 100 years.

It is a great pity that there is still no real intellectual synthesis of trauma in the 20th century—nor how and why the culture of trauma was transformed in the past two or three decades of the last century. Too often trauma studies that delve into history rely on literature as a primary sources, rather than history. The experiences of Sassoon and Owen were hardly typical of the management of psychiatric injury in the First World War, and their accounts in fiction or poetry were little known the immediate postwar years. Captain W E Johns, the inventor of Biggles, was far more popular and gave a heroic narrative that people wanted to hear. Field Marshall Haig was genuinely mourned when he died, and the fact that he still seats on his horse at the top of Whitehall, looking down on the Cenotaph is not an example of postmodern irony, but a mark of the fact that he was credited with masterminding Britain's military victory. When the now classic First World War play, "Journey's End" was premiered in 1928 its author, RC Sherriff, was shocked when he realized that the production was going to be "antiwar," protesting that he had never intended it to be anything of the sort.(5, 6, 7)

True, the publication of "All Quiet on the Western Front" in Germany in 1929 and then in Britain the following signaled the start of a change. Lloyd George's memoirs started the trashing of Haig's reputation in the 1930s, but the real turning point came in the 1950s and 1960s with Alan Clark's "The Donkeys" followed by the premier of "Oh What a Lovely War" in 1963. The way was then clear for the apotheosis of our current views of the Great War in the person of arguably its now most famous participant, Captain Edmond Blackadder, and in particular the poignant last episode, recently voted the nation's most favorite TV episode.

Our own views on our history have I would suggest also been influenced by the same narratives changes that influenced Richard Curtis and Ben Elton when they created Captain Blackadder. It is time for historians not comedy script writers to reclaim the history of trauma and for us as practitioners and researchers to engage with the real history of PTSD, one free from our own modern conceptions of how it "should have been," but instead how it was. How do we account for the very different view of children's resilience in war time given by Melanie Klein to that of our modern commentators? What about the work of pioneering sociologists such as Quarantarelli whose findings on the outcome of disasters reads so differently from our own? Why, for example, did studies from the First World War seem to report that prisoners of war were largely free from anxiety symptoms, whereas now the same group are seen as particularly at risk?

Just before Ben Shephard published his history of war and psychiatry (8) he agreed to talk about it at a major conference on psychological trauma. I recall the buzz of anticipation before he spoke and then the almost palpable shock once the audience started to realize that he was "not one of us." True, he isn't—but the field needs to engage with historians such as Ben Shephard and Mark Micale (9) just as much as with neuroscientists.

One more new chapter deserves mention. Presumably in response to increasing concerns about the increasing scope and spread of PTSD, and/or its increasingly prominence in the Courts, the editors have requested a new chapter on symptom exaggeration, and a very good one it is. But by focusing on exaggeration, inevitably the agenda has to reflect what are often overstated concerns about the malingering of PTSD (not unknown, but not common either) at the expense of the more interesting and relevant topic of the influences on symptom reporting, both positive and negative.

For example, whenever I interview a soldier, there are always contextual effects on what he, or occasionally she, is prepared to admit to at any given time. On my first trip to an operational theatre I witnessed a Royal Marine trying to board the flight with a broken leg and continuing to deny there was anything wrong even when rumbled. He was a rather more blatant example of the symptom minimization that we encounter each time we visit a base shortly before a deployment to administer health questionnaires. Most soldiers have joined the modern professional armies of the developed world because they want to deploy—for the excitement, challenge, and desire to put their training into reality, and also if they have any career ambitions. It is in their interest to minimize any symptom or problem that might result in them being refused permission to deploy, one more reason why predeployment screening for mental health problems is doomed to fail.(10)

We also see minimization of symptoms if personnel are screened directly on their return from deployment. Military personnel are not stupid, and know that if they endorse too many symptoms then they will be held back in order to be interviewed by a psychologist or psychiatrist, and thus miss their postoperational tour leave. So why should we surprised that in another circumstance, perhaps a year later, when they are planning on leaving the military and/or not wanting to return to Iraq or wherever (been there, done that, time to move on), their thoughts now turn to what happens next and how they might guarantee future health care.

In each and every instance, context is intervening to decide what symptoms will be endorsed, when, to whom, and for what purpose. Soldiers, like everyone else, are not disinterested academic observers of their own condition.(11)

It is evidence like this that calls into question one assumption that underlies a few chapters—that there exists the "real" or "true" level of symptoms, which can be determined either with sophisticated questionnaires now or neuroimaging and/or neurophysiology in the future. I am doubtful if this is possible. Not just reporting, but perhaps even experiencing symptoms might be better understood as a pair of scales, in which there are factors promoting expression, and factors promoting suppression, and what happens at any given time is the result of the balance of the forces operating at any given moment. The fact that that rear-end shunts cause whiplash in Sweden but not in Lithuania is also of relevance to PTSD.(12)

And what about the future? As in the first edition, the editors point to promising avenues of research in the neurosciences and to the prospects of new pharmacological agents. However, a new departure is the discussion of possible pharmacological prevention, as opposed to treatment, of PTSD. This is a topic in which the "man in the street" (at least if journalists are to be believed) expresses doubts, usually because of concerns that this in some way diminishes our humanity, often linked to vague analogies with "Brave New World." If the man in the street knew more about epidemiology and public health he might also point out the differences between treating those who clearly have psychiatric disorders and have come forward for treatment, and treating those who have been exposed to a trauma, most of whom won't develop psychiatric disorder, especially when we as yet we have no robust way of separating out that majority from the minority who will. The balance between risk and harm is very different, something which this author believes will take a long time and some pretty heavy evidence to change. Talk of the "golden hour" in major trauma or stroke care needs to done cautiously, as the analogy is far from exact.

Anyway, the reader who opens this volume can be guaranteed a fascinating, scholarly but still accessible account of PTSD in 2010. A warm welcome then for the second edition, a brief rest for the editors, but then it will be time to start on the third.

Professor Simon Wessely
King's Centre for Military Health Research
Department of Psychological Medicine
Institute of Psychiatry
King's College London

REFERENCES

1. Brewin CR, Scragg P, Robertson M et al. Promoting mental health following the London bombings: a screen and treat approach. J Trauma Stress 2008; 21(1): 3–8.
2. Iversen A, Dyson C, Smith N et al. "Goodbye and Good Luck"; the mental health needs and treatment experiences of British Veterans. submitted for publication. Br J Psychiatry 2005; 186: 480-486
3. Wessely S. Ten Books. Britsh J Psychiatry 2002; 181: 81–4.
4. Furedi F. Therapy Culture: Cultivating Vulnerability In An Anxious Age. Routledge, 2003.
5. Bond B. The Unquiet Western Front: Britain's Role in Literature and History. Cambridge: Cambridge University Press; 2002.
6. Todman D. "San Peur and Sans Reproche": The retirement, death and mourning of Sir Douglas Haig: 1918–1928. J Mil Hist 2003; 67: 1083–106.
7. Sheffield G. 'Oh! What a Futile War: Perceptions of the First World War in Modern British Media and Culture', in War, culture and the media: representations of the military in 20th century Britain, S. Carruthers, Stewart I, ed. Flicks Books: Wiltshire, 1996. 54–74.
8. Shephard B. A War of Nerves, Soldiers and Psychiatrists 1914-1994. London: Jonathan Cape; 2000.
9. Micale M, Lerner P, eds. Traumatic Pasts: History, Psychiatry and Trauma in the Modern Age, 1860-1930. Cambridge University Press: Cambridge, 2001: 140–71.
10. Rona RJ, Hooper R, Jones M et al. Mental health screening in armed forces before the Iraq war and prevention of subsequent psychological morbidity: follow-up study. BMJ 2006; 333(7576): 991.
11. Wessely S. War Stories. British J Psychiatry 2005; 186: 473–5.
12. Schrader H, Obelieniene D, Bovim G et al. Natural evolution of late whiplash syndrome outside the medicolegal context. Lancet 1996; 347: 1207–11.

1 | Posttraumatic stress disorder: Diagnosis, history, and longitudinal course

Arieh Y Shalev

WHAT IS POSTTRAUMATIC STRESS DISORDER?

Posttraumatic stress disorder (PTSD) is an anxiety disorder defined by the co-occurrence in survivors of extreme adversity reexperiencing avoidance and hyperarousal symptoms.(1) Unlike most other mental disorders, the diagnosis of PTSD relies on associating concurrent symptoms with a previous "traumatic" event. The association is both chronological (symptoms starting after the event) and content related: PTSD reexperiencing and avoidance symptoms involve recollections and reminders of the traumatic event. Individuals who suffer from PTSD continuously and uncontrollably relive the very distressing elements of the traumatic event in the form of intrusive recollection and a sense of permanent threat. They avoid places, situations, and mental states that can evoke such recollections.

The image of men and women condemned to repeatedly relive a traumatic event has always captured human imagination. It was immortalized in ancient legends, such as that of Lot's wife, petrified into a column of salt, as she looked backward to the chaos of Sodom. This metaphor of being frozen by looking back at the trauma served as inspiration for generations of artists (see adjacent figures)

More recent expressions depict combat soldiers as ones for whom "the war does not end when the shooting stops" (2) or the holocaust survivors who experience the components of the horror decades after liberation.(3)

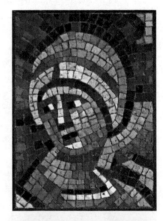

Beyond reminders of the traumatic event, PTSD symptoms include pervasive alterations in one's emotional life, in the form of depressed mood, tension, restlessness, and irritability (Box 1.1). PTSD, therefore, encompasses trauma-related symptoms, anxiety symptoms and symptoms otherwise found in depression. PTSD is also the common outcome of all types of traumatic events, from most horrifying and protracted (e.g., child abuse) to shorter events or incidents (e.g., rape, assault, combat event, accidents). The latter have been referred to as Type I Trauma, whereas the former, or Type II Trauma, have been associated with complex PTSD and other psychological difficulties (e.g., mistrust, subjective sense of emptiness, relational difficulties). The construct of PTSD has replaced, in fact, several event-related syndromes that preexisted its definition (e.g., "concentration camp syndrome," "war neurosis" or "rape victim syndrome"). The configuration of PTSD symptoms is the same in all these occurrences, whereas the specific mental content differs, reflecting the particularities of each person's experience.

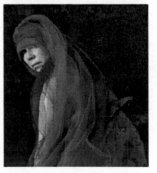

PTSD is not seen in every survivor of a potentially traumatic event. Exposure, therefore, is not a sufficient cause of the disorder. Instead, the traumatic event is currently viewed as "triggering" a reaction, to which prior and posterior (postevent) factors contribute at least as much (4–6 and see below).

BOX 1.1 *DSM-IV* DIAGNOSTIC CRITERIA FOR POSTTRAUMATIC STRESS DISORDER (PTSD).

2 Posttraumatic stress disorder

A. The person has been exposed to a traumatic event in which both of the following were present:
    (1) The person experienced, witnessed, or was confronted with an event or events that involved actual or threatened death or serious injury, or a threat to the physical integrity of self or others.
    (2) The person's response involved intense fear, helplessness, or horror.

B. The traumatic event is persistently reexperienced in one (or more) of the following ways:
    (1) Recurrent and intrusive distressing recollections of the event, including images, thoughts, and perceptions;
    (2) Recurrent distressing dreams of the event;
    (3) Acting or feeling as if the traumatic event were recurring;
    (4) Intense psychological distress at exposure to internal or external cues that symbolize or resemble an aspect of the traumatic event;
    (5) Physiological reactivity on exposure to internal or external cues that symbolize or resemble an aspect of the traumatic event.

C. Avoidance of stimuli associated with the trauma and numbing of general responsiveness (not present before the trauma) as indicated by three (or more) of the following:
    (1) Efforts to avoid thoughts, feelings, or conversations associated with the trauma;
    (2) Efforts to avoid activities, places, or people that arouse recollections of the trauma;
    (3) Inability to recall an important aspect of the trauma;
    (4) Markedly diminished interest or participation in significant activities;
    (5) Feeling of detachment or estrangement from others;
    (6) Restricted range of affect (e.g., unable to have loving feelings);
    (7) Sense of a foreshortened future (e.g., does not expect to have a career, marriage, children, or a normal life span).

D. Persistent symptoms of increased arousal (not present before the trauma) as indicated by two (or more) of the following:
    (1) Difficulty falling or staying asleep
    (2) Irritability or outbursts of anger
    (3) Difficulty concentrating
    (4) Hypervigilance
    (5) Exaggerated startle response

E. Duration of the disturbance (symptoms in criteria B, C, and D) is more than one month.

F. The disturbance causes clinically significant distress or impairment in social occupational or other important areas of functioning

DIAGNOSIS, HISTORY, AND LIFE COURSE

Along with other novel diagnostic entities (e.g., panic disorder), PTSD was first defined and included in the American Psychiatric Association's third *Diagnostic and Statistical Manual* (*DSM-III*; (7)). Though received with significant scepticism, the disorder has nonetheless won a central place in the current discourse on life stresses and mental disorders. Among the many reasons for such a "success" are (a) the growing attention to nonpsychotic disorders in modern psychiatry; (b) increased social awareness of, and aversion for, human rights violations, war, and violence; and (c) the growing interest, by neurobehavioral scientists, in emotions, memory, brain plasticity, and gene environment interaction. Triggered by an external event, and involving both emotional deregulation and memory disturbance, PTSD is the prototype of environmentally induced disorder.

As with other disorders in *DSM-III*, PTSD was essentially defined by its overt and reliably observable expressions (as opposed to mental dispositions, psychological conflicts, or patterns of subjective experiences). *DSM-III* attempted to increase the reliability of psychiatric diagnoses by defining mandatory "diagnostic criteria" for each disorder. These criteria are states of mind, activities, and dispositions that the patient can readily communicate and the clinician can rather easily recognize and confirm. Trauma survivors often report other symptoms (e.g., a sense of inner change, loneliness, despair), but these do not count for the diagnosis of PTSD. Numerous rating scales and structured interviews have been validated for PTSD and are routinely used in studies of this disorder.

It has been argued, though, that some PTSD symptoms might be too easily perceived and communicated and thus may create an impression of an "epidemic of PTSD" following major, spectacular, and socially contagious events. Studies of the prevalence of PTSD following the September 11, 2001 attacks on the Twin Towers in New York have been criticized for overestimating the rate of PTSD on the basis of commonly reported symptoms (e.g., (8)). Most such cases of PTSD have, in fact, recovered within few months of the attacks (9).

Nevertheless, the definition of PTSD has enabled an ever-growing stream of empirical studies of comparable groups of trauma survivors. Thus, while the boundaries of PTSD and the accuracy of the diagnosis made shortly after a traumatic event are a still matter of debate, it is currently clear that this "man-made" definition of the disorder is a good enough object for scientific enquiry. Clinicians, however, should be aware of the significant variability of individual experiences and symptoms within this diagnostic entity and of the major role of the particularities of each trauma in shaping survivors behaviour and recovery paths.

Despite the link to a traumatic event, *DSM IV* and the related World Health Organization's 10th edition of International Classification of Diseases (10) do not posit a pathogenic mechanism for PTSD. Putative mechanisms have been proposed for PTSD others, including "fear conditioning," an abnormality of "fear processing," or "shattered cognitive assumptions."(11–13) These theories established a basis for theory-based interventions for PTSD, such as cognitive-behavioural therapy (CBT) or pharmacotherapy by agents that interfere with the early stress responses.

This chapter will address the disorder's boundaries, that is, its frequent coexistence with major depression and other mental disorders, and the difficulties to discern PTSD from a normal response to traumatic events at the early aftermath of the latter. It will also present arguments for and against assuming a complex PTSD resulting from Type II trauma. As a starter, the chapter will briefly examine the history of PTSD, evaluate the evidence for the syndrome's reliability and validity, and discuss the changes in the definition of PTSD over time. A detailed historical review of trauma-related disorders before 1980 is beyond the scope of this chapter (but see 14–16).

A brief history

Traumatic syndromes resembling PTSD have been described and harshly debated during the 20th century. Rescuers of survivors of ship explosions in Toulon in 1907 and 1911, for example, exhibited "recapitulation of the scene, terrifying dreams, diffuse anxiety, fatigue, and various minor phobias" ((14) p. 247). A debate concerning the nature and the therapy of "shell shock" raged during most of World War I, at which time three different approaches to treating the disorder were used: (a) a social environment approach, exemplified by treating soldiers in military installations, close to the frontline, and expecting their full return to military duty (17); (b) a behaviouristic approach, exemplified by directly addressing avoidance and bodily (i.e., conversion) symptoms (e.g., (18)); and (c) a psychotherapeutic approach, exemplified by exploring the content and the personal meaning of traumatic experienced as a means of recovery (e.g., (19)).

The burden of compensation for World War I–combat neuroses resulted in restrictive administrative decisions, such as *not* to compensate financially for battle shock during World War II (in the United Kingdom), or to use the neutral term "battle fatigue" for stress disorders among combatants of the U.S. army, instead of implying a mental disorder.(14)

Under such different titles, the clinical observations repeated themselves quite systematically. Symptoms of "operational fatigue" included (16) irritability, fatigue, difficulties falling asleep, startle reaction, depression, tremor and evidences of sympathetic overreactivity, difficulties in concentration and mental confusion, preoccupation with combat experiences, nightmares and battle dreams, phobias, personality changes, and increased alcoholism. (p. 210). A "traumatic neurosis" (11) comprised "Fixation on the trauma, typical dream life, contraction of general level of functioning, irritability and proclivity to explosive aggressive reactions" (p. 86). These descriptions clearly resemble those currently used for PTSD.

Despite clinical observations during World War I and II, traumatic stress disorders were not included in *DSM-I* (1952-1968) and *DSM-II* (1968-1980). DSM I included a category of "gross stress reaction" of a maximum duration of two months, thereby implying that genuine reactions to major stressors are transient, and prolonged illness reflects more basic disturbances. Those who remain chronically ill after a traumatic exposure essentially express another underlying disorder (e.g., childhood neurosis, depressive illness) possibly revealed by trauma. *DSM-II* eliminated the gross stress reaction category altogether and provided no alternative diagnosis for reactions to major stressors.

The introduction of PTSD into *DSM-III* followed the realization of the profound psychological effect of the Vietnam War, (20, 21) and concurrent studies of rape victims. A major force behind the delineation of PTSD was Vietnam Veterans Working Group (VVWG), a heterogeneous association of professionals and activists formed in 1974 and supported by the American Orthopsychiatric Association and the National Council of Churches. The VVWG drew the attention of the American Psychiatric Association (APA) Task Force on Nomenclature (the *DSM-III* Task Force) to the need for stress-related syndromes to be recognized. It further compiled 724 observations of psychologically disabled veterans and provided a tentative list of syndrome, closely resembling Kardiner's description of "traumatic neuroses" among World War I veterans. These and other observations were submitted to the Committee of Reactive Disorders appointed by the APA task force and the latter decided to include PTSD in *DSM-III* as one based on "consensus" rather than "empirically validated" disorder.(20)

Empirical findings have somewhat refined PTSD diagnostic criteria in subsequent editions of the DSM. The definition of a "traumatic event" (PTSD criterion A) was modified (see the following). A requirement for a minimal one-month duration was included. Survivor guilt, which appeared in *DSM-III*, was omitted because studies have shown that it was infrequent. The item "physiological reaction to reminders of the trauma" was moved from the "hyperarousal" (D) criterion to the "intrusion" (B) criterion. Finally *DSM-IV* has introduced a requirement for clinically significant distress or impairment (Criterion F). *DSM-IV* (1994) also added an associated syndrome—acute stress disorder (ASD) that will be discussed as follows.

The syndrome

The current (*DSM-IV*) diagnostic criteria for PTSD differ from those originally included in *DSM-III* in several ways. Unlike *DSM-III*, *DSM-IV* definition of a traumatic event does not require an outstanding stressor that "would evoke significant symptoms of distress in almost everyone." Milder and more common stressors, such as road traffic accidents or sudden traumatic loss, have been shown to induce prolonged PTSD symptoms in a proportion of survivors.(22–28) Accordingly, traumatic events occur quite frequently, with different proportions of survivors developing PTSD after each trauma type. Table 1.1 summarizes the likelihood of being exposed to a traumatic event, as recorded in several studies of civilian adults.

Traumatic events in *DSM-IV* also include instances of witnessing trauma to others (such as witnessing an execution or being involved in rescue operations). The requirement of direct exposure to the stressful event is not required any more: suffice it to be *confronted* with an event. The definition of the *event* currently includes an emotional reaction while exposed. The latter involves intense fear, helplessness, or horror. In U.S. studies using the liberal *DSM-IV* "trauma" criteria (7, 23–25) the probability of experiencing a traumatic event during one's life is very high indeed, reaching 97% of male adults. Interestingly, the rates of exposure to a traumatic event and subsequent PTSD were found to be much lower in a European and an Australian study.(26, 27)

The World Health Organization's ICD-10 has kept the original perception of a traumatic event as outstanding and universally distressing: "event or situation (either short or long lasting) of an exceptionally threatening or catastrophic nature, which is likely to cause

Table 1.1 Likelihood of exposure to traumatic events in the general population.

Author & publication year	Study Population (n)	Sample	PTSD among Males (%)	PTSD among Females (%)	Trauma type
Kessler et al., 1995	USA (5877)	General population	61%	51%	Any trauma
Breslau et al., 1991	USA (1007)	Young adults (age=21–30)	43%	37%	Any trauma
Norris et al., 1992	USA (1000)	Adults	74%	65%	Ten selected events
Stein et al., 1997	Canada (1000)	Adults	81%	74%	List of traumatic events
Breslau et al., 1998	USA (2181)	Adults	97%	87%	DSM IV events
Perkonigg et al., 2000	Europe (3021)	Adults	Male = 26% Female = 17.7%	Male = 1% Female = 2.2%	Any trauma

pervasive distress in almost anyone." Virtually, all current studies of PTSD use *DSM-IV* diagnostic criteria, thereby including in their sample survivors of an array of major and minor events, the major defining element of which has become the subjective reaction to the event rather than its "objective" appearance.

Consistency of PTSD Symptoms

PTSD symptoms may be seen within hours of a traumatic event.(29) At the other end, nightmares and intrusive recollections can be found, decades after exposure, in survivors of prolonged adversities who are minimally disturbed. Avoidance alone may develop as well, in the form of specific phobia, reluctance to evoke specific topics, or avoidance of places and activities without the associated hyperarousal and intrusive recollections. It is typical of phobic subjects not to be distressed as long as they can successfully avoid the object of their phobia. Irritability can also be an isolated outcome of a trauma, particularly upon homecoming from military conflicts. Abnormal irritability is often felt by survivors families and may lead misuse of alcohol as a "tranquilizer."

Partial PTSD is a subthreshold condition in which some but not all PTSD symptoms criteria are formally met. Partial PTSD is often as frequent as PTSD (30) and similarly unremitting.(31, 32) Not meeting the PTSD Criterion C (avoidance) is the most frequent reason for having partial PTSD. As can be seen in Box 1.1 one has to experience at least three symptoms in order to meet the C criterion (compared with *one* reexperiencing symptom and *two* hyperarousal symptoms). Moreover, only three of Criterion C's seven items (Items one to three) are directly related to avoiding reminders of the traumatic event. The other four items (diminished interest, detachment and estrangement, restricted range of affect, and sense of foreshortened future) reflect "psychological numbing," a construct borrowed from the literature on grief and bereavement. More important, the four numbing symptoms resemble those seen in depression (e.g., anhedonia)—a disorder that frequently co-occurs with PTSD.

PTSD Criterion D includes several expressions of increased arousal (insomnia, irritability, bursts of anger) and exaggerated startle response. Exaggerated startle has been described among trauma survivors throughout history. For example, '"stragglers" who ceased to function as soldiers during the American Civil War were "trembling, staring into the middle distance and jumping at any loud noise."(33) Kardiner (11) similarly recognized "auditory hypersensitiveness" as one of the core features of traumatic neurosis in World War I veterans (p. 95). Startle reaction was among the frequent symptoms seen in airmen with "operational fatigue" ((16); p. 210). Exaggerated startle is reported by up to 88% of PTSD patients.(34)

Several studies evaluated the construct validity of PTSD (e.g., (22, 35, 36)) and found it to be very good and generally matching the subdivision into reexperiencing, avoidance, and hyperarousal. Despite somewhat fluctuating longitudinal trajectories in individuals, symptom severity in cohorts of chronic PTSD patients remains stable over time.(37)

The time course of PTSD

PTSD symptoms are very frequently in the immediate aftermath of trauma exposure (e.g., in 94% of rape victims, within a week of the trauma; 38). PTSD symptoms decrease with time in most of those who initially express them—and so does the prevalence of diagnosable PTSD (e.g., 39%, 17% at six months and 10% at one year on a cohort of Israeli civilians admitted to a general hospital ER (e.g., (39)). In a seminal epidemiological study, Kessler et al. (40) described 60% recovery in trauma survivors with early PTSD. The National Vietnam Veterans Readjustment Study (NVVRS) showed 30% lifetime prevalence and 15.2% point prevalence of PTSD, more than 20 years after the war.(41) A reanalyses of the NVVRS study, in which combat exposure was independently ascertained, from military records, yielded lower lifetime (18.7%) and point prevalence (9.7%) of PTSD, (42) but similar ratio of lifetime to chronic PTSD.

Most cases of spontaneous recovery occur within a year from the traumatic event.(40) Survivors who recover later often have partial PTSD and are vulnerable to subsequent exposure to analogous events.(43, 44)

Because they frequently decline, early PTSD symptoms should be seen as sensitive and nonspecific predictors of the chronic disorder.(43) Indeed, the negative predictive value of early symptoms (i.e., the likelihood that someone who *does not* have symptoms will develop PTSD) is more reliable than their positive predictive value. The clinician's dilemma, therefore, is to identify, among those who express high levels of symptom, those at risk of keeping these symptoms.

The presence of early dissociation symptoms, such as detachment, time distortion, feeling "on automatic pilot" or out-of-the-body experience or frank episodes of dissociation signal a high risk for chronic PTSD.(4) Similarly early and severe depression (44) and elevated heart rate levels shortly after the traumatic event (45) have been linked with higher risk of PTSD. Past history of mental illness, previous traumatic experiences, and dysfunctional families also contribute to PTSD. Finally, events and conditions that follow the traumatic event have a major effect on the likelihood of recovery from early symptoms.(46) The subjective appraisals of the event, and of one's reactions to the event, contribute significantly to the persistence of PTSD symptoms (e.g., (47)) as do societies responses, where people close to the victim provide support; for example, family friends can be protective. Cognitive-behavioural therapies specifically address these distortions and hence are effective as treatments for PTSD.(48–50)

Severity and Comorbidity

The severity of chronic PTSD is subject to fluctuations.(37) Exacerbations in the severity of PTSD symptoms are often due to life pressures, exposure to reminders of the traumatic event, or failure in an area of living (e.g., family or work). Thus, many PTSD sufferers see their symptoms exacerbated when they retire from work, develop serious illness, or lose stabilizing elements of their lives.

PTSD patients are very sensitive to ongoing stressors, to which they often react by becoming distraught, angry, or inappropriately using sedatives or alcohol. For the clinician, this feature of PTSD suggests that the environment within which chronic PTSD patients live should be a target for monitoring and intervening. It is somewhat easier to help a recovered PTSD patient keep his or her work, by guidance and advice, than to medically or psychologically address the symptoms and the complications of a severe recurrence of symptoms. While such "tertiary" prevention is recommended for most chronic mental illnesses, PTSD patients should be seen as particularly reactive to stressors and negative events, and especially lonely, frustrated, and isolated.

PTSD often co-occurs with other mental disorders, particularly with major depression, anxiety disorders, and substance abuse. The U.S. National Comorbidity Study, for example (41), has shown that 88.3% of male PTSD subjects and 79% of women with PTSD have at least one other mental disorder. Depression was experienced by about one-half of all PTSD subjects (48.5% in women and 47.9% in men). Anxiety disorders were seen in more than one-third, and drug and alcohol abuse by a third of all women and half of all men. Other studies (51–55) have confirmed the frequent co-occurrence of PTSD and depression—at levels between 34% to 51% (current) and 95% (lifetime).

Boundaries and subtypes

Acute stress disorder

In an attempt better to differentiate the early and normal responses to traumatic events from "pathological" ones, *DSM-IV* proposed a diagnostic category of acute stress disorder (ASD; Box 1.2). ASD includes PTSD symptoms and symptoms of dissociation, appearing immediately after a traumatic event and up to four weeks later. ASD is a robust predictor of chronic PTSD, yet most PTSD patients do not have an initial ASD.

BOX 1.2   SYMPTOM CRITERIA FOR ACUTE STRESS DISORDER.

A.   A traumatic event—as in PTSD

B.   Dissociative symptoms (at least three required):
1.   A subjective sense of numbing, detachment, or absence of emotional responsiveness;
2.   A reduction in awareness of his or her surroundings (e.g., "being in a daze");
3.   Derealization;
4.   Depersonalization;
5.   Dissociative amnesia (i.e., inability to recall an important aspect of the trauma).

C.   The traumatic event is persistently reexperienced in at least one of the following ways: recurrent images, thoughts, dreams, illusions, flashback episodes or a sense of reliving the experience or distress on exposure to reminders of the traumatic event.

D.   Marked avoidance of stimuli that arouse recollections of the trauma (e.g., thoughts, feelings, conversations, activities, places, people).

E.   Marked symptoms of anxiety or increased arousal (e.g., difficulty sleeping, irritability, poor concentration, hypervigilance, exaggerated startle response, motor restlessness).

F.   The disturbance causes clinically significant distress or impairment in social, occupational, or other important areas of functioning or impairs the individual's ability to pursue some necessary task, such as obtaining necessary assistance or mobilizing personal resources by telling family members about the traumatic experience.

G.   The disturbance lasts for a minimum of two days and a maximum of four weeks and occurs within four weeks of the traumatic event.

Dissociation symptoms do not significantly to improve predictions made from other early symptoms. Moreover, numerous trauma survivors who do not show dissociation symptoms and who do not qualify for the diagnosis of ASD develop PTSD. For these reasons, ASD has been criticized as being of little value.(56) Nevertheless, when it can be diagnosed, ASD signals a very high likelihood (between 34% and 72%) of developing chronic PTSD.(57, 58)

Clinicians may wish to use this diagnostic category with great caution and, specifically, not to exclude individuals without ASD, and who are otherwise distressed, from receiving early treatment. Interestingly, ICD-10 defines an acute response to stress as starting at the time of the traumatic events and lasting for up to two or three days. ICD-10 acute response differs, therefore, from ASD in that it only pertains to the very early reaction—and is not properly a "disorder"—but rather a reaction.

Acute PTSD and chronic PTSD

Another controversial matter is the subdivision of PTSD into acute (duration of symptoms less than three months) and chronic (duration of symptoms exceeds three months) subtypes. The two subtypes are identical, save for the duration and timing. The "chronic" condition is diagnosed after three months, which is truly exceptional in psychiatry, and medicine in general. Many of those with acute PTSD (60% e.g., 40) may recover with or without treatment. Most important, both conditions require similar therapies. Clinicians may wish to identify and treat survivors with high levels of early PTSD symptoms, anxiety, or depression without paying much attention to the current subdivisions.

Delayed-onset PTSD

This condition consists of delayed appearance of PTSD more than six months after a traumatic event. Such delayed appearance has been linked with seeking compensation and malingering. Yet one sometimes encounters individuals who have been coping well with the consequences of a traumatic event and who developed PTSD at a distance from the traumatic event, often as a result of another event. A systematic study of 150 combat veterans with delayed PTSD (first referral to treatment between six months and six years following trauma (59) has shown that 90% of these individuals had been symptomatic prior to seeking help. Some 40% of the cases were identified as "delayed referral," that is, subjects who suffered without seeking help; 33% had subsyndromal PTSD since the traumatic event, 13% had reactivated previously recovered PTSD, and 4% had been given other psychiatric diagnoses before being identified as suffering from PTSD.

Thought to be an exception, new data on American veterans of the war in Iraq and Afghanistan (e.g., (60)) show a paradoxical increase in the prevalence of PTSD during the year that follows deployment. These findings may reflect a growing concern about going back to combat zone among those who remain in the force, a progressive realization of how one's reactions were abnormal during deployment (i.e., while being on a survival mode of living) or an increased saliency of symptoms in a context of nonmilitary life (e.g., troubles concentrating and irritability may become very obvious when one has to go back to work—or play with one's children). It is also possible that the delayed expression of PTSD is more typical of survivors of prolonged adversities (e.g., captivity, abuse) who fail to adjust to the highly competitive society within which most of us live.

Trauma-induced personality changes

Survivors of Type 2 trauma may show a particularly severe form of PTSD, associated with profound personality changes. The degree to which traumatic events can affect personality structures has been the subject of a heated debate, which ended by not including in the *DSM-IV* the diagnostic category of "disorders of stress not otherwise specified" (DESNOS, *DSM-IV* draft criteria, 1991). DESNOS was found to be consistently associated with PTSD, and therefore, was not granted an independent status in *DSM-IV*. Interestingly, ICD-10 recognizes enduring personality changes resulting from exposure to "catastrophic stress" such as concentration camp experiences, torture, or hostage situation. Traumatic personality changes must be present for at least two years and include the following symptoms: permanent hostile or distressful attitude toward the world, social withdrawal, feeling of emptiness, enduring feeling of being "on edge" and estrangement (a permanent feeling of being changed or being different from others).

Clearly, the discussion of trauma-induced personality change is hampered by our current view of mental disorders. Specifically, the boundary between "personality" and the very chronic mental disorders is not well traced. Moreover, PTSD symptoms of pervasive avoidance, irritability, increased stimulus response, and restriction to one's life are very likely to be perceived, by the patient and by the family, as involving permanent personality changes. Indeed, one of the most frequent complaints of PTSD patients is "I am not the same." Understandably, childhood trauma, abuse, and neglect may lead to severe developmental difficulties, which often present as personality disorders.

CONCLUSION

The uniqueness of PTSD among mental disorders is that this condition develops after salient events, and therefore, can be detected at an early stage and, to some extent, prevented. Despite its "political" origins and despite the admixture of various symptoms in this manmade syndrome, PTSD has proved to be robust, persistent, reliably diagnosable, and clearly linked with substantial distress and dysfunction. Indeed, similar constellations of symptoms have been described in trauma survivors throughout history. Biologically, the disorder has been associated with consistent, converging, and replicable findings, particularly in the areas of startle physiology and neuroendocrinology and some recent brainimaging studies. Several recent treatment studies, including pharmacology and psychological therapies, are quickly reversing a previous image of a hopeless condition. PTSD, therefore, is a story of success.

Yet PTSD is also a matter of debate, mainly because the disorder is used and abused in compensation claims, in ideological debates (e.g., the false memory debate) and in introducing some of the worse forms of therapies to the clinical arena. The main threat to the survival of this condition is, therefore, its misuse and overextension to include any and all illnesses that follow trauma. Intrinsic inconsistencies, however, do exist. First, the co-occurrence of PTSD and depression is a major area for future research—particularly when the contribution of early depression to chronic PTSD is considered. Second, the boundary with normal reactions to traumatic stress, particularly at the early aftermath of traumatic events, needs better definition. Finally, the complex causation of chronic PTSD, and particularly the role of postevent factors in maintaining the disorder, should make us rethink about the nature of the link between the triggering traumatic event and the subsequent psychological, biological, and genomic events. PTSD, therefore, faces an exciting future as subject of clinical and scientific investigation. PTSD is also likely to be at the center of future debates concerning human nature, human resilience to stress, and the role of culture in defining what is disordered and what is not.

REFERENCES

1. American Psychiatric Association, Diagnostic and Statistical Manual of Mental Disorders, 4th edition (DSM-IV) (American Psychiatric Press: Washington, DC, 1994).
2. Solomon Z, Combat Stress Reaction: The Enduring Toll of War (Plenum: New York, 1993).
3. Eitinger L, Concentration Camp Survivors in Norway and Israel (Allen & Unwin: London, 1964).
4. Shalev AY, Peri T, Canneti L, Schreiber S, Predictors of PTSD in recent trauma survivors: a prospective study, Am J Psychiatry (1992) 153:219–25.
5. King LA, King DW, Fairbank JA et al, Resilience and recovery factors in post-traumatic stress disorder among female and male Vietnam veterans: hardiness, postwar social support, and additional stressful life events, J Pers Soc Psychol (1998) 74:420–34
6. Yehuda R, McFarlane AC, Conflict between current knowledge about posttraumatic stress disorder and its original conceptual basis, Am J Psychiatry (1995) 152:1705–13.
7. American Psychiatric Association, Diagnostic and Statistical Manual of Mental Disorders, 3rd edn (DSM-III) (American Psychiatric Press: Washington, DC, 1980).
8. North CS, Pfefferbaum B, Research on the Mental Health Effects of Terrorism JAMA. 2002;288:633-636.
9. Galea S, Vlahov D, Resnick H, Ahern J, Susser E, Gold J, Bucuvalas M, Kilpatrick D. Trends of probable post-traumatic stress disorder in New York City after the September 11 terrorist attacks. Am J Epidemiol. 5:158:514-524, 2003
10. World Health Organization, The ICD 10 Classification of Mental and Behavioural Disorders: Diagnostic Criteria for Research (WHO: Geneva, 1993).
11. Kardiner A, The Traumatic Neuroses of War (Hoeber: New York, 1941).
12. Pitman RK, Post-traumatic stress disorder, conditioning, and network theory, Psychiatric Annals, 18:182–9.
13. Janoff Bulman R, The aftermath of victimization: rebuilding shattered assumptions. In: Figley CR, ed, Trauma and its Wake, the Study and Treatment of Post-traumatic Stress Disorder (Brunner-Mazel: New York, 1985) 15–36.
14. Trimble MR. Posttraumatic Neurosis. From Railway Spine to the Whiplash. John Wiley: Chichester; 1981.
15. Merskey H. Shell shock. In: Berrios EG, Freedman H, eds. 150 years of British Psychiatry. Gaskell: London; 1991.
16. Grinker RR, Spiegel JP. Men under stress. Backiston: Philadelphia; 1945.
17. Salmon TW. The care and treatment of mental diseases and war neuroses ('shell shock') in the British Army. Ment Hyg 1917; 1: 509–47.
18. Jones E, Thomas A, Ironside S. Shell shock: an outcome study of a First World War 'PIE' unit. Psychol Med 2007; 37: 215–23.
19. Rivers WHR. The repression of war experiences. Proc R Soc Med 1918; 11: 1–20.
20. Bloom SL. Our hearts and our hopes are turned to peace: origins of the International Society for traumatic stress. In: Shalev AY, Yehuda R, McFarlane AC, eds. International Handbook of Human Response to Trauma. Kluwer Academic/Plenum: New York, 2000: 27–50.

21. Young A. An alternative history of traumatic stress. In: Shalev AY, Yehuda R, McFarlane AC, eds. International Handbook of Human Response to Trauma. Kluwer Academic/Plenum: New York; 2000.

22. Keane TM. Symptomatology of Vietnam veterans with posttraumatic stress disorder. In: Davidson JRT, Foa E, eds. Posttraumatic Stress Disorder: DSM IV and Beyond. American Psychiatric Press: Washington, DC, 1993: 99–111.

23. Breslau N, Davis GC. Posttraumatic stress disorder: the etiologic specificity of wartime stressors. Am J Psychiatry 1988; 144: 578–83.

24. Breslau N, Davis GC, Andreski P, Peterson E. Traumatic events and posttraumatic stress disorder in an urban population of young adults. Arch Gen Psychiatry 1991; 48: 216–22.

25. Breslau N, Kessler RC, Chilcoat HD et al. Trauma and posttraumatic stress disorder in the community: the 1996 Detroit Area Survey of Trauma. Arch Gen Psychiatry 1998; 55: 626–32.

26. Perkonigg A, Kessler RC, Storz S, Wittchen HU. Traumatic events and posttraumatic stress disorder in the community: prevalence, risk factors and comorbidity. Acta Psychiatr Scand 2000; 101(1): 46–59.

27. Creamer M, Burgess P, McFarlane AC. Posttraumatic stress disorder: findings from the Australian National Survey of mental health and well-being. Psychol Med 2001; 31(7): 1237–47.

28. Resnick HS, Kilpatrick DG, Dansky BS et al. Prevalence of civilian trauma and posttraumatic stress disorder in a representative national sample of women. J Consult Clin Psychol 1993; 61: 984–91.

29. Norris FH. Epidemiology of trauma: frequency and impact of different potentially traumatic events on different demographic groups. J Consult Clin Psychol 1992; 60: 409–18.

30. Stein MB, Walker JR, Hazen AL, Forde DR. Full and partial posttraumatic stress disorder: findings from a community survey. Am J Psychiatry 1997; 154: 1114–9.

31. Carlier IV, Lamberts RD, Fouwels AJ, Gersons BP. PTSD in relation to dissociation in traumatized police officers. Am J Psychiatry 1996; 153: 1325–8.

32. Carlier IV, Gersons BPR. Partial posttraumatic stress disorder (PTSD): the issue of psychological scars and the occurrence of PTSD symptoms. J Nerv Ment Dis 1995; 183: 107–9.

33. Marlowe DH. Psychological and psycho-social consequences of combat and deployment with special emphasis on the Gulf War. Rand: Santa Monica, CA; in press.

34. Davidson JRT, Kudler HS, Smith RD. Assessment and pharmacotherapy of posttraumatic stress disorder. In: Giller EL, ed. Biological Assessment and Treatment of Posttraumatic Stress Disorder. American Psychiatric Press: Washington, DC, 1990; 203–21.

35. Fawzi MC, Pham T, Lin L et al. The validity of posttraumatic stress disorder among Vietnamese refugees. J Trauma Stress 1997; 10: 101–8.

36. Kilpatrick DG, Resnick HS. Posttraumatic stress disorder associated with exposure to criminal victimization in clinical and community populations. In: Davidson JRT, Foa E, eds. Posttraumatic Stress Disorder: DSM IV and Beyond. American Psychiatric Press: Washington, DC, 1993; 113–43.

37. Niles BL, Newman E, Fisher LM. Obstacles to assessment of PTSD in longitudinal research. In: Shalev AY, Yehuda R, McFarlane AC, eds. International Handbook of Human Response to Trauma. Kluwer Academic/Plenum: New York, 2000; 213–22.

38. Rothbaum BO, Foa EB, Riggs DS, Murdock T, Walsh WA: prospective examination of post-traumatic stress disorder in rape victims. J Traumatic Stress, 1992;5:455–75.

39. Shalev AY, Freedman S, Brandes D et al. Predicting PTSD in civilian trauma survivors: prospective evaluation of self report and clinician administered instruments. Br J Psychiatry 1997; 170: 558–64.

40. Kessler RC, Sonnega A, Bromet EJ et al. Posttraumatic stress disorder in the National Comorbidity Survey. Arch Gen Psychiatry 1995; 52: 1048–60.

41. Kulka RA, Schlenger WE, Fairbank JA et al. Trauma and the Vietnam War generation: report of findings from the National Vietnam Veterans readjustment study. Brunner/Mazel: New York; 1990.

42. Dohrenwend BP, Turner JB, Turse NA et al. The psychological risks of Vietnam for U.S. veterans: a revisit with new data and methods. Science 2006; 313(5789): 979–82.

43. Freedman SA, Peri T, Brandes D, Shalev AY. Predictors of chronic PTSD – a prospective study. Br J Psychiatry 1999; 174: 353–9.

44. Shalev AY, Freedman S, Peri T et al. Prospective study of posttraumatic stress disorder and depression following trauma. Am J Psychiatry 1998; 155: 630–7.

45. Shalev AY, Sahar T, Freedman S et al. A prospective study of heart rate responses following trauma and the subsequent development of PTSD. Arch Gen Psychiatry 1998; 55: 553–9.

46. Brewin CR, Andrews B, Valentine JD. Meta-analysis of risk factors for posttraumatic stress disorder in trauma-exposed adults. J Consult Clin Psychol 2000; 68(5): 748–66.

47. Ehlers A, Mayou RA, Bryant B. Psychological predictors of chronic posttraumatic stress disorder after motor vehicle accidents. J Abnorm Psychol 1998; 107: 508–19.

48. Bryant RA, Harvey AG, Dang ST et al. Treatment of acute stress disorder: a comparison of cognitivebehavioral therapy and supportive counseling. J Consult Clin Psychol 1998; 66: 862–6.

49. Bryant RA, Sackville T, Dang S et al. Treatment of acute stress disorder: an evaluation of cognitive behavioral therapy and supportive counseling techniques. Am J Psychiatry 1999; 156: 1780–6.

50. National Collaborating Centre for Mental Health. Posttraumatic stress disorder: the management of PTSD in adults and children in primary and secondary care. London (UK): National Institute for Clinical Excellence (NICE), 2005: 167.

51. Green BL, Grace MC, Lindy JD et al. Risk factors for PTSD and other diagnoses in a general sample of Vietnam veterans. Am J Psychiatry 1990; 147: 729–33.

52. Engdahl BE, Speed N, Eberly RE, Schwartz J. Comorbidity of psychiatric disorders and personality profiles of American World War II prisoners of war. J Nerv Ment Dis 1991; 179: 181–91.

53. McFarlane AC, Papay P. Multiple diagnoses in posttraumatic stress disorder in the victims of a natural disaster. J Nerv Ment Dis 1992; 180: 498–504.

54. North CS, Smith EM, Spitznagel EL. Posttraumatic stress disorder in survivors of a mass shooting. Am J Psychiatry 1994; 151: 82–8.

55. Bleich A, Koslowsky M, Dolev A, Lerer B. Posttraumatic stress disorder and depression. An analysis of comorbidity. Br J Psychiatry 1997; 170: 479–82.

56. Marshall RD, Spitzer R, Liebowitz MR. Review and critique of the new DSM-IV diagnosis of acute stress disorder. Am J Psychiatry 1999; 156: 1677–85.

57. Bryant RA. Early predictors of posttraumatic stress disorder. Biol Psychiatry 2003; 53(9): 789–95.

58. Harvey AG, Bryant RA. The relationship between acute stress disorder and posttraumatic stress disorder: a prospective evaluation of motor vehicle accident survivors. J Consult Clin Psychol 1998; 66: 507–12.

59. Solomon Z, Kotler M, Shalev A, Lin R. Delayed posttraumatic stress disorders, Psychiatry 1989; 52: 428–36.

60. Milliken CS, Auchterlonie JL, Hoge CW. Longitudinal assessment of mental health problems among active and reserve component soldiers returning from the Iraq war. JAMA 2007; 298(18): 2141–8.

2 | Epidemiology of traumatic events and posttraumatic stress disorder

Tracie O Afifi, Gordon JG Asmundson, and Jitender Sareen

EPIDEMIOLOGY OF TRAUMATIC EVENTS AND POSTTRAUMATIC STRESS DISORDER

Many people experience traumatic events through their lifetime. After an exposure to a traumatic event, some individuals may develop posttraumatic stress disorder (PTSD). Studies using community samples provide information on the epidemiology of traumatic events and PTSD in the general population. Using the current literature primarily on general population samples, this chapter reviews: (a) definitions of traumatic events, (b) methods of assessing traumatic events and PTSD in epidemiologic studies, (c) epidemiologic studies on traumatic events and PTSD, (d) epidemiology of traumatic events, (e) epidemiology of PTSD, and (f) mental and physical health comorbidities of PTSD.

DEFINITIONS OF TRAUMATIC EVENTS

The Diagnostic and Statistical Manual of Mental Disorders' (DSM) first criterion for PTSD requires that a person be exposed to a traumatic event. *DSM-III* and *DSM-III-R* criteria defined a traumatic event as an event outside the range of usual human experience and one that would be distressing for almost anyone.(1, 2) The definition of what constitutes a traumatic event was expanded in the *DSM-IV* criteria. According to the current *DSM-IV* diagnostic criteria for PTSD, a traumatic event is an event that is experienced or witnessed and involves the actual or threatened death, serious injury, or threat of physical integrity of oneself or others and invokes a response of fear, helplessness, or horror.(3) Many different types of traumatic events are included under the *DSM-IV* definition such as war-related events, natural disasters, physical assault, sexual assault or violence, threats with weapons, serious accidents, illness, and the unexpected death of loved ones. Many individuals will experience a traumatic event or several events throughout their lifetime. Some people who are exposed to a traumatic event will develop symptoms of PTSD and may meet criteria for a PTSD diagnosis.

METHODS OF ASSESSING TRAUMATIC EVENTS AND PTSD IN EPIDEMIOLOGIC GENERAL POPULATION STUDIES

Several epidemiologic studies on traumatic events and PTSD have been conducted using general population samples. Most of these studies have used samples from the United States. The first studies were conducted in the 1980s using *DSM-III* and later *DSM-III-R* criteria. In the mid-1990s, studies using *DSM-IV* criteria began to be published. The prevalence of exposure to traumatic events and PTSD reported in epidemiologic studies varies depending on the method and criteria used for assessing traumatic events.(4)

With regard to method, earlier studies using *DSM-III* criteria inquire about traumatic events using a single question, while studies using *DSM-IV* criteria provide respondents with a list of qualifying traumatic events. The list method and the use of longer versus shorter lists results in higher prevalence estimates of exposure to traumatic events and number of traumatic events experienced compared to a single-question method.(4) In addition, the expansion of the definition of traumatic events in the *DSM-IV* criteria indicates that studies using *DSM-IV* criteria include a greater number of qualifying traumatic events compared to earlier studies using *DSM-III* or *DSM-III-R* criteria, which also has an impact on the prevalence of traumatic event exposure and PTSD.(4, 5)

Methods in studies also differ when respondents endorse experiencing more than one traumatic event. When respondents have experienced multiple traumatic events, some studies will require the respondent to identify the worst traumatic event, while other studies will use a random method to select a traumatic event for assessing PTSD symptoms. Kessler et al. (1995) stated that studies using the worst event method will likely overestimate the associations of that event with PTSD, while using a random method to select an event may provide more accurate information regarding a trauma.(6) Direct comparison of both methods has indicated that prevalence of PTSD based on the worst event method and random event method was 13.6% and 9.2%, respectively.(7) However, further investigation determined that both methods provided similar findings with regard to identifying sex differences and traumatic events with the highest likelihood of PTSD.(8)

In addition, studies have also differed in the year in which data were collected, location of data collection, ages of the respondents, interviewing methods (face-to-face versus telephone interviewing), and the representativeness of the community samples. All these factors may play a role in why variation in the prevalence estimates of traumatic events and PTSD has been reported in different epidemiologic studies and may limit comparability of estimates in some studies. Also, because most of the earlier studies were conducted in the United States, results may not be generalizable to other countries.

EPIDEMIOLOGIC GENERAL POPULATION STUDIES ON TRAUMATIC EVENTS AND PTSD

Details of epidemiologic surveys that assess traumatic events and the prevalence of PTSD using general population samples have been summarized in Table 2.1. The first two large-scale epidemiologic surveys on PTSD using *DSM-III* criteria and general population samples were conducted in the early 1980s with data from St. Louis using the Epidemiologic Catchment Area (ECA) survey (9) and the Piedmont region of North Carolina (10). In 1989, Breslau et al. (1991) conducted the first investigation of traumatic events and PTSD using *DSM-III-R* criteria in a community sample of young adults from southeast Michigan.(11) Following this study, *DSM-III-R* criteria were used to assess traumatic events and PTSD in a U.S. sample from Southeastern cities (Charleston, Greenville, Charlotte, and Savannah) (12), a national sample of young adult females (13), the first nationally representative sample of males and females using the National Comorbidity Survey (NCS) (6), a community sample of mothers from southeast Michigan (14), and a community sample from three cities in Chile using the Chile Psychiatric Prevalence Study (CPPS) (15).

Following these studies, *DSM-IV* criteria was used to assess traumatic events and PTSD in several samples including a community sample from Winnipeg, Canada (16); a community sample from Lubeck, Germany (17); a community sample from Detroit (7); a national sample from Australia (18); a sample of older adults from the Netherlands (19); a community sample from Mexico (20); a national sample from Sweden (21); a national sample from the United States (22, 23); and a European study including six countries (Belgium, France, Germany, Italy, the Netherlands, and Spain).(24) Details of the prevalence of exposure to traumatic events and PTSD from each study will now be discussed.

EPIDEMIOLOGY OF TRAUMATIC EVENTS

Prevalence of Traumatic Events
Epidemiologic research has indicated that experiencing a traumatic event in the general population is not a rare occurrence. The first general population sample assessing traumatic events conducted in 1989 was from southeast Michigan using a sample of young adults.(11) The data indicated that 39.1% (95% CI = 36.1% to 42.2%) of the respondents reported experiencing at least one traumatic event in their lifetime. The most common traumatic events reported were sudden injury or serious accident (9.4%), physical assault (8.3%), seeing someone seriously hurt or killed (7.1%), and news of the sudden death or injury of a close friend or relative (5.7%).

Table 2.1 Lifetime and current prevalence of PTSD in the general population (Posttraumatic Stress Disorder).

Dataset and/or place of collection (Authors)	Type of Sample	Year of Data Collection	n (response rate)	Age in years	Diagnostic Tools	Current prevalence %	Lifetime prevalence %
(ECA) USA (Helzer et al) (9)	Community sample	1981–1982	2,493 (67%)	Adult	DIS/*DSM-III*	N/A	1.0%
North Carolina, USA (Davidson et al) (10)	Community sample	N/A	2,985 (79%)	18–95	DIS/*DSM-III*	six month 0.44%	1.3%
Michigan, USA (Breslau et al) (11)	Community sample	1989	1,007 (84%)	21–30	DIS/*DSM-III-R*	N/A	9.2%
Southeastern cities, USA (Norris et al) (12)	Community sample	1990	1,000 (71%)	18+	TSS based on *DSM-III-R*	5.1%	N/A
USA (Resnick et al) (13)	National sample	1989	4,008 ♀ only (N/A)	18–34	DIS/*DSM-III-R*	six month 4.6% (♀)	12.3% (♀)
(NCS) USA (Kessler et al) (6)	National sample	1990–1992	5,877 (82.4%)	15–54	DIS/CIDI/*DSM-III-R*	N/A	7.8%
Michigan, USA (Breslau et al) (14)	Community sample	1990–1992	801 mothers (75%)	Mean 33.1	DIS/*DSM-III-R*	N/A	13.8%(♀)
(CPPS) Chile (Zlotnick et al) (15)	Community sample	1992–1999	2,390 (90.3%)	15+	DIS/*DSM-III-R*	N/A	4.4%
Winnipeg, Canada (Stein et al) (16)	Community sample	1994	1,002 (72%)		Modified PTSD Symptom Scale/*DSM-IV*	one month 2.7 (♀) 1.2 (♂)	N/A
Detroit, USA (Breslau et al) (7)	Community sample	1996	2,181 (86.8%)	18–45	DIS/CIDI/*DSM-IV*	N/A	9.2%[a]
Lubeck Germany (Hapke et al) (17)	Community sample	1996–1997	4,075	18–64	M-CIDI/*SDM-IV*	12 month 0.7%	1.4%
(NSMHWB) Australia (Creamer et al) (18)	National sample	1997	10,641 (78%)	18+	CIDI/*DSM-IV*	12 month 1.33%	N/A
(LASA) Netherlands (van Zelst et al) (19)	National sample	1998–1999	422 (N/A)	61–95	CIDI-*DSM-IV*	six month 0.9%	N/A
Mexico (Norris et al) (20)	Community sample	1999–2001	2,509 (79%)	18–92	CIDI/*DSM-IV*	N/A	11.2%
Sweden (Frans et al) (21)	National sample	N/A	1,824 (60.8%)	18–70	*DSM-IV*	N/A	5.6%
(NCS-R) USA (Kessler et al at 2005) (22, 23)	National sample	2001–2003	5,692 (70.9%)	18+	WHM-CIDI/*DSM-IV*	12 month 3.5%	6.8%
(ESEMeD) Europe (24)	National sample	2001–2003	21,425 (61.2%)	18+	WMH-CIDI/*DSM-IV*	12 month 0.9%	1.9%

[a] Conditional probability of PTSD after exposure.
N/A = Not available.

Another community sample from the United States assessing 10 traumatic events indicated that 21% (SE = 1.3%) and 69% (SE = 1.5%) of the total sample had experienced any past year and lifetime traumatic event, respectively.(12) The most commonly experienced traumatic events were tragic death, robbery, and car accident. In a representative sample of females from the United States, 69% reported experiencing a lifetime traumatic event with 36% of females experiencing any crime-related event (e.g., sexual assault, physical assault, homicide of friend, or family member) and 33% of females experiencing a noncrime event (e.g., accident, natural disaster, fear of death or injury, witnessing death or injury) only.(13)

Using the NCS, Kessler (1995) found that exposure to traumatic events were high in the general U.S. population with 60.7% of males and 51.2% of females endorsing any lifetime traumatic event.(6) In a community sample of mothers from southeast Michigan, the prevalence of one or more traumatic events was 40%.(14) The prevalence of traumatic events was similar in the sample from Chile, with 39.7% of the sample reporting a traumatic experience.(15) A representative community sample from Detroit found the prevalence of lifetime traumatic events to be much higher, with 89.6% (SE = 0.8%) of the sample endorsing experiencing a lifetime traumatic event.(7) The most commonly experienced event in this study was the sudden unexpected death of a relative or friend.

Data from the Winnipeg community sample also found that many individuals had been exposed to a lifetime traumatic event, with 74.2% endorsement among females and 81.3% endorsement among males.(16) The violent death of a friend or family member and being physically attacked were the two most common traumatic events among both males and females. The prevalence of traumatic events were also prevalent in the national sample from Australia, with 64.6% of males and 49.5% of females reporting at least one traumatic event.(18) In the community sample from Mexico, 76% of the sample reported experiencing a lifetime traumatic event.(20) These data also indicated that traumatic bereavement, witnessing someone killed or injured, and life-threatening accident were the three most common traumatic events among males and females. Similarly, 80.8% of the national sample from Sweden reported experiencing at least one traumatic event.(21)

Prevalence of Multiple Traumatic Events

Research has indicated that exposure to more than one traumatic event is also common in the general population. A study by Breslau et al. (1991) indicated that out of all the young adults from the community sample who were exposed to a traumatic event, 67.3% experienced one traumatic event, 23.3% experienced two traumatic events, and 9.4% experienced three traumatic events.(11) Among the representative sample of females experiencing crime-related traumatic events (rape, sexual assault, physical assault, homicide of a family member), 67.5% reported experiencing one event, 23.7% reported experiencing two different crime events, 8.8% experienced three or more different crime events, and 41% of those experiencing a crime event experiencing multiple incidents of the same event.(13) The NCS data indicated that 34.2% of males and 24.9% of females experienced two or more lifetime traumatic events.(6) Canadian data using *DSM-IV* criteria found an even higher prevalence of multiple lifetime traumatic events reported among males and females (55.4% among males and 45.8% among females).(16) Finally, Breslau et al. (1998) reported a mean number of 4.8 (SE = 0.1) distinct events among those experiencing trauma in the community sample from Detroit.(7)

When assessing the prevalence of one or more lifetime traumatic events reported in general population samples, studies using *DSM-IV* criteria tended to report higher estimates. As previously mentioned, *DSM-IV* criteria expanded the definition of traumatic events, increasing the number of events qualifying as trauma. This may partly explain the increased prevalence in traumatic events reported in more recent studies. Differences in year and location of data collection and age range of the sample may also influence the prevalence of traumatic events reported within a sample.

Sex Differences in Exposure to Traumatic Events

Research has generally found that males are more likely to experience lifetime traumatic events compared to females.(6, 11, 12, 16, 21) However, some sex differences have been found when investigating specific traumatic events among males and females. For example, Breslau et al. (1991) found that the traumatic experience of rape was only reported among females. (11) Norris et al. (1992) found that males were more likely than females to be physically assaulted, be in a motor vehicle crash, and be exposed to combat, while females were more likely than males to be sexually assaulted.(12) No other sex differences were detected in this study with regard to lifetime exposure to robbery, fire, other disaster or hazard, and tragic death. Kessler et al. (1995) reported numerous sex differences with regard to lifetime prevalence of traumatic events.(6) More specifically, males relative to females were more likely to experience physical attack, combat, threat with a weapon, life-threatening accident, natural disaster with fire, and witnessing someone badly injured or killed. However, females were more likely to experience rape, molestation, child physical abuse, and childhood neglect relative to males. Breslau et al. (1998) found similar results using a community sample from Detroit, which indicated that males compared to females were more likely to be mugged or threatened with a weapon, shot or stabbed, and badly beaten, while females relative to males were more likely to experience rape and other sexual assault.(7) In the community sample from Germany, females were more likely to experience rape and sexual abuse than were males, but when considering lifetime prevalence of any traumatic event, gender differences were not found.(17) In the national sample from Australia, males were significantly more likely to experience being physically attacked, threatened with a weapon, and to be exposed to combat, while females were more likely to be exposed to rape and sexual molestation.(18) Sex differences were also noted in the community sample from Mexico, with males being more likely to experience traumatic bereavement, witnessing someone killed or injured, life-threatening accident, physical assault, being threatened with a weapon, combat, and torture or terrorism, while females were more likely to experience sexual assault.(20)

The most consistent findings among all general population studies of traumatic events with regard to sex differences is that females are more likely to experience sexual traumatization involving sexual assault, rape, or molestation, while males are more likely to experience combat and assaultive violence such as physical attacks and threats with a weapon. However, comparing sex differences across studies is challenging because not all studies include the same qualification for traumatic events.

Risk Factors for Traumatic Events

Some studies using general population samples have identified certain factors that increase the risk for experiencing a traumatic event. In addition to sex being a risk factor for certain traumatic events, as discussed above, other risk factors have been identified in the literature. Norris et al. (1992) found race differences, with White respondents being significantly more likely than Black respondents to experience lifetime traumatic events in a community sample of Southeastern United States cities.(12) Contrary to this finding, Breslau et al. (1998) found in a community sample from Detroit that being non-White was associated with increased odds of assaultive violence and trauma to others compared to being White.(7) This research also indicated that lower educational attainment and household income was associated with increased odds of assaultive violence.

Among young adults from southeast Michigan, risk factors for exposure to traumatic events included being male, having less than a college education, a history of three or more early conduct problems, a family history or psychiatric problems, neuroticism, and extraversion.(11) These young adults were reinterviewed three years later, and results revealed that neuroticism and extraversion remained prospective predictors of exposure to traumatic events. (25) Another prospective study from southeast Michigan that assessed externalizing problems, anxiety, and intelligence at age six and exposure to traumatic events at age 17 found that high externalizing problems increased the odds of exposure to assaultive violence, while IQ above 115 lowered the odds of exposure to assaultive and other types of trauma.(26) Only a few studies have assessed risk factors for traumatic events. However, results from these studies indicate that such events are not random occurrences.(4) In fact, research using twin pairs from the general population found that genetically based personality factors may increase the likelihood of experiencing certain traumatic events.(27) More specifically, it was found that antisocial personality traits predicted exposure to violent assaultive traumatic events.

EPIDEMIOLOGY OF POSTTRAUMATIC STRESS DISORDER

Prevalence of PTSD

Table 2.1 provides a summary of the lifetime and current (past one month, six months, 12 months) prevalence rates of PTSD based on several general population samples. As previously mentioned, differences in PTSD prevalence estimates reported in general population samples may be due to the method and diagnostic criteria for assessing traumatic events and PTSD symptoms and differences in study samples, including year and location of data collection, age of respondents, and interviewing methods. Regardless of study differences, epidemiologic investigations are able to provide estimates of how prevalent PTSD is in the general population.

The two earliest studies of PTSD conducted in the early 1980s using general population samples and *DSM-III* criteria provided similar estimates of the prevalence of lifetime PTSD. The first study using ECA data indicated that only 1% of the total sample met full *DSM-III* criteria for a lifetime PTSD diagnosis.(9) However, 15% of males and 16% of females had a least one PTSD symptom after experiencing a traumatic event. Similarly, data from a community sample from North Carolina reported that 1.3% of the sample met *DSM-III* criteria for lifetime PTSD.(10)

Later general population samples using *DSM-III-R* criteria produced larger prevalence estimates for PTSD. The Breslau study (1991), using a sample of young adults from Michigan, found that 9.2% (95% CI = 7.6% to 11.2%) of the total sample met criteria for lifetime PTSD.(11) However, 23.6% of individuals exposed to traumatic events developed PTSD. Similarly, the community sample from four Southeast United States cities found that 5.1% of the sample met criteria for current PTSD.(12) In a national U.S. sample of females only, the lifetime and past six-month prevalence of PTSD was 12.3% and 4.6%, respectively.(13) Similarly, results from a community sample of mothers from southeast Michigan found the prevalence of lifetime PTSD to be 13.8%.(14) The results from a national U.S. sample of males and females using NCS data estimated lifetime prevalence of PTSD to be 7.8% (SE = 0.5%).(6) The prevalence of lifetime PTSD in the representative sample from Chile was 4.4% (SE = 0.5%), slightly lower than figures from the United States.(15)

Studies using general population samples and *DSM-IV* criteria also found higher PTSD prevalence estimates. A Canadian study by Stein et al. found that 2.7% of females and 1.2% of males met *DSM-IV* criteria for a past month diagnosis of PTSD.(16) The study also indicated that an additional 3.4% of females and 0.3% of males had a past month subthreshold PTSD diagnosis. Subthreshold or partial PTSD has been defined in different ways, but generally speaking, it is applicable only when an individual lacks one or more specified criteria required to meet the full *DSM* diagnosis. Breslau et al. (1998) reported the conditional probability of PTSD after traumatic event exposure to be 9.2% in a community sample from Detroit.(7) The community sample from Germany indicated that lifetime, past year, and conditional probability of PTSD was 1.4% (SE = 0.18), 0.7% (SE = 0.13%), and 6.9% (SE = 0.89), respectively (17). The national sample from Australia reported that 1.3% (SE = 0.12%) of the sample met criteria for past 12-month diagnosis of PTSD.(18) A representative sample from the Netherlands reported that 0.9% (95% CI = 0.7–1.1) of the older adult sample met criteria for a past six-month PTSD diagnosis, while 13.1% (95% CI = 12.7–13.6) met criteria for subthreshold PTSD.(19) The prevalence of lifetime PTSD was 11.2% (SE = 0.6) in the community sample from Mexico.(20) Results from the National Comorbidity Survey Replication (NCS-R), a nationally representative study from the United States, indicated that past year and lifetime prevalence of PTSD was 3.5% (SE = 0.3%) and 6.8% (SE =0.4%), respectively.(22, 23) Findings from the study of six European countries reported a much lower prevalence of lifetime PTSD of only 1.9% (95% CI = 1.7–2.1).(24)

Collectively, studies dated from the early 1980s to the present indicate that the lifetime prevalence of PTSD in general population samples of males and females ranges from 1% to 11%. Factors decreasing comparability of studies, such as selected *DSM* criteria and study methods, have already been mentioned. However, it should be noted that the large range of PTSD prevalence estimates may be partly explained by the studies being conducted in different cities and in different countries. The prevalence of traumatic events, and thereby PTSD, may depend on crime, poverty, politics, violence and other factors, which differ in different parts of the world. For example, Zlonick et al. (2006) speculate that differences in the prevalence of PTSD found in Mexico and Chile may in part be due to greater crime and poverty rates in Mexico compared to

Chile.(15) Regardless of the range in PTSD prevalence reported in general population samples, findings from these epidemiologic studies have determined that PTSD is prevalent in the general population and is considered an important public health concern.

Duration of PTSD Symptoms

PTSD has been found to be a chronic condition for many individuals. A standard definition of PTSD chronicity does not exist in the research literature. However, many studies require that the duration of PTSD symptoms must last at least six months to be considered a chronic case. ECA data have indicated that, among individuals with PTSD symptoms, symptoms lasted less than six months for 49% of individuals, but persisted for more than six years for one-third of symptomatic persons.(9) These data also indicated that long duration of symptoms occurred for males who experienced combat and for females who were physically attacked. In the community sample from North Carolina, approximately 50% of individuals with PTSD were considered to be chronic cases as measured by symptoms lasting more than six months.(10) In the sample of young adults from Detroit, 57% of those with PTSD had symptoms lasting for more than one year.(28) These data also indicated that a family history of antisocial behavior and female sex were specific risk factors for chronic PTSD. The nationally representative NCS data also found that PTSD is chronic, with one-third of individuals not recovering from their symptoms even after many years and regardless of treatment.(6) Breslau et al. (1998) found that 26% and 40% individuals with PTSD remitted after six months and 12 months, respectively.(7) These data also indicated that duration of symptoms lasted longer in females (median duration 48.1 months) compared to males (median duration 12.0 months). The community sample from Mexico indicated that 62% of those with PTSD had symptoms lasting longer than one year and were considered chronic PTSD cases.(20)

Results from a prospective longitudinal study of adolescents and young adults (aged 14–24 years) indicated that 48% of individuals with full or subthreshold PTSD at baseline continued to experience full or subthreshold PTSD during the two follow-up periods (approximately 20 and 42 months after baseline) and were classified as chronic PTSD cases.(29) Also, the experience of new traumatic events after the baseline assessment, higher avoidant symptoms, more help seeking, and lower self-competence were predictors of chronic PTSD in this sample. In another study investigating predictors of chronic PTSD in the sample recruited from an emergency room, depressive symptoms measured at one week, one month, and four months after the traumatic event were the best predictors of chronicity.(30) Furthermore, a study of monozygotic veteran pairs indicated that 15 years after the Vietnam War, the prevalence of PTSD among the twin pair serving in the military in Southeast Asia remained substantially increased compared to the nonserving twin pair.(31)

Sex Differences in Prevalence of PTSD

Epidemiologic investigations of PTSD have indicated that females are more likely than males to develop PTSD after the exposure to a traumatic event.(6, 7, 9–11, 15, 16, 19, 20). More specifically, several studies report that PTSD is approximately twice as prevalent among females compared to males.(6, 7, 11, 15, 16, 20) Breslau et al. (1997) examined sex differences of PTSD in detail using the southeast Michigan community sample of young adults and found that males and females did not differ on the cumulative incidence of traumatic events or the number of traumatic exposures, yet females were two times more likely to experience PTSD after a traumatic event.(32) The risk factors that partially explained the sex differences in these data were preexisting anxiety disorders or major depressive disorders and greater exposure to traumatic events in childhood. Another study using a representative sample from Detroit of adults aged 18 to 45 years indicated that sex differences were primarily due to females' risk of PTSD following exposure to assaultive violence (36%), compared to males (6%).(33, 34) These data also indicated that assaultive trauma was associated with increased risk of PTSD following a later traumatic event.(35) This trauma sensitization hypothesis finding was replicated in another community sample of young adults from a mid-Atlantic U.S. city, indicating that when assaultive violence preceded a subsequent nonassaultive traumatic event the risk for PTSD increased significantly among females (relative risk = 4.9, 95% CI =2.1–11.11), but not among males (relative risk = 1.6, 95% CI = 0.9–3.0).(36) The data from the Canadian sample from Winnipeg showed that females did not experience a greater number of traumatic events compared to males; however, females were more likely to experience full or subthreshold PTSD after experiencing any trauma and nonsexual assaultive violence.(37)

It is noteworthy that sex differences have not been found in all epidemiological studies. Results from the national sample in Australia indicated that the past 12-month prevalence of PTSD among males and females was similar (1.2% versus 1.4%).(18) Also, data from the community sample from Germany indicated that the female gender was not an independent risk factor for PTSD.(17) The authors suggest that the increased risk of PTSD among females may be due to their greater likelihood of experiencing trauma events most associated with PTSD (i.e., rape and sexual abuse) and having preexisting disorders associated with increased risk of PTSD, compared to males. Generally speaking, however, females do not have a greater vulnerability to PTSD.

A review of 25 years of research does confirm the increased likelihood of females developing PTSD, compared to males, but indicates that females' higher prevalence of PTSD is not solely a result of higher exposure to sexual trauma.(38) The current literature seems to indicate that the type of traumatic events, preexisting psychiatric disorders, and childhood events may also account for some of the variance in the relationship between sex and PTSD. Further research in this area is warranted.

Traumatic Events Exposure and PTSD

The prevalence of PTSD has been found to vary depending on the type of traumatic event experienced. Also, males and females experience specific traumatic events at different rates, which has an impact on the relationship between traumatic event exposure and the development of PTSD. In the early study by Helzer et al. (1987), the only two experiences associated with PTSD among males were combat and seeing someone hurt or die, while a serious accident, physical attack, seeing someone hurt or die, and threat or close call were associated with PTSD among females.(9) Of these traumatic events, PTSD was the most common among females who were physically attacked. These data also indicated that experiencing a natural disaster did not account for any of the PTSD cases among males or females. In the general sample of young adults from southeast Michigan, the lowest rate of PTSD was associated with sudden injury or serious accident (11.6%) and was significantly greater for threat of death (24.0%), seeing someone killed or seriously hurt (23.6%), physical assault (22.6%), and news of sudden death or accident of a close relative or friend (21.1%).(11) These data also indicated that 80% of females reporting rape (rape only reported among females) met criteria for PTSD. Kessler et al. (1995) found that the traumatic events most commonly associated with PTSD among males were combat exposure (28.8%) and witnessing someone badly injured or killed (24.3%), while rape (29.9%) and sexual molestation (19.1%) were the most common traumatic events associated with PTSD among females.(6) However, this study also indicated that rape had the highest conditional probability associated with PTSD for both males and females, with 65% of males and 46% of females meeting criteria for PTSD when reporting rape as the most upsetting traumatic event. In the national U.S. sample of females, the prevalence of PTSD was the highest among those reporting physical assault and rape.(13) In the national Australian sample, sexual trauma (rape and molestation) was associated with the greatest likelihood of developing PTSD among both males and females.(39)

Not all studies investigate the relationship between exposure to traumatic events and prevalence of PTSD separately for males and females. In a combined sample of males and females, Norris et al. (1992) found that the types of traumatic events with the highest association with PTSD were sexual assault (14%), physical assault (13%), and motor vehicle crash (12%).(12) Breslau et al. (1998) found that 31% of all PTSD cases were attributable to the single traumatic event of an unexpected death of a loved one, while collectively the traumatic event category of assaultive violence accounted for 39.5% of PTSD cases.(7) When looking at the combined male and female community sample from Mexico, sexual assault or molestation was the most highly associated traumatic event with PTSD.(20) In a representative sample of active Canadian military personnel (n = 8,441, age = 16 to 54 years), exposure to combat (adjusted odds ratios = 2.10, 95% CI = 1.28–3.45), and witnessing atrocities or massacres (adjusted odds ratios = 4.33, 95% CI = 2.79–6.72) were associated with increased odds of past year (*DSM-IV*) PTSD (relative to no past year mental disorder) after adjusting for sex, age, marital status, income, education, military rank, type of force, and other deployment-related traumatic events.(40)

Research has identified numerous traumatic events that are highly associated with increased prevalence of PTSD. Arguably, the most consistent finding in the literature on exposure to traumatic events and PTSD is the relationship between sexual violence leading to PTSD among females and combat exposure leading to PTSD among males.

Risk Factors for PTSD

As previously mentioned, female sex is associated with a greater risk of PTSD. In addition, research has identified other important risk factors that increase the likelihood of PTSD after the exposure to a traumatic event. Childhood behavior problems (i.e., lying, vandalism, fighting) before the age of 15 have been found to be associated with PTSD, which may reflect a greater likelihood of exposure to traumatic events and/or a predisposition to experiencing symptoms after the trauma.(9) Other childhood and family factors were identified in another community sample, which indicated that individuals with PTSD were more likely to have experienced childhood poverty, family history of psychiatric illness, parental divorce or separation before the age of 10, and child abuse.(10) A study using the NCS found that, after adjusting for individual type of trauma, only a history of affective disorders among females and a history of anxiety disorders and parental mental disorder among males predicted PTSD.(41) In a study of young adults, PTSD was associated with neuroticism, separation from parents in childhood, preexisting psychiatric anxiety or depression, and a family history of anxiety or antisocial behavior.(11) Similarly, in a study of older adults (61 years to 95 years), neuroticism and early adverse childhood events were found to be risk factors for PTSD.(19) In a nationally representative U.S. sample using NCS data, neuroticism was found to be significantly associated with PTSD among females, while neuroticism and self-criticism were associated with PTSD among males after adjusting for specific traumatic events, lifetime anxiety disorders, and parental mental disorders.(42) Interestingly, in a prospective study from southeast Michigan, externalizing problems and anxiety at age six increased the odds of PTSD following an exposure to a traumatic event at age 17, while IQ of greater than 115 at age six decreased the odds of PTSD.(26) Similarly, a longitudinal study using a New Zealand birth cohort found that children's externalizing disorders, family history of mental health difficulties, family adversities, low IQ, and chronic environmental stressors assessed before the age of 11 were risk factors for PTSD up to the age of 32.(43) Similar results from a U.S. sample indicated that high levels of depressed and anxious feelings reported in Grade 1 were associated with 1.5 times increased risk of developing PTSD after a traumatic event in early adulthood.(44)

A meta-analysis of 77 studies published between 1980 and 2000 identified 14 risk factors for PTSD.(45) More specifically, the results of the meta-analysis collectively indicate that psychiatric history, reported child abuse, and family psychiatric history are the most uniform risk factors for predicting PTSD regardless of the study population and methods.

MENTAL AND PHYSICAL HEALTH COMORBIDITIES OF PTSD

Mental Health

Comorbidity of other psychiatric disorders is common among individuals with PTSD. Helzer et al. (1987) found that individuals with PTSD were twice as likely to have a comorbid psychiatric disorder, with obsessive-compulsive disorder (OCD), dysthymia, and manic-depressive disorder being the most prevalent comorbid diagnoses.(9) Davidson et al. (1991) found that when compared to individuals without PTSD individuals with PTSD were more likely to have somatization disorder, schizophrenia, panic disorder, social phobia, OCD, drug abuse or dependence, major depression, agoraphobia, simple phobia, and generalized anxiety disorder (GAD).(10) Breslau et al. (1991) found in the general population sample of young adults that 82.8% of those with PTSD had one or more comorbid psychiatric disorders, including OCD, agoraphobia, dysthymia, mania, panic, major depression, GAD, drug abuse or dependence, and alcohol abuse or dependence.(11) Similarly, results from the NCS indicated that 88.3% of males and 79% of females with PTSD had at least one other comorbid psychiatric diagnosis. (6) The prevalence of comorbid lifetime mental disorders was equally as high in the Chilean sample with 90.4% of individuals with PTSD reporting a comorbid mental health disorder.(15) Results from the national Australian sample also found comorbidity of PTSD and other Axis I disorder to be prevalent, with 85.2% of males and 79.7% of females with PTSD meeting criteria for at least one other Axis I disorder.(18) Another study using the same data found that 34.4% of individuals with PTSD also met criteria for a substance use disorder.(46) In a nationally representative Canadian sample, PTSD (assessed using a single item asking whether the respondent had been given a diagnosis of PTSD from a health care professional) was associated with major depression, mania, panic attacks, agoraphobia, social phobia, alcohol dependence, and drug dependence.(47) These data indicated that major depression was the comorbid disorder with the largest effects.

Many PTSD studies do not assess order of onset of psychiatric disorders, either due to the cross-sectional design of the study or the lack of data on age of onset of each disorder. However, in a sample of mothers from southeast Michigan, it was determined that PTSD increased the risk of first onset major depression and alcohol abuse/dependence and that preexisting major depression increased the risk of experiencing trauma and vulnerability to PTSD following traumatic events.(14) In addition, a survival analysis using NCS data indicated that individuals with a current diagnosis of PTSD were more likely to develop secondary other anxiety, mood, and substance use disorder compared to those without PTSD.(48) This increased risk was not found when PTSD was in remission. A review of the comorbidity literature indicates that PTSD may have a causal role in the onset of some secondary psychiatric diagnoses, while preexisting psychiatric disorders may also increase vulnerability of PTSD after exposure to a traumatic event.(49) Prospective studies on the PTSD and comorbidity are necessary to further understand the temporal sequence of disorder onset and the causal relationship among commonly comorbid psychiatric disorders.

Suicidal Behavior
Research has found a significant relationship between PTSD and suicidal ideation and attempts using general population samples. An earlier study found that individuals with PTSD were 14.9 times (95% CI = 5.10–43.66) more likely to attempt suicide compared to individuals without PTSD.(10) The odds ratios were attenuated when comorbidity of major depression was controlled, yet the relationship between PTSD and suicide attempts remained statistically significant (Adjusted odds ratio = 8.2, 95% CI = 5.49–12.21). Results from the NCS indicated that PTSD was associated with increased odds of subsequent suicidal ideation (odds ratio = 5.1, 95% CI = 3.9–6.8) and suicide attempts (odd ratio = 6.0, 95% CI = 3.4–10.7) after controlling for person–year and sociodemographic variables.(50) In another investigation of females using the NCS data, PTSD was associated with 2.5 times greater odds of suicidal ideation after adjusting for the effects of sociodemographic variables, sexual assault history, psychosocial characteristics, alcohol symptoms, and depression.(51) Using a national Canadian sample, those with current self-reported, physician-diagnosed PTSD were 2.35 times more likely to have attempted suicide in the past year, even after controlling for sociodemographic variables, numerous psychiatric disorders, and medical morbidity.(47) The current body of literature supports the relationship between PTSD and increased likelihood of suicidal ideation and attempts, which highlights the possible utility of screening those with PTSD for suicidal behavior.

Physical Health Conditions
PTSD has been found to have significant associations with physical health conditions. An early community study found that individuals with PTSD compared to those without PTSD were more likely to have bronchial asthma (13.5% versus 4.8%, $p = 0.02$), peptic ulcer (12.8% versus 4.1%, $p = 0.02$), and hypertension (31.4% versus 18.5%, $p = 0.04$).(10) These data did not reveal any other significant relationships between PTSD and other physical health conditions assessed (emphysema, diabetes, heart disease, arthritis, cerebrovascular disease, cancer, arteriosclerosis, and neurological disorder). Chronic PTSD, defined as symptoms lasting at least one year, has also been found to be associated with an increased likelihood of arthritis, bronchitis, migraine, and gynecologic problems (among females) compared to nonchronic PTSD.(28) In a prospective study, it was found that PTSD at baseline was associated with more gastrointestinal, cardiopulmonary, conversion or pseudoneurological, and sexual symptoms.(52) In addition, these data indicated that those with PTSD reported more somatic symptoms compared to individuals with other psychiatric disorders. In a nationally representative sample using NCS data, it was found that among anxiety disorders, PTSD had the strongest associations with physical disorders, including neurological conditions, vascular conditions, gastrointestinal disease,

metabolic/autoimmune conditions, and bone and joint conditions, after adjusting for socio-demographic variables, major depression, dysthymia, bipolar disorder, alcohol use disorder, substance use disorder, and other anxiety disorders.(53) Another study using NCS data found that individuals with PTSD were more likely to report having a physical condition after adjusting for sex, health perceptions, stress, health-related behaviors, insurance coverage, number of trauma exposures, number of psychiatric disorders, and neuroticism.(54) In a national Canadian sample, individuals with current self-reported, physician-diagnosed PTSD were more likely to have a higher prevalence of all physical health problems assessed in the survey compared to those reporting no PTSD diagnosis.(47) These data also indicated that PTSD was associated with increased odds of respiratory diseases, cardiovascular diseases, chronic pain conditions, gastrointestinal illnesses, cancer, chronic fatigue syndrome, and multiple chemical sensitivities after adjusting for sociodemographic variables and psychiatric disorders. Research has also indicated that PTSD commonly co-occurs with chronic pain, which may be due to factors that predispose individuals to both conditions (shared vulnerability) and/or aspects of chronic pain maintaining or complicating PTSD and vise versa (mutual maintenance).(55)

The relationship between PTSD and physical health has also been reported in military samples. In an American sample of Iraq war veterans, numerous physical health symptoms (i.e., pain symptoms, dizziness, fainting, indigestion problems) were found to be more prevalent among those with PTSD compared to those without PTSD one year after serving in Iraq.(56) In a sample of female veterans, medical conditions were more prevalent in females with a history of PTSD compared to females with depression or females reporting neither depression nor PTSD.(57) Similarly, in a Canadian sample of male veterans, PTSD symptoms directly influenced diagnosable physical symptoms when controlling for the effects of depression and alcohol dependence and indirectly influenced physical health symptoms through depression only.(58) In a population-based survey of Gulf War veterans, those who screened positive for a PTSD diagnosis were more likely to have more self-reported physical health symptoms and medical conditions compared to those without PTSD.(59) More information on PTSD and the military can be found in a later chapter of this book. Using several general population and military samples, research has confirmed that a significantly association between PTSD and physical health problems exists.

CONCLUSIONS

Traumatic events and PTSD are prevalent in the general population. Research has identified certain factors that increase the risk of exposure to traumatic events and vulnerability to PTSD. PTSD is an important public health problem not only due to the high prevalence found in the general population but also because of its morbidity and the significant relationships found between PTSD and other psychiatric disorders, suicidal behavior, and physical health problems. Knowledge of the epidemiology of traumatic events and PTSD will help inform prevention efforts and increased ability to screen for PTSD and its associated conditions in populations that have been exposed to its known risk factors.

REFERENCES

1. American Psychiatric Association. Diagnostic and Statistical Manual of Mental Disorders. 3rd ed. Washington, DC: American Psychiatric Press, Inc; 1980.
2. American Psychiatric Association. Diagnostic and Statistical Manual of Mental Disorders. 3rd ed. Washington, DC: American Psychiatric Press, Inc; 1987.
3. American Psychiatric Association. Diagnostic & Statistical Manual for Mental Disorders (DSM). 4th ed. Washington, DC: American Psychiatric Press, Inc; 1994.
4. Breslau N. Epidemiological studies of trauma, posttraumatic stress disorder, and other psychiatric disorders. Can J Psychiatry 2002; 47: 923–9.
5. Breslau N, Kessler RC. The stressor criterion in DSM-IV posttraumatic stress disorder: An empirical investigation. Biol Psychiatry 2001; 50: 699–704.
6. Kessler RC, Sonnega A, Bromet E, Hughes M, Nelson CB. Posttraumatic stress disorder in the national comorbidity survey. Arch Gen Psychiatry 1995; 52: 1048–60.
7. Breslau N, Kessler RC, Chilcoat HD et al. Trauma and posttraumatic stress disorder in the community: the 1996 Detroit area survey of trauma. Arch Gen Psychiatry 1998; 55: 626–32.

8. Breslau N, Peterson EL, Poission M, Schultz LR, Lucia VC. Estimating post-traumatic stress disorder in the community: lifetime perspective and the impact of typical traumatic events. Psychol Med 2004; 34: 889–98.

9. Helzer J, Robins L, McEvoy L. Post-traumatic stress disorder in the general population: findings of the epidemiologic catchment area survey. N Engl J Med 1987; 317: 1630–4.

10. Davidson JRT, Hughes D, Blazer D, George LK. Posttraumatic stress disorder in the community: an epidemiological study. Psychol Med 1991; 21: 1–19.

11. Breslau N, Davis GC, Andreski P, Peterson EL. Traumatic events and posttraumatic stress disorder in an urban population of young adults. Arch Gen Psychiatry 1991; 48: 216–22.

12. Norris FH. Epidemiology of trauma: Frequency and impact of different potentially traumatic events on different demographic groups. J Consult Clin Psychol 1992; 60: 409–18.

13. Resnick HS, Kilpatrick DG, Dansky BS, Saunders BE, Best CL. Prevalence of civilian trauma and posttraumatic stress disorder in a representative national sample of women. J Consult Clin Psychol 1993; 61: 984–91.

14. Breslau N, Davis GC, Peterson EL, Schultz L. Psychiatric sequelae of posttraumatic stress disorder in women. Arch Gen Psychiatry 1997; 54: 81–7.

15. Zlotnick C, Johnson J, Kohn R et al. Epidemiology of trauma, post-traumatic stress disorder (PTSD) and co-morbid disorders in Chile. Psychol Med 2006; 36: 1523–33.

16. Stein MB, Walker JR, Hazen AL, Forde DR. Full and partial posttraumatic stress disorder: findings from a community survey. Am J Psychiatry 1997; 154: 1114–9.

17. Hapke U, Schumann A, Rumpf H-J, John U, Meyer C. Post-traumatic stress disorder: the role of trauma, pre-existing psychitric disorders, and gender. Eur Arch Psychiatry Clin Neurosci 2006; 256: 299–306.

18. Creamer M, Burgess P, Mcfarlane AC. Post-traumatic stress disorder: findings from the Australian national survey of mental health and well-being. Psychol Med 2001; 31: 1237–47.

19. Van Zelst W, De Beurs E, Beekman ATF, Deeg DJH, Van Dyck R. Prevalence and risk factors of posttraumatic stress disorder in older adults. Psychother Psychosom 2003; 72: 333–42.

20. Norris FH, Murphy AD, Baker CK et al. Epidemiology of trauma and posttraumatic stress disorder in Mexico. J Abnorm Psychol 2003; 112: 646–56.

21. Frans O, Rimmo PA, Aberg L, Fredrikson M. Trauma exposure and post-traumatic stress disorder in the general population. Acta Psychiatr Scand 2005; 111: 291–9.

22. Kessler RC, Chiu WT, Demler O, Walters EE. Prevalence, severity, and comorbidity of 12-month DSM-IV disorders in the national comorbidity survey replication. Arch Gen Psychiatry 2005; 62: 617–27.

23. Kessler RC, Berglund P, Demler O, Jin R, Walters EE. Lifetime prevalence and age-of-onset distributions of DSM-IV disorders in the national comorbidity survey replication. Arch Gen Psychiatry 2005; 62: 593–602.

24. Alonso J, Angermeyer MC, Bernert S et al. Prevalence of mental disorders in Europe: results from the European study of the epidemiology of mental disorders (ESEMeD) project. Acta Psychiatr Scand Suppl 2004; (420): 21–7.

25. Breslau N, Davis GC, Andreski P. Risk factors for PTSD-related traumatic events: a prospective study. Am J Psychiatry 1995; 152: 529–35.

26. Breslau N, Lucia VC, Alvarado GF. Intelligence and other predisposing factors in exposure to trauma and posttraumatic stress disorder. Arch Gen Psychiatry 2006; 63: 1238–45.

27. Jang KL, Stein MB, Taylor S, Asmundson GJG, Livesley WJ. Exposure to traumatic events and experiences: aetiological relationships with personality function. Psychiatry Res 2003; 120: 61–9.

28. Breslau N, Davis GC. Posttraumatic stress disorder in an urban population of young adults: risk factors for chronicity. Am J Psychiatry 1992; 149: 671–5.

29. Perkonigg A, Pfister H, Stein MB et al. Longitudinal course of posttraumatic stress disorder and posttraumatic stress disorder symptoms in a community sample of adolescents and young adults. Am J Psychiatry 2005; 162: 1320–7.

30. Freedman SA, Brandes D, Peri T, Shalev A. Predictors of chronic post-traumatic stress disorder. Br J Psychiatry 1999; 174: 353–9.

31. Goldberg J, True WR, Eisen SA, Henderson WG. A twin study of the effects of the Vietnam War on posttraumatic stress disorder. JAMA 1990; 263: 1227–32.

32. Breslau N, Davis GC, Andreski P, Peterson EL, Schultz LR. Sex differences in posttraumatic stress disorder. Arch Gen Psychiatry 1997; 54(11): 1044–8.

33. Breslau N. Gender differences in trauma and posttraumatic stress disorder. J Gend Specif Med 2002; 5: 34–40.

34. Breslau N, Chilcoat HD, Kessler RC, Lucia VC. Vulnerability to assaultive violence: further specification of the sex differences in post-traumatic stress disorder. Psychol Med 1999; 29: 813–21.

35. Breslau N, Chilcoat HD, Kessler RC, Davis CG. Previous exposure to trauma and PTSD effects of subsequent trauma: results from the Detroit area survey of trauma. Am J Psychiatry 1999; 156: 902–7.

36. Breslau N, Anthony JC. Gender differences in the sensitivity to posttraumatic stress disorder: an epidemiological study of urban young adults. J Abnorm Psychol 2007; 116: 607–11.

37. Stein MB, Walker JR, Forde DR. Gender differences in susceptibility to posttraumatic stress disorder. Behav Res and Ther 2000; 38: 619–28.

38. Tolin DF, Foa EB. Sex differences in trauma and posttraumatic stress disorder: a quantitative review of 25 years of research. Psychol Bull 2006; 132: 959–92.

39. Rosenman S. Trauma and posttraumatic stress disorder in Australia: findings in the population sample of the Australian national survey of mental health and wellbeing. Aust N Z J Psychiatry 2002; 36: 515–20.

40. Sareen J, Cox BJ, Afifi TO et al. Combat and peacekeeping operations in relation to prevalence of mental disorders and perceived need for mental health care: findings from a large representative sample of military personnel. Arch Gen Psychiatry 2007; 64: 843–52.

41. Bromet E, Sonnega A, Kessler RC. Risk factors for DSM-III-R posttraumatic stress disorder: findings from the national comorbidity survey. Am J Epidemiol 1998; 147(4): 353–61.

42. Cox BJ, MacPherson PSR, Enns MW, McWilliams LA. Neuroticism and self-criticism associated with posttraumatic stress disorder in a nationally representative sample. Behav Res Ther 2004; 42: 105–14.

43. Koenen KC, Moffitt TE, Poulton R, Martin J, Caspi A. Early childhood factors associated with the development of post-traumatic stress disorder: results from a longitudinal birth cohort. Psychol Med 2007; 37: 181–92.

44. Storr CL, Ialongo NS, Anthony JC, Breslau N. Childhood antecedents of exposure to traumatic events and posttraumatic stress disorder. Am J Psychiatry 2007; 164: 119–25.

45. Brewin CR, Andrews B, Valentine JD. Meta-analysis of risk factors for posttraumatic stress disorder in trauma-exposed adults. J Consult Clin Psychol 2000; 68(5): 748–66.

46. Mills KL, Teesson M, Ross J, Peters L. Trauma, PTSD, and substance use disorders: findings from the Australian national survey of mental health and well-being. Am J Psychiatry 2006; 163: 651–8.

47. Sareen J, Cox BJ, Stein MB et al. Physical and mental comorbidity, disability, and suicidal behavior associated with posttraumatic stress disorders in a large community sample. Psychosom Med 2007; 69: 242–8.

48. Kessler RC. Posttraumatic stress disorder: The burden to the individual and to society. J Clin Psychiatry 2000; 61: 4–12.

49. Brady KT, Killeen TK, Brewerton T, Lucerini S. Comorbidity of psychiatric disorders and posttraumatic stress disorder. J Clin Psychiatry 2000; 61: 22–32.

50. Kessler RC, Borges G, Walters EE. Prevalence of and risk factors for lifetime suicide attempts in the national comorbidity survey. Arch Gen Psychiatry 1999; 56(7): 617–26.

51. Ullman SE, Brecklin L. Sexual assault history and suicidal behavior in a national sample of women. Suicide Life Threat Behav 2002; 32: 117–30.

52. Andreski P, Chilcoat H, Breslau N. Post-traumatic stress disorder and somatization symptoms: a prospective study. Psychiatry Res 1998; 79: 131–8.

53. Sareen J, Cox BJ, Clara I, Asmundson GJG. The relationship between anxiety disorders and physical disorders in the U.S. national comorbidity survey. Depress Anxiety 2005; 21: 193–202.

54. Lauterbach D, Vora R, Rakow M. The relationship between posttraumatic stress disorder and self-reported health problems. Psychosom Med 2005; 67: 939–47.

55. Asmundson GJ, Coons MJ, Taylor S, Katz J. PTSD and the experience of pain: research and clinical implications of shared vulnerability and mutual maintenance models. Can J Psychiatry 2002; 47(10): 930–7.

56. Hoge CW, Terhakopian A, Castro CA, Messer SC, Engel CC. Association of postraumatic stress disorder with somatic symptoms, health care visits, and absenteeism among Iraq war veterans. Am J Psychiatry 2007; 164: 150–3.

57. Frayne SM, Seaver MR, Loveland S et al. Burden of medical illness in women with depression and posttraumatic stress disorder. Arch Intern Med 2004; 164(12): 1306–12.

58. Asmundson GJG, Stein MB, McCreary DR. Posttraumatic stress disorder symptoms influence health status of deployed peacekeepers and nondeployed military personnel. J Nerv Ment Dis 2002; 190: 807–15.

59. Barrett DH, Doebbeling CC, Schwartz DA et al. Posttraumatic stress disorder and self-reported physical health status among U.S. military personnel serving during the gulf war period. Psychosomatics 2002; 43: 195–205.

3 | Diagnostic dilemmas in assessing post traumatic stress disorder

Berthold PR Gersons and Miranda Olff

INTRODUCTION

The introduction of the Third Diagnostic and Statistical Manual (*DSM-III* (1)), International Classification of Diseases of the World Health Organization version 10 (ICD-10) (2) and Fourth Diagnostic and Statistical Manual (*DSM-IV* (3)) has helped psychiatrists to become more precise in assessing psychiatric disorders. In *DSM-III* the posttraumatic stress disorder (PTSD) has been introduced for the first time in psychiatry as a coherent profile of signs and symptoms related to the experience of a traumatic incident. Large epidemiological studies have contributed to the validity of this disorder.(4, 5, 6) In the assessment of PTSD two flaws however can interfere with the correct establishing of the diagnosis of PTSD. The first flaw is people do not tell easily about their traumatic experiences and doctors do not like to hear the terrible details. The accuracy of the information generated during the psychiatric interview concerning trauma depends on the level of skills used to establish a trustful relationship with the patient and a willingness to listen to horrifying details. Also, the patient is often unaware of any relationship between the symptoms of PTSD and the experience of the trauma. As we know in psychiatry the accuracy of the information that we get during the interview depends strongly on our willingness to listen. A nonjudgmental attitude in the interview is a necessary prerequisite. The second flaw in assessing PTSD is the overwhelming affect that accompanies the report of someone who experienced trauma. For the listener, therefore, it sometimes seems self-evident traumatic experiences must result in some kind of disorder, especially PTSD. Asking about symptoms after listening to the details of a traumatic incident can look like an unneeded burden. Here the epidemiology of PTSD (4, 5) helps us enormously to understand the limited relationship between the experience of trauma and the development of PTSD. While between 50% and 90% of the general population experience trauma at least once during lifetime, the lifetime prevalence of PTSD lies between seven and eight (6, 7), which still means a huge burden on society. Men and women differ in terms of risk to develop PTSD after trauma; for men it is between 8% and 13%, and for women, between 20% and 30%.(6, 7) Differences in appraisal and coping mechanisms as well as psychobiological response patterns have been related to these differences.(8)

The initial response to a trauma can be characterized as a "normal reaction" toward an "abnormal" event that relates to sleep, nightmares, concentration, emotionality, and flashbacks. "Watchful waiting" is recommended when symptoms are mild and have been present for less than four weeks after the trauma. Early psychological intervention, often called debriefing, has no effect in preventing PTSD (9)—despite the high satisfaction. Instead, public information on psychological reactions and crisis intervention combined with practical support is useful for people to regain control over their situation.

Treatment is needed when severe early posttraumatic symptoms arise or when the disorder of PTSD is diagnosed. It should be noted that other disorders like depression, anxiety, or addictive disorders may also occur and are also often comorbid to PTSD. Before starting treatment, it is essential first to assess the diagnosis of PTSD. It is equally necessary to evaluate the effectiveness of the intervention after the treatment as well; here comes a dilemma: For patients it is often already very satisfactory to have experienced the intense emotions related to the trauma in the trusted setting with the therapist. The patient rarely judges the result of the treatment by evaluating the disappearance of symptoms. Whereas, for the therapist, sometimes the cathartic expression of emotions by the patient is often taken as proof of a well-established working through the traumatic experience. Also therapists do not always evaluate the treatment in a more objective fashion. Studies of debriefing after traumatic experiences, for instance, have shown a high satisfaction by the debriefed patients and by the therapist themselves (10, 11, 12, 13), and those who were debriefed showed higher symptom profiles in the follow up compared to the nondebriefed.(14, 15) Therefore, the precise assessment of symptoms is important for the assessment of PTSD. It also helps the patient to understand that he or she is not only suffering from traumatic experiences but also from symptoms resulting from the experience.

The assessment skill sets for PTSD consist of the skills to assess trauma in all its gruesome details and to assess symptoms resulting from the traumatic incident(s). In this chapter, we will first pay attention to the assessment of trauma and its pre- and post-treatment dilemmas. Then we will continue with the symptoms of PTSD. There are specific structured interviews and self-report instruments developed for the assessment of PTSD. The chapter will only highlight these instruments but not discuss them in detail. There are also other techniques to help to establish the diagnosis of PTSD with psychophysiologic measures and neuroimaging and neurohormonal measures. These techniques will not be discussed here, however. Then we will discuss the issue of the trauma-spectrum disorders and comorbidity in PTSD.

DILEMMAS IN THE ASSESSMENT OF TRAUMA

In *DSM-IV*[1] diagnostic criteria for PTSD trauma is described as follows:

The person has been exposed to a traumatic event in which both of the following were present:

(1) The person experienced, witnessed, or was confronted with an event or events that involved actual or threatened death or serious injury, or a threat to the physical integrity of self or others
(2) The person's response involved intense fear, helplessness, or horror.

What follows from the definition is the distinction between the actual traumatic event and the person's reaction.

Traumatic event

The definition does not describe exactly what a traumatic event means. There are characteristics concerning the actual role of the person involved in the event:

•   The person must be exposed to an event.
•   The event can be an experience of the person him or herself.
•   The event can be an experience of others in which the person is a witness.

The conditions that result from the definition, for instance, give the following examples. A person who has been a victim of an automobile accident and who lost consciousness for the incident itself did not consciously experience the traumatic incident. However, for instance, when the same person later on learns that her husband died in the incident and, as was the case in our hospital, also experienced her leg was broken has to cope with two traumatic events following the incident. This is important to understand because the reexperienced symptoms of the event can only evolve when someone consciously went through the incident. Another example was a police officer who could not work because of illness at a specific day, and another officer who worked in her place for that day was killed in the police car. She developed quite similar symptoms to PTSD and she tried to reconstruct the event. She felt guilty because she thought she should have been the one to be killed and not her fellow police officer. This assessment of the actual involvement in the incident is important in treatment when this implies imaginal exposure. It is another question if such exposure can be helpful in such situations, but the nature of reexperiencing is essentially different. For the assessment, it is important to analyze very precisely the actual involvement in the traumatic situation with the patient.

---

[1] Because DSM-IV favors a more precise description of symptoms compared to ICD-10 we will quote from the DSM-IV definition of PTSD.

In the *DSM-IV* definition of trauma the examples mentioned are as follows:

- Actual death
- Threatened death
- Serious injury
- Threat to the physical integrity to self
- Threat to the physical integrity of others.

These events can become traumatic for the person who experienced, witnessed, or was confronted with the event. From our police studies (16, 17) we, therefore, made the distinction between *threatening* and *depressive* experiences. The threatening ones are those incidents in which the patient him or herself is the victim. The depressive experiences are those events in which the patient witnesses the traumatic incident. This distinction is important because it makes the traumatic experience very different. In a threatening experience, one's fight–flight stress responses are activated to reach safety. This is important, for instance, for survivors of fires, robberies, and rapes. But in the same instances, those who were not directly threatened but only witness the incident become overwhelmed by the helplessness to see others hurt, die, or suffer any other trauma. Here also the fight–flight responses can become activated but more to flee from the horrible experience and from the intense feeling of helplessness. An 18-year-old girl witnessed a robbery in daylight. Her office manager asked her to accompany her to put a cassette with the money of the day into the deposit box of the bank. The box was located outside the bank. When they approached the bank one of the two boys put a gun on the head of the office manager. She gave the cassette to the boy and the boys disappeared in the crowd. The girl was not threatened at all by the boys who actually did not take notice of her. But she witnessed the threat and later on started to get reexperiences of this scene. She was not used at all to such events. Ursano (18), for instance, wrote about the risk factor for emergency workers, for example, they seem to be more at risk to develop PTSD when the corpses resembled their family or children. The confrontation with death and destruction is in itself a frequent experience for rescue workers but when they associate the victims with their close ones the traumatic experience can result in PTSD. Here we are reminded of an aspect of the definition of the stressor criterion mentioned in the *DSM-IIIR* description of PTSD: ". . . an event outside the range of usual human experience and that would be markedly distressing to almost anyone. . . ." This criterion has been abandoned in *DSM-IV* because the stressors as we know from epidemiology are much more common human experiences, which is in contrast to what was thought before. However, it still is important because even one usual experience can make the difference.

By focusing on the definition of (threatening) death or injury, too much attention is sometimes only paid to the result of some act. In fact in the reexperiencing we know that not only the result of the act comes back in memory, for example, a dead body, but also the details of the actual happenings themselves. A man survived an air crash. The plane crashed on the landing lane because of storm. This was accompanied by an enormous noise. The plane turned around. Then the walls of the cabin started to crumble. One of the stewardesses felt over him. So the air crash in itself is of course a traumatic event. But the traumatic experiences, which can come back as symptoms in PTSD, are these specific aspects of the threatening happening. In this case, for instance, the trembling of the plane, the noise of the crash, the falling down of the stewardess, and the view of a crumbling cabin became the traumatic details. Also violent behavior of someone else can become the reminder of the incident. Here also specific moments are often reexperienced. This is also meant by the adjunctive serious to injury. Here the threat is the most important aspect of the event. A significant aspect of an incident is often that it is unexpected. A person driving came along an accident. He saw a tractor with a white stick behind it. A moment later he found out it was someone's leg with its flesh stripped of. Also, the adjective *serious,* in medical parlance, denotes the critical condition of the victim. To make a critical inquiry into a traumatic experience and to make an effective assessment, it is mostly the unexpected, unwelcome details that are essential. For instance, someone tried reanimation to keep an old man alive. However, under the pressure of the act, the rescuer had broken the ribs of the person he was trying to save. In the reexperiencing, he relives the noise of the moment the ribs broke, and the persons reaction—intense fear, helplessness, and horror.

In contrast to *DSM-III* not only the experience of a traumatic event is necessary for the diagnosis but also the response of intense fear, helplessness, and horror. For instance, threat to one's physical integrity will specifically result in these intense reactions, for example, in rape, sexual abuse in childhood, and torture of any kind. Rape is always accompanied by threat and some kind of violence. Here also the reminders give a clue to the traumatic aspects of the experience, like the use of a knife or the threat, "I will kill you when you tell someone else." Here fear also plays an important role in the aftermath of the event. Though not mentioned for all traumatic events, shame is one factor that is usually very strongly felt in the three types of events. Here the assessment skills are important. Questioning about trauma not only involves facts but also extreme emotions associated with the incident. The traumatized person tries often to suppress the intense emotional reminders. The victim also protects the interviewer from being confronted with the repulsive details and the extreme emotions. For instance, a woman who has been raped by a group of youngsters had lots of difficulties telling all the terrible details of the experience. There had been moments that one of the boys had put the gun into her vagina and at other moments to her head. It is extremely difficult to not only tell these horrid details but also listen to them. These elements are most important in treatment. However, for the patient, it is important that the therapist listens without hesitation to these details. So one has to ask questions, for example, as given below:

- Did you feel fear?
- What were the most fearful experiences?
- Did you feel helpless?
- At which moments you felt most helpless?
- Did you feel horror?
- At which moments you felt most horror?
- Do you feel ashamed to tell these things?

Abuse in childhood is also often connected with violence and neglect. Here also shame and helplessness play an important role in the traumatization of the person. A critical factor in the assessment of sexual traumas is the trust to be established between the patient and the therapist. This is of course not self-evident. Judith Herman (19) calls our attention for a "stabilization phase" in which the patient can test the therapist about the safety of the treatment situation. It is good to realize the assessment phase can be complicated by the need for safety. The traumatized person not only suffers from the event that resulted in his or her trauma but also from the disappearance of trust he or she had in other human beings before the event. This is also the case with torture victims, whereas the safety of the consulting room for other trauma victims can resemble too much the torture room, disconnected from the outside world, sitting in the consulting room. Basoglu et al. (20) has paid attention to the development of psychological preparedness for torture. This office of the therapist can repeat this experience as well.

Horror is also an emotion that is often difficult to share. An example of such horror is the following example: In 1992, in Amsterdam, a plane crashed on a neighborhood.(21) This caused a fire as high as the apartment buildings that were struck by the plane. Eyewitnesses not only experienced this unbelievable scene but also heard the shouting and crying of burning people, some of them jumping off the balconies; thus, these details are horrible and difficult to tell. Such extreme emotions are characteristic of traumatic experiences. Fear is often presented this way, "I felt the adrenaline flow through my body." One remembers fear as a somatic experience of increased heartbeat, the trembling of the legs, being rooted to the ground, being unable to speak, cold hands, and so on.

For the therapist, there are risks connected to the listening about the events, especially when confronted with having to observe the extreme emotions of the patient in session. This is called secondary traumatization or vicarious traumatization.(22) It is well known in psychiatry, and it is also essential for a good interview that an empathic, understanding relationship with the patient is developed . The patient tells his or her story and details of symptoms only when he or she can trust the therapist. The right attitude, therefore, is one of willingness to listen and of acceptance. Such attitudes stimulate the patient to continue to tell; however, with trauma histories, this is much more complicated. The patient might worry that the interviewer will not take his or her story and the complaints serious or be afraid that the disclosure of gruesome details of the traumatic incident could scare the therapist him or herself. For instance, after listening to the story of burning people jumping from the balconies, even the therapist might be prone to dreaming about it. Treatment of a survivor of a plane crash can make the therapist fearful of flying. Secondary traumatizing refers to a sort of 'infectious' effect of listening to trauma stories. One feels saddened and helpless. Especially the listening to the details can cause the interviewer to develop nightmares of such incidents. So PTSD can endanger the mental health of the interviewer. It is, therefore, advised to limit the number of trauma patients one has to interview or to treat. Also regular intervision between trauma-therapists is highly recommended to limit their risk of secondary traumatisation.

Another dilemma lies in the discussion on whether the emotional response (A2 criterion) to trauma should get more weight than the type of event (A1).(23)

While some have argued that this definition is too narrowly defined and should be broadened to even include experiences that are distressing, but not necessarily directly associated with physical threat or injury (23, 24), others have been critical, stating that this definition is too inclusive.(25) The "conceptual bracket creep" (25) refers to the broadening of the stressor criterion in *DSM-IV*, especially to the inclusion of "second-hand exposure," such as learning about the unexpected death of a close friend/relative or watching atrocities on television . This seems to increase the eligible events by about 20%.(26) However, what is more important in this case is the question addressed in *DSM-IV*, that is, "whether or not to include reactions to the numerous stressors that are upsetting, but not life threatening or even to eliminate the stressor criterion altogether." The fear that more inclusive definitions will vastly increase the frequency of the diagnosis seems to be unrealistic. More minor stressors simply will not result in the other diagnostic criteria for PTSD.

SYMPTOMS ASSESSMENT

A variety of common symptoms are already covered in the assessment of the traumatic event. The symptom profile of PTSD has been divided into three sections:

1   Reexperiencing symptoms
2   Avoidance symptoms
3   Hyperarousal symptoms.

In the interview, a person often realizes the reexperience symptoms are related to the traumatic event. So they are more easily reported. The other two groups of symptoms are less well known to the sufferer and, therefore, are connected to the experience of the event. In the context of *DSM-IV* guidelines, a clear problem the therapist is faced with while asking about the different symptoms is a lack of frequency and intensity of the symptom mentioned. In the structured interviews for PTSD this is mostly better defined.

Reexperience symptoms
These are as follows:
B. The traumatic event is persistently reexperienced in one (or more) of the following ways:

1   Recurrent and intrusive distressing recollections of the event, including images, thoughts, or perceptions;
2   Recurrent distressing dreams of the event;
3   Acting or feeling as if the traumatic event were recurring (includes a sense of reliving the experience, illusions, hallucinations, and dissociative flashback episodes, including those that occur on awakening or when intoxicated);
4   Intense psychological distress during exposure to internal or external cues that symbolize or resemble an aspect of the traumatic event;
5   Physiological reactivity on exposure to internal or external cues that symbolize or resemble an aspect of the traumatic event.

In the reexperience symptoms there are some important characteristics:

*   The person involved does not have control over the occurrence of the symptoms.
*   The reexperience is a perceptional one that resemble actual experience.
*   The perceptional quality of the remembrance is essentially different from telling a story.

When a symptom is regarded persistent it means that nearly every week it occurs, and it is quite typical that the symptoms reoccur. Mostly specific episodes of the traumatic scene come back again and again. At moments of rest, for example, before sleep, when someone is most relaxed, he or she can be taken by surprise in reliving and seeing the terrible happening. They also come back in dreams. For instance, the partner can tell the bedclothes were wet and disordered or the person was talking and behaving in his sleep. The confrontations of cues that symbolize or resemble an aspect of the traumatic event are characteristic. Someone who survived an air crash bends down every time when a plane crosses the sky. After a rape by a colored person every time a woman sees a colored person she feels frightened even when knowing there is no real danger. Every element of the traumatic incident, such as sound, color, scene, and so on, can act as the trigger of the conditioned fear response, which is accompanied by some kind of reminder or reliving. It is hypothesized that this impaired extinction of fear conditioning may lie at the core of the development of PTSD and other anxiety disorders.(27)

The physiological reactivity means that the confrontation with cues result in increased heartbeat, transpiration, feeling cold, trembling, and so on. In psychobiological research trauma scripts are often used to examine, for instance, the heart rate response or changes in brain activation in response to the patient's own trauma story.(28, 29)

Avoidance symptoms

These are as follows:

C. Persistent avoidance of stimuli associated with the trauma and numbing of general responsiveness (not present before the trauma) as indicated by three (or more) of the following:

1 Efforts to avoid thoughts, feelings, or conversations associated with the trauma;
2 Efforts to avoid activities, places, or people that arouse recollections of the trauma;
3 Inability to recall an important aspect of the trauma;
4 Markedly diminished interest or participation in significant activities;
5 Feeling detachment or estrangement from others;
6 Restricted range of affect (e.g., unable to have love feelings)
7 Sense of a foreshortened future (e.g., does not expect to have career, marriage, children, or a normal life span).

Here two kinds of reactions are described: actual avoidance or numbing of general responsiveness. These symptoms strongly relate to the general fight–flight response to stress. The numbing seems related to a third kind of response, which is known from animals: acting as if one is dead. In the interview one has to rigorously pursue and probe for avoidance behavior. Often a patient is so used to the avoidance that it is not perceived as an active strategy. In fact much of the normal activities before the traumatic events are not taking place anymore. Certain neighborhoods will not be visited anymore. Those who suffered war and camps avoid the scenes of endless streams of refugees on television. So in assessing avoidance symptoms one has to understand that the traumatic cue brings back the perceptual remembrances of the trauma. Also, the intense pain, grief, and helplessness are felt again. It feels like "an open wound." The wound will never completely close. Also fear is intense again, and behind it often extreme feelings of aggression are hiding. The avoidance can also involve (like in C1) social withdrawal. Here the following question helps: "Do others perceive you as being changed after the incident?" The answer is often this: "Yes, I was always actively involved but now I do not like to go out." An example of how complicated this can be is the following. An officer who shot a person was complemented after returning to the police station. He was seen as a hero. However, he felt terrible because he did not want to kill anybody. He felt guilty not withstanding the rightness of the act in the terrible situation. He realized his colleagues had no idea about how lousy he felt. They could not understand his withdrawal and in a certain way they did not like to see their hero withdrawn. For the assessment of the inability to recall an important aspect of the trauma one has to investigate very carefully the traumatic incident. The traumatized person is not always aware of this symptom. A woman survived a killing in daylight while sitting in good weather with friends outside a cafe. She could only remember seeing coming near a group of men and then she remembers being in the hospital crying. She was not hurt herself.

But the actual traumatic moment has been lost because of dissociation. Another well-known aspect of the remembrance of traumatic incidents is the fact the one involved feels very convinced of the details of the happening. For instance I treated three persons who survived the same crash; each presented a different version in terms of recounting the incident and presenting the details of the incident. But they felt threatened after being faced with the probability their memory was not totally accurate. In the face of danger one must rely on few cues, which activates the stress response. From the work of le Doux (30) we know our brains work to perceive these threatening cues after which our fight–flight behavior becomes activated. Certain details are not taken into consideration or are lost. This is also defined by what is called "tunnel vision." The perception is restricted to endangering elements.

The symptoms listed under C4, 5, 6, and 7 overlap strongly with symptoms of depression. The interest in initiating activities or participation in something can be lost. The world that seemed normal and safe before the incident is no longer perceived that way and seems far less important after the incident. Here we see that the appreciation of the world, of what is important, can have changed tremendously. A UN military officer went to Bosnia to identify the corpses of killed inhabitants. In one month he saw a 300 bodily remains of the dead in a devastated surrounding complete with burned and destroyed houses. Before this, in his homeland, the solder was an active participant in local activities in the area where he was living with his family. After this trip, he felt everything was unimportant. He also felt detached from his partner and even his children, which is a terrible feeling. In the treatment it became clear as to what was the reason for this detachment; he felt he is no longer capable of safeguarding his family and he internally anticipated the possibility of losing them. Also, this symptom of detachment is difficult to express because the person involved feels very guilty about it. The restricted range of affect also becomes clear from the fact that the "shine" of normal experience has been lost. The sense of a foreshortened future relates to the loss of control over one's life and over the lives one feels responsible for.

A dilemma within the *DSM IV* classification is that research indicates that the avoidance cluster may need to be split into two distinct factors.(31) The first factor consists of actively avoiding thoughts or feelings about the event or doing things that remind the person of the event. The second factor describes emotional numbing as in having difficulty enjoying things or having sad or loving feelings, feeling distant from other people, or finding it hard to imagine fulfilling future goals. Foa et al. (32) already suggested that avoidance and numbing represent two separate factors reflecting different mechanisms. Previous models attempted to characterize PTSD based on the theoretical position that the clinical manifestations of PTSD follow a pattern of oscillations.(32, 33) Avoidance would be an effortful and strategic process following distress associated with intrusive thoughts or episodes of reexperiencing the traumatic event, whereas numbing, that is, a lack of emotional responsiveness and social withdrawal, is a consequence of uncontrollable arousal as in hypervigilance and anger.

Hyperarousal symptoms
These are as follows:

D. Persistent symptoms of increased arousal (not present before the trauma) as indicated by two (or more) of the following:

1   Difficulty falling or staying asleep;
2   Irritability or outburst of anger;
3   Difficulty concentrating:
4   Hypervigilance;
5   Exaggerated, startled response.

These symptoms are more easy to assess. The sleeping problem can relate to the fear that the traumatic incident can happen again. After the air crash in Amsterdam, we saw people who could only sleep with the light and TV on. Here the stimuli came in place of the increased need to scan the environment for endangering cues. Also waking up after two hours is common, as it seems dangerous to be not awake. To have no control over one's reactions becomes clear in the symptom irritability or outburst of anger. A shopkeeper was robbed at gun point just before closing time. He developed PTSD. One of the symptoms was his hypervigilance. He was afraid the robbery would happen again. He had much difficulty in being patient with his clients. His normal humor had faded away. People no longer liked to visit his cheese shop. This change affected the family front as well; he became quite irritable toward his wife and children. He changed, so partners often told us. Children suffered because of the irritability of their parent. One can easily understand this irritability. The traumatized person seems to be constantly distinguishing dangerous stimuli from "unimportant" stimuli. This is in fact the description of hypervigilence. Also one sees this in the behavior. A person has taken the chair as close to the wall as possible that his back was against the wall and to feel safe that no one can between him and the wall. A person who had been attacked very violently constantly slowed down when bicycling because he feared the persons bicycling behind him. Also normal stimuli like the closing of a door can startle the person extremely. The difficulty in concentrating corresponds also to this "scanning behavior." For example, recalling and describing the danger experienced is not difficult; on the contrary, a person might actively recall all sorts of details associated with the danger experienced. But if the same person were to read two pages of a book, he will likely forget the contents and start all over again. One might forget to what to buy during shopping. One needs to write down at home a list before going to the shop.

The hyperarousal symptoms are quite invalidating. Normal relations and normal activities become disordered. We see the person involved to cope with it in less adaptive ways by avoiding and withdrawal.

Dissociative symptoms

Apart from the symptoms B3, "dissociative flashback episodes," and C3, "inability to recall an important aspect of the trauma," dissociative symptoms are not very well specified in the DSM-IV description of PTSD. Spiegel and others (34) have argued that PTSD is a disorder of memory. From this viewpoint, more symptoms similar to the two mentioned above can be seen as distorting normal memory functions like encoding, storage, and retrieval of traumatic memories. Bremner et al. (35) have argued that dissociation is the main mechanism in the development of PTSD; an example is the lack of emotions while remembering traumatic events. Without such accompanying emotions, the incident according to the definition is not a traumatic one. Here we have a problem; dissociation could have negated such emotions. Thus, the person remembers the incident but cannot remember the intense emotions he felt while it happened. Brewin (36) has described different forms of memory: (1) verbally accessible memory (VAM) involving explicit, conscious, and hippocampally dependent memories, such as ordinary autobiographical memories, and (2) situational assessable memory systems (SAM), which involve implicit, image-based, cue-dependent, and nonhippocampally dependent memories at the amygdala level as when sensory memories of the traumatic event are reexperienced after being triggered by external cues. One of the aims of treatment is integrating the memories of the trauma into the totality of a person's memory system.

A specific accompanying symptom is often the depersonalization or derealization, which are dissociative symptoms. Especially from sexual child abuse, it is well known that the traumatic incident can be forgotten. This is part of a heavy debate, especially because some accuse that therapists "implant such memories." One has to be very careful in the interview not to suggest such experiences. But one cannot leave them out, particularly because when the therapist detects long periods of amnesia during childhood phase, as becomes evident during the session, the possibility that that there was a childhood trauma must indeed be taken seriously.

Marmar et al (37) has described a set of specific dissociative features of the traumatic experience that are quite common. These symptoms are called peritraumatic dissociation. These symptoms are part of the traumatic experience of a person and come back while remembering the event. For instance, a traumatic situation feels "endless" in time, whereas it could have lasted only for a short moment. Also the incident can be experienced as a "slow-motion" scene in which the sound associated with the actual event can change or even be absent. Peritraumatic dissociation describes the changes in perception, especially in time–space relation. A police officer who was sitting in his car shot through the windscreen at a man who took a woman as the hostage. The window-screen splintered into thousand particles. He, however, saw them falling down slowly, as if they were water drops. It sounded like "Christmas bells." The traumatic value of an incident can, therefore, change the perception; thus, the perception concerning time, sound, place of the incident may not only vary but may instead regard the incident as unreal, as if it never happened.

STRUCTURED INSTRUMENTS

Structured interviews and self-report instruments have a definite advantage because they don't need much clinical skills while using them, as outlined before. Also they make the validity of assessment between groups better. Many instruments have been developed for epidemiological purposes and for research on PTSD. We will summarize a few here. The *Impact of Events Scale (IES)* of Horowitz et al (38) is not only well known but is also the oldest one in its category. It is more often used because it gives a fine presentation of the reexperience and avoidance characteristics. However, the disadvantage is it has been developed far before the formulation of PTSD in *DSM-III* and *IV* and may not cover many of the symptoms as presented in *DSM-III* and *IV*; for example, the hyperarousal symptoms are not part of this scale. The revised version now includes these hyperarousal symptoms (IES-R), though. The Structured Clinical Interview for *DSM-IV* (39)) is also available with a PTSD part. Furthermore, in current research, the Clinician Administered PTSD Scale for *DSM-IV (CAPS-DX)* is also very often used. (40) For epidemiological research with trained lay interviewers (not clinicians), the Composite International Diagnostic Interview (41) is available for PTSD assessment. Breslau et al. (42) reported about a 7-item symptom list to discover PTSD in the community and later Brewin et al. (43) developed a 10-item instrument to screen for the presence of PTSD. Also, self-report instruments have been used in research and are sometimes recommended for use in clinical practice as well. These are the Davidson Trauma Scale (DTS) (44), the Self-Rating Scale for PTSD (SRS-PTSD) (45), the Self-Rating Inventory for Posttraumatic Stress Disorder (SID) (46) and the Posttraumatic Diagnostic Scale (PDS) (47). Most of the self-report instruments have been developed for special trauma populations, like Vietnam veterans (CAPS), police and disaster victims (46) and rape victims (47).

TRAUMA SPECTRUM AND COMORBIDITY

The ICD-10 classification (2) mentions that PTSD is often accompanied by anxiety, depression, or even obsessive–compulsive disorder. The consequence is that when a patient comes for assessment, one should not restrict assessment to only focus on PTSD but must instead look for other accompanying symptoms described previously. Comorbidity of PTSD with other disorders, including the dissociative ones, is quite common. Therefore, some have argued for the need of a so-called trauma spectrum of disorders (48, 49, 50). There are important overlaps with depression, other anxiety disorders and with dissociative disorders. Also, PTSD can become complicated by addiction. Acute stress disorder (ASD) has been recognized in *DSM-IV* (3). There is also much interest in subthreshold manifestations of PTSD-symptoms described as partial PTSD (51). Herman (52) and van der Kolk (53) have pleaded for adding complex PTSD to *DSM-IV* items of measure. Much attention has been given to a partial relationship between the borderline personality disorder and early trauma. Complex PTSD has been developed to describe the long-term effect of PTSD on the personality.

For future research, it will be necessary to pay more attention to trauma spectrum disorders, which, in the meantime, should not, however, stop clinicians from assessing PTSD alone.

CONCLUSION

In the assessment of the diagnosis of PTSD many dilemmas have been mentioned. Psychiatrists are mostly familiar with the difficulty of assessing, for instance, psychotic symptoms because having such skills is usually associated with one's bearing a professionally accomplished persona and professional pride, whereas for other doctors such assessment turns out to be extremely difficult. The disorders like PTSD that are related to traumatic events may at first seem more easy to detect. The improved classification of disorders in DSM and ICD over time has tremendously increased the in between reliability of making diagnosis of different disorders. However, behind the short descriptions, definitions, and sentences, much clinical expertise is hidden, which helps with precise diagnosis of PTSD and other disorder. A special aspect in the skills for assessing PTSD is the impact of any unpleasant stories divulged during the diagnosis. It is important to understand that the patient often does not want to share his or her terrible experiences with the therapist, which he or she feels acts sometimes as a protection so that the therapist does not get bogged down with such details and extreme emotions. For the clinician, it is, therefore, necessary to realize how one should be prepared with knowledge and skills to start assessing PTSD. Those who argue for seeing PTSD as a dissociative disorder help us to understand the symptoms from the view of a memory disorder. The use of structured instruments and self-rating inventories can be helpful, but to what extent is not yet well known. The risk of secondary traumatization has to be taken very seriously.

REFERENCES

1. American Psychiatric Association. Diagnostic And Statistical Manual of Mental Disorders, third edition (DSM-III). Washington, DC: APA; 1980.
2. World Health Organization. The ICD-10 Classification of Mental and Behavioural Disorders; Clinical Descriptions and the Diagnostic Guidelines. Geneva; 1992.
3. American Psychiatric Association. Diagnostic and Statistical Manual of Mental Disorders, fourth edition (DSM-IV). Washington, DC: APA; 1994.
4. Kessler, RC, Sonnega A, Bromet E, Nelson CB. Posttraumatic stress disorder in the national comorbidity survey. Arch Gen Psychiatry 1995; 52, 1058–60.
5. Breslau N, Kessler RC, Chilcoat HD et al. Trauma and posttraumatic stress disorder in the community; the 1996 Detroit area survey of trauma. Arch Gen Psychiatry 1998; 55: 626–32.
6. Olff M, de Vries G-J. The epidemiology of PTSD in the Netherlands. 9th European Conference on Traumatic Stress, Stockholm. Stockholm: Sweden, 2005: 106.
7. Breslau N, Davis GC, Andreski P, Peterson EL, Schultz LR. Sex differences in posttraumatic stress disorder. Arch Gen Psychiatry 1997; 54(11): 1044–8.
8. Olff M, Langeland W, Draijer N, Gersons BPR. Gender differences in posttraumatic stress disorder. Psychol Bull 2007; 133(2): 183–204.
9. National Institute for Clinical Excellence. The management of PTSD in primary and secondary care. London: NICE; 2005.
10. Kenardy JA, Webster RA, Lewin TJ et al. Stress debriefing and patterns of recovery following a natural disaster. J Trauma Stress 1996; 9: 37–50.
11. Bisson JI, Jenkins PL. Psychological debriefing for victims of acute burn trauma. Br J Psychiatry 1997; 171: 583.
12. Bisson JI, Jenkins PL, Alexander J, Bannister C. Randomized controlled trial of psychological debriefing for victims of acute burn trauma. Br J Psychiatry 1997; 171: 78–81.
13. Carlier IVE, Van Uchelen JJ, Lamberts RD, Gersons BPR. Disaster-related posttraumatic stress in police officers; a field study of the impact of debriefing. Stress Med 1998b; 14: 143–8.
14. van Emmerik AA, Kamphuis JH, Hulsbosch AM, Emmelkamp PM. Single session debriefing after psychological trauma: a meta-analysis. Lancet 2002; 360: 766–71.
15. Sijbrandij EM, Olff M, Reitsma JB, Carlier IVE, Gersons BPR. Emotional or educational debriefing after psychological trauma: Randomised controlled trial. Br J Psychiatry 2006; 189, 150–5.
16. Carlier IVE, Gersons BPR. Partial PTSD; the issue of psychological scars and the occurrence of the PTSD symptoms. J Nerv Ment Dis 1995; 183, 107–9.
17. Carlier, I.V.E., Lamberts, R.D., Gersons, B.P.R., Risk factors for posttraumatic stress symptomatology in police officers: a prospective analysis. J Nerv Ment Dis 185(8):498-506, 1997.
18. Ursano RJ, Fullerton CS, Vance K, Kao TC. Posttraumatic stress disorder and identification in disaster workers. Am J Psychiatry 1999; 156, 353–9.
19. Herman J. Trauma and Recovery; the Aftermath of Violence - From Domestic Abuse to Political Terror. Basic Books; 1992.
20. Basoglu M, Mineka S, Paker M et al. Psychological preparedness for trauma as a protective factor in survivors of torture. Psychol Med 1997; 27: 1421–33.
21. Carlier IVE, Gersons BPR. Stress reaction in disaster victims following the Bijlmermeer plane crash. J Trauma Stress 1997; 10: 329–35.
22. Figley CR. Compassion fatigue as secundary stress disorder: An overview. In: Figley CR, ed. Compassion fatigue: Secundary Traumatic Stress Disorder in Treating the Traumatized. New York: Brunner/Mazel, 1995: 1–20.
23. Avina C, O'Donohue W. Sexual harassment and PTSD: is sexual harassment diagnosable trauma? J Trauma Stress 2002; 15: 69–75.
24. Olff M, Gersons BPR. What is a traumatic event? Br J Psychiatry 2005; 187, 189–90.
25. McNally RJ. Progress and controversy in the study of posttraumatic stress disorder. Annu Rev Psychol 2003; 54: 229–52.

26. Breslau N, Kessler RC. The stressor criterion in DSM^IV posttraumatic stress disorder, an empirical investigation. Biol Psychiatry 2001; 50: 699–704.

27. Knight DC, Smith CN, Cheng DT, Stein EA, Helmstetter FJ. "Amygdala and hippocampal activity during acquisition and extinction of human fear conditioning", Cogn Affect Behav Neurosci 2004; 4(3): 317–25.

28. Lindauer RJL, Van Meijel EPM, Jalink M et al. Heart rate responsivity to script-driven imagery in posttraumatic stress disorder: specificity of response and effects of psychotherapy. Psychosom Med 2006; 68(1); 33–40.

29. Lindauer RJL, Booij J, Habraken JBA et al. Cerebral blood flow changes during script-driven imagery in police officers with posttraumatic stress disorder. Biol Psychiatry 2004; 56(11): 853–61.

30. LeDoux J. The emotional brain. The mysterious underpinnings of emotional life. New York: Simon and Schuster; 1996.

31. Olff M, Sijbrandij M, Opmeer BC, Carlier IV, Gersons BP, The structure of acute posttraumatic stress symptoms: 'Reexperiencing', 'Active avoidance', 'Dysphoria', and 'Hyperarousal', J Anxiety Disord, 2009 Jun;23(5):656-9.

32. Foa EB, Riggs DS, Gershuny BS. Arousal, numbing, and intrusion: symptom structure of PTSD following assault. Am J Psychiatry 1995; 152(1): 116–20.

33. Litz BT. Emotional Numbing in combat-related posttraumatic-stress-disorder - a critical-review and reformulation. Clin Psychol Rev 1992; 12(4): 417–32.

34. Butler LD, Spiegel D. Trauma and memory, in: American Psychiatric Press, Washington. Review of Psychiatry 1997; 16(2): 13–53.

35. Bremner JD, Marmar CR. Trauma, memory, and dissociation. American Psychiatric Press, Washington; 1998.

36. Brewin CR. A cognitive neuroscience account of posttraumatic stress disorder and its treatment. Behav Res Ther 2001; 39: 373–93.

37. Marmar CR, Weiss DS, Schlengen WE et al. Peritraumatic dissociation and posttraumatic stress in male Vietnam theater veterans. Am J Psychiatry 1994; 151: 902–7.

38. Horowitz MJ, Wilner N, Alvarez W. Impact of event scale: a measure of subjective stress. Psychosom Med 1979; 41: 209–18.

39. Spitzer RL, Williams JBW, Gibbon M. Structured clinical interview for DSM-III-R, Version NP-V. New York: Biometrics Research Department, New York State Psychiatric Institute; 1987.

40. Blake D, Weathers F, Nagy D. A clinician administered PTSD scale for the assessing current and lifetime PTSD: the CAPS-I. Behav Ther 1990; 18: 187–8.

41. Kessler RC, Andrews G, Mroczek D, Ustun B, Wittchen HU. The world health organization composite international diagnostic interview short-form (CIDI-SF). Int J Methods in Psychiatry Res 1998; 7: 171–85.

42. Breslau N, Peterson EL, Kessler RC, Schultz LR. Short screening scale for DSM-IV posttraumatic stress disorder. Am J Psychiatry 1999; 156: 908–11.

43. Brewin CR, Rose S, Andrews B et al. Brief screening instrument for post-traumatic stress disorder. Br J Psychiatry 2002; 181: 158–62.

44. Davidson JR, Book SW, Colket JT et al. Assessment of a new self-rating scale for posttraumatic stress disorder. Psychol Med 1997; 27: 153–60.

45. Carlier IVE, Lamberts RD, van Uchelen JJ, Gersons BPR. Clinical utility of a brief diagnostic test for posttraumatic stress disorder. Psychosom Med 1998a; 60: 42–7.

46. Hovens JE, Van der Ploeg HM, Bramsen I. The development of the self-rating inventory for posttraumatic stress disorder. Acta Psychiatrica Scandinavica 1994; 90: 172–83.

47. Foa EB, Hearst-Ikeda D, Perry KJ. Evaluation of a brief cognitive-behavioral program for the prevention of chronic PTSD in recent assault victims. J Consult Clin Psychol 1995a; 63: 948–55.

48. Bremner JD. Editorial: Acute and chronic responses to psychological trauma: where do we go from here? Am J Psychiatry 1999; 156(3): 349-351.

49. Horowitz MJ. Stress-response Syndromes (2nd ed.). Northvale, NJ: Jason Aronson; 1986.

50. Van der Kolk BA, McFarlane AC, Weiseath L, eds. Traumatic Stress: the Effects of Overwhelming Experience on Mind, Body, and Society. New York: Guilford Press; 1996.

51. Carlier IVE, Gersons BPR. Partial posttraumatic stress disorder (PTSD): The issue of psychological scars and the occurrence of PTSD symptoms, J Nerv Ment Dis 1995; 183(2): 107–9.

52. Herman JL. Sequelae of prolonged and repeated trauma: evidence for a complex posttraumatic syndrome (DESNOS). In: Davidson JRT, Foa EB, eds. Posttraumatic Stress Disorder: DSM-IV and Beyond. Washington, DC: APA; 1993.

53. Van der Kolk B.A, McFarlane AC, Weiseath L eds. Traumatic Stress: the Effects of Overwhelming Experience on Mind, Body, and Society. New York: Guilford Press; 1996.

4 | Neuroimaging and posttraumatic stress disorder

Sarah N Garfinkel and Israel Liberzon

INTRODUCTION

Neuroimaging provides a powerful way to investigate the structural and functional abnormalities associated with posttraumatic stress disorder (PTSD) and PTSD vulnerability. It can be used to identify mechanisms that mediate emotional processing in healthy individuals as well as the dysregulation of these processes in posttraumatic stress disorder (PTSD). Reviewed are neuroimaging findings in PTSD, with a focus on studies utilizing symptom provocation, cognitive activation, and functional connectivity. These studies identify neurocircuitry associated with PTSD, highlighting the role of the medial prefrontal cortex (mPFC), insula, amygdala, sublenticular extended amygdala (SLEA), and hippocampus, in mediating symptom formation in PTSD. In addition, psychological processes presently emerging as new foci in neuroimaging research relevant to PTSD, such as fear conditioning, habituation, extinction recall; cognitive–emotional interactions are also discussed. Findings linking neurocircuitry subserving these processes to the abnormalities associated with PTSD are highlighted, suggesting that mPFC is implicated in a number of these processes. Finally, a section on receptor imaging will discuss the differences in functional neurochemistry associated with PTSD.

The last decade saw the emergence of neurocircuitry models of PTSD, (1–3), which were inspired by both basic animal research and a growing number of human neuroimaging studies. These models conceptualize PTSD as a state of heightened responsivity to threatening stimuli and/or a state of insufficient inhibitory control over exaggerated threat sensitivity. They emphasize the centrality of threat-related processing in the pathophysiology of PTSD and hence account for the "hypersensitivity to threat" that is highly characteristic of PTSD (such as hypervigilence and hyperarousal). It is becoming increasingly apparent, however, that the "hypersensitivity to threat" models do not fully capture the full complexity of PTSD or the complexity of changes associated with, trauma exposure and PTSD development. For instance, important phenomena associated with PTSD, such as intrusive thoughts and memories, avoidance and numbing, generalization, vulnerability, and resilience factors, all need to be further understood in terms of underlying psychological mechanisms and their neurobiological substrates. There is presently a growing appreciation that additional mechanisms, other than hyperresponsivity to threat, must be involved in PTSD pathophysiology. Lines of research have begun exploring neurobiological and psychological processes seemingly relevant to the development, maintenance and/or recovery of PTSD, including conditioning, habituation, stimulus generalization, extinction resistance, and (impaired) extinction recall. In addition, processes (and underlying neurocircuitry) involving higher order cognitive–emotional interactions, appraisal, reappraisal, and metaawareness may also play an important role in PTSD vulnerability, pathophysiology, and resilience. In recent years, a growing body of literature has examined these processes both in healthy and PTSD subjects. This chapter will first review what is currently known on the basis of functional neuroimaging in PTSD, with a particular emphasis on symptom provocation studies, cognitive activation studies and functional connectivity analyses. The second part of the chapter focuses on specific psychological processes that have been implicated in PTSD symptom generation or pathophysiology. These include neuroimaging studies of fear-conditioning phenomena (with a particular emphasis on extinction and extinction recall) and also cognitive–emotional interactions. Finally, potential future directions for PTSD research are discussed.

PART I: NEUROIMAGING STUDIES IN PTSD

Different neuroimaging modalities, such as single-photon emission tomography (SPECT), positron emission tomography (PET), and functional magnetic resonance imaging (fMRI), have all been used in conjunction with PTSD research. This chapter will incorporate many of these modalities, with a particular emphasis on fMRI.

Symptom provocation studies

Studies utilizing symptom provocation to investigate PTSD do so by employing autobiographical stimuli that are trauma related (e.g., narrative scripts of personal trauma) or alternatively are more general in nature, employing generally evocative but not necessarily autobiographically relevant pictures and sounds. Such studies were the first to emerge, were the first to provide relatively stable and replicable findings, and are still the most common studies in the PTSD functional neuroimaging literature. In one of the first functional imaging symptom provocation studies, Rauch and colleagues (4) used individualized trauma scripts and [15O] H2O PET, in a small and heterogeneous group of eight PTSD subjects. They demonstrated increased regional cerebral blood flow (rCBF) in anterior paralimbic (right posterior medialorbito frontal cortex [OFC], insular, anterior temporal polar, and medial temporal cortex) and limbic structures (amygdala) in the provoked versus control contrast. In a following study, the same group then used combat-related, emotionally negative and neutral pictures paired with verbal descriptions (imagery) in combat veterans with and without PTSD. Combat veterans with PTSD had increased rCBF in ventral anterior cingulated cortex (ACC) and right amygdala when generating mental images of combat-related pictures but had deceased rCBF in the ACC in the combat image viewing versus neutral image viewing contrast.(5) Though these early studies had methodological limitations, such as a small and heterogeneous sample size, as well as a lack of adequate control groups that limited the generalization of their findings, they set the stage for more detailed studies into the neural substrate of the symptomatic PTSD state.

In an ensuing study, our group exposed three groups of subjects (14 combat PTSD subjects, 11 combat-exposed subjects without PTSD, and 11 combat unexposed healthy subjects) to combat sounds or white noise in two counterbalanced sessions and studied rCBF with 99mTc hexamethylpropyleneamineoxime (HMPAO) SPECT. Only the PTSD group showed increased rCBF in the left amygdaloid region.(6) Another study using combat-related pictures and sounds and PET in 10 combat veterans with and 10 without PTSD, revealed decreased blood flow in medial prefrontal cortex (mPFC) (Area 25) and other areas in response to traumatic pictures and sounds in PTSD patients, while non-PTSD control subjects activated the anterior cingulate (Area 24) to a greater degree than PTSD patients.(7) The same group also studied childhood sexual abuse (CSA) subjects (22 women, 10 of whom had PTSD) with exposure to traumatic and neutral scripts and PET. The PTSD group showed rCBF increases in posterior cingulate (Area 31) and superior and middle frontal gyri bilaterally in Brodmann Areas 9 and 10. The PTSD group also showed deactivation in the subcallosal anterior cingulate (Area 25) and decreased activation in an adjacent portion of anterior cingulate (Area 32).(7) Using PET and script-driven imagery in 16 subjects with CSA (eight subjects with PTSD), Shin and colleagues also reported deactivation of the medial prefrontal and as well as left inferior frontal (Broca's) areas in the PTSD group.(8)

Lanius and colleagues reported two fMRI studies where they used a script-driven symptom provocation paradigm. They also observed significantly decreased blood oxygen level–dependent method (BOLD) signal in the ventral ACC (Brodmann's area 32) and the thalamus in the PTSD group to both the traumatic and nontraumatic emotional states conditions, suggesting that the earlier neuroimaging findings related to these areas in PTSD may not be specific to traumatic stimuli.(9, 10) Hendler and colleagues studied processing of repeated versus novel visual presentations in an fMRI study of combat veterans with and without PTSD. Repeated presentations resulted in less decrease in BOLD signal in the lateral occipital cortex in PTSD subjects, interpreted as impaired visual habituation to trauma-related stimuli.(11) A more recent PET script-driven imagery study of 17 Vietnam veterans with PTSD and 19 without PTSD replicated rCBF decreases in the medial frontal gyrus in the PTSD group. This activity was inversely correlated with rCBF changes in the left amygdala and the right amygdala–periamygdaloid cortex. Interestingly, only the male subgroup showed increased rCBF in left amygdale.(12) We recently reported the results of a [15O] H2O PET, script-driven imagery study of emotionally evocative and neutral autobiographic events in 16 combat veterans with PTSD (PTSD patients [PP], 15 combat veterans without PTSD (combat controls [CC]) and 14 healthy, age-matched, control subjects; (noncombat controls [NC]) that allow to isolate changes that are trauma related (PP vs. NC and CC vs. NC) and PTSD specific (PTSD vs. CC). While all subjects deactivated the mPFC and activated the insula for traumatic scripts, the PP deactivated the rostral anterior cingulate cortex (rACC) more than both control groups (CC and NC) but did not demonstrate ventromedial PFC (vmPFC) deactivation observed in controls. The findings observed only in the PTSD group (deactivation of the rACC and higher vMPFC activity) may reflect neural substrates specific to PTSD.(13)

Neural activation in response to symptom provocation in PTSD has been shown to differ, in part, as a function of comorbid depression.(14) In one recent study, 15 traumatized subjects with PTSD and major depression (MDD), 11 traumatized subjects with PTSD and no MDD, and 16 subjects who met criterion A for PTSD but did not reach full diagnosis, were subjected to script-driven imagery (both traumatic and neutral scripts). Commonalities in brain activation between PTSD subjects with and without MDD were revealed in the dorsal and ventral ACC, where reduced activation was observed in response to traumatic scripts relative to traumatized control subjects. In addition, reduced blood flow, relative to healthy controls, was also observed in the two PTSD groups in the ventrolateral prefrontal cortex. After controlling for differences in PTSD severity, the PTSD group with MDD displayed *less* activity than the PTSD group without MDD in the left anterior insula (BA 13). PTSD group with MDD had *increased* activation in the anterior and posterior cingulated gyri relative to the PTSD without MDD subjects. Given the frequent occurrence of comorbidites, such as MDD, with PTSD, these latter findings highlight the necessity to delineate what activation variations are a function of PTSD and what are attributable to comorbidities.(14)

To date, though the vast majority of studies have been performed in adult PTSD populations, only limited studies have been performed in children and/or adolescents with PTSD to investigate the neural correlates induced by symptom provocation. One small study examined brain responses during visual perception and imaginary recollection of traumatic reminders in adolescents (aged 12–14 years) who developed PTSD versus those who did not after experiencing an earthquake.(15) Sample size was limited (five with PTSD vs. six trauma exposed PTSD negative individuals). During earthquake imagery (as compared with neural imagery), the PTSD group was found to have activation in the bilateral visual cortex, bilarteral cerebellum, and left parahippocampal gyrus, relative to the control group. During earthquake perception relative to neutral perception, the control group showed activation of the ACC, but the PTSD group did not. Additional analyses demonstrated that intergroup differences were significant, providing preliminary evidence that neurobiological alternation of PTSD in adolescence are similar to those occurring in adult PTSD populations.(15)

Correlation with Cross-sectional Symptom Severity

Another way of investigating symptom genesis in PTSD is to correlate imaging findings with measures of symptom severity. Such an approach allows a quantitative assessment of whether changes in brain function are related to the magnitude of specific PTSD symptoms. Osuch and colleagues correlated rCBF response with flashback intensity in a personalized, script-driven imagery PET paradigm in eight chronic PTSD subjects. rCBF correlated directly with flashback intensity in the brain stem, insula, and hippocampus, and inversely in the prefrontal, right fusiform, and medial temporal cortices.(16) Similarly, in an fMRI study, Lanius and colleagues reported that seven CSA subjects with PTSD and concomitant dissociative responses to symptom provocation by scripts had increased activation in the ACC, mPFC, and several other cortical areas compared to 10 control subjects.(17) However, none of these activations correlated with either dissociative or flashback intensity. The small samples and significant comorbidity limit the interpretation of these findings. In a script-driven imagery and PET study (8), Shin and colleagues reported that symptom severity in the PTSD group (as measured by the total score on the clinician-administered PTSD scale [CAPS]) was positively related to rCBF in the right amygdala and negatively related to rCBF in medial frontal gyrus after controlling for depression severity score. In a recent block design fMRI study, investigators examined the time course of amygdala responses to trauma-relevant negative words, panic-relevant negative words (negative control condition), positive/safety words, and neutral words, in nine predominantly sexual assault PTSD patients and 14 healthy controls.(18) The PTSD group showed an increased left amygdala response to trauma-relevant negative versus neutral stimuli compared to controls in the first two (but not last two) runs, and this response correlated with the symptom severity (CAPS total score). Healthy controls showed the opposite pattern.

Hypoactive mPFC
(e.g. reduced mPFC responses
to overt fear vs. happy faces).

Impaired ACC
(e.g. reduced activation during
counting Stroop).

Hyperactive amygdala
(e.g. in response to subliminal fear faces).

Impaired hippocampal function
(e.g. Impaired spatial memory).

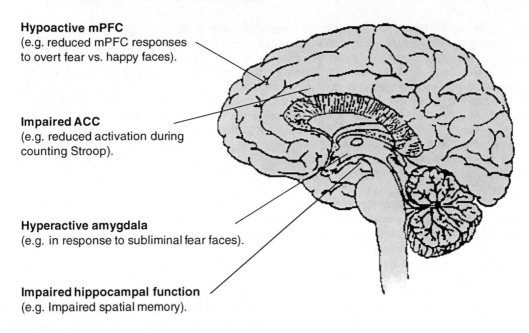

Figure 4.1   A summary of key functional neuroanatomical impairments associated with PTSD and examples of cognitive activation paradigms that expose these deficits.

In summary, symptom provocation studies have implicated a number of structures in the genesis of PTSD, particularly anterior paralimbic and limbic structures, such as the medial orbital frontal cortex (OFC), the insula, and the medial temporal cortex. One of the more consistent and reliable findings, is decreased or failure of activation in subregions of the mPFC and ACC, and this was demonstrated by a number of studies, though was not universally found. Increased responsivity of the amygdala has been observed in some studies, but has not been a consistent finding. Design and/or methodological factors may contribute to these divergent findings, including the method of symptom provocation (trauma imagery vs. external stimuli), experimental tasks (passive viewing vs. active recall), scanning methodology, and relatively small samples, all of which may affect the ability to activate and/or detect amygdala response.

Cognitive activation studies

One way to assess specific impairments in neuronal processing associated with PTSD is via cognitive activation studies. These studies utilize a neurocognitive task (a "probe") that is expected to selectively activate neural circuits implicated in task-related processing. Selectively activating a circuit without eliciting symptoms has a substantial advantage in that this overcomes the confound of eliciting a large number of more general or nonspecific trauma-related responses. Investigators have used cognitive activation strategies to further examine a number of regions implicated in PTSD by symptom provocation studies, such as the mPFC, amygdala, ACC, and hippocampus (see Figure 4.1).

The ACC is a region that has been implicated in PTSD, where symptom provocation studies have revealed it to be hypofunctioning, or failing to activate, relative to unaffected controls. The ACC is a region that has been activated by many functional neuroimaging studies and has been implicated in different processes involving cognitive–emotional interactions. A variety of evidence supports the existence of functional subdivisions in the ACC, with dorsal ACC supporting cognitive control and error-related processing, while rACC is involved in the assessment of salience of emotional information and the regulation of emotional responses. (19) Bremner et al. (2004) used the modified Stroop task (color Stroop, emotional Stroop, and control task) and [15O] H2O PET to probe ACC function in 12 women with early CSA-related PTSD and nine CSA women without PTSD. The PTSD group demonstrated a relative decrease in ACC blood flow during the emotional but not the color Stroop task, which elicited increased rCBF in the ACC (BA 24 and 32) in both groups.(20) Shin et al. (2001) also investigated ACC functioning in 16 Vietnam combat veterans (eight with PTSD) using fMRI and an emotional counting Stroop paradigm. Subjects were asked to count the number of combat-related, generally negative, and neutral words while being scanned. In the comparison of combat-related words with generally negative words, the non-PTSD group showed significant BOLD signal increases in rACC but the PTSD group did not.(21) In addition, to assess interference processing and inhibitory control, tasks commonly associated with ACC function, a version of the counting Stroop task incorporating only affectively neutral words also demonstrated hypoactivation of the ACC in patients with PTSD. This task requires participants to count the number of identical words presented on the screen and to press a button corresponding to the correct number. In the interference condition, the presented word—a numerical value, is an "incorrect" response (e.g., four words on the screen all read "two"); in the neutral condition, the words do not include numbers (e.g., four words on the screen all read "cat"). This task was performed in 26 trauma-exposed men, 13 of whom met diagnosis for PTSD. The PTSD group exhibited less deactivation in subgenual ACC and more deactivation in the insula as compared to controls during the interference minus neutral task.(22)

The amygdala is integral to the generation and maintenance of emotional responses, and this has been shown in both animal and human studies.(23–25) The amygdala is a region implicated in rapidly assessing the salience of emotional and especially threat-related stimuli. (26) A number of studies have presented fearful faces to individuals with PTSD, using various exposure durations, and these have converged upon increased amygdala responsivity in PTSD (especially when stimulus presentation is rapid (27–29)). Rauch et al. (2000) compared amygdala responses in nine PTSD subjects versus eight combat-exposed, non-PTSD subjects using a previously validated masked emotional faces paradigm. Contrasting fearful versus happy masked faces revealed exaggerated amygdala responses in the PTSD subjects. Furthermore, the magnitude of these responses distinguished PTSD subjects with 75% sensitivity and 100% specificity.(29) These findings suggest that PTSD is associated with increased amygdala responsivity to threat-related (but not necessarily trauma-related) stimuli. Another group used a similar masked emotional faces paradigm to examine 13 subjects with acute, rather than chronic PTSD.(27) There was a positive correlation between the severity of PTSD and the difference in amygdala responses between masked fearful and happy faces. These findings suggest that functional abnormalities in brain responses to emotional stimuli observed in chronic PTSD might be apparent already in the acute phase. In a recent study, Bryant et al., (2008) exposed 15 patients with PTSD and 15 age and sex-matched nontraumatized controls to fearful stimuli (16.7 ms), followed by a 163.3 ms neutral mask. They found significantly greater left amygdala activity in the PTSD relative to the control group.(30)

Regarding overt presentation of fearful faces, heightened amygdala activity does not appear to be particularly robust during this type of processing of fear stimuli, though differences have been obtained in some studies.(28) In one study, Shin et al. (2005) used overtly presented emotional facial expressions and fMRI to compare BOLD responses in 13 men with PTSD and 13 trauma-exposed men without PTSD. The PTSD group showed increased amygdala responses and decreased mPFC responses to overt fearful (vs. happy) facial expressions.(31) The amygdala is known to be involved with the rapid assessment of threat, and hence it appears amydgala-related hypoactivation associated with PTSD is more sensitive to subliminal exposure durations in the region of 12 to 30 ms. Overt, longer duration exposure might lead to signal that integrates repeated stimulation and the habituation processes, and thus it might be less sensitive in picking up changes involving a specific process.

Another region implicated in PTSD is the hippocampus, which plays a role in explicit memory processes as well as contextual learning.(32, 33) Individuals with PTSD perform poorly on neuropsychological memory tasks.(34,35) A number of structural MRI studies reported decreased hippocampal volumes in individuals with PTSD (34, 36–39), and Magnetic resonance spectroscopy (MRS) studies have reported decreased N-acetylaspartate (NAA) levels in the hippocampus, interpreted as reflecting decreased neuronal integrity.(40, 41) Reductions in hippocampal volumes have ranged from 5% to 26% and have tended to be found bilaterally across studies.(42) It should be noted, however, that a number of studies have not replicated the finding of decreased hippocampal volumes in PTSD.(43–45) These discrepancies suggests that smaller hippocampi may be restricted to subgroups of PTSD, may be secondary to comorbid conditions, or that hippocampal pathology may be subtle and not always detectable using standard morphometric MRI procedures.(42) Furthermore, it has not been clear whether reported hippocampal changes are acquired signs of PTSD or potential predisposing factors.

Work done in twin studies helps to clarify what are the predisposing factors relative to acquired signs of PTSD. Gilbertson et al. (2002) studied monozygotic twins discordant for trauma exposure, with and without PTSD, and found that both twins with PTSD and their trauma-unexposed twin had smaller hippocampi relative to trauma-exposed, non-PTSD twins and their cotwin.(46) Moreover, the same group, both PTSD and trauma–nonexposed cotwin, showed impaired hippocampus-mediated spatial processing, using a cue configuration task. (47) These findings offer compelling evidence for reduced hippocampal size and function serving as a vulnerability or predisposing factor for PTSD.

To investigate impaired hippocampal functioning associated with PTSD, Shin et al. (2004) used PET in 16 firefighters (eight with PTSD) using a word stem completion task. Subjects completed a three-letter word stem with deeply encoded/high-recall and shallow encoded/low-recall words learned during a preceding training session. Somewhat surprisingly the PTSD group demonstrated greater rCBF in the hippocampi (bilateral) across conditions, and symptom severity was positively associated with rCBF in hippocampus and parahippocampal gyrus. In the comparison of high- versus low-recall conditions, however, PTSD showed smaller rCBF increases in the left hippocampus. This was interpreted as potentially reflecting reduced efficiency of hippocampus during the performance of an explicit memory task.(42)

Functional connectivity analyses

There is a growing awareness that complicated cognitive and emotional processes rely on the orchestrated interactions of distributed brain networks, rather than, or at least in addition to, activation of individual brain regions. Consequently, functional connectivity analysis, which refers to the application of specific statistical methods to functional neuroimaging data sets to identify correlated brain activity across various regions (48, 49), is a particularly relevant and useful technique. Several recent studies have applied functional connectivity analysis to neuroimaging studies of PTSD. Gilboa et al. (2004) studied 20 individuals with a history of civilian trauma (10 with PTSD), using symptom provocation (autobiographical trauma-related and neutral scripts), and [15O] H2O PET. A multivariate analysis technique (partial least squares) was used to identify brain regions whose activity covaried with two reference ("seed") voxels, one in right PFC (BA 10) and the other in right amygdala. Amygdala activity was found to significantly influence activity in the visual cortex, subcallosal gyrus, and anterior cingulate in the PTSD subjects but not in the trauma-exposed controls.(50) These findings indicate that blood flow measures reflect influence of the amygdala on medial frontal regions in PTSD, rather than a failure of mPFC inhibition of the amygdala. In addition, correlational analyses did not lend support for the failure of inhibition of the ACC over the amygdala.

Lanius et al. (2004) used functional connectivity analyses on data gathered during fMRI script-driven symptom provocation experiments in 11 subjects with PTSD from sexual abuse/ assault or motor vehicle accident (MVA) and 13 trauma-exposed subjects without PTSD. In the case of PTSD subjects (vs. controls) connectivity maps for right ACC showed greater correlations in the right posterior cingulate cortex (PCC) (BA 29), right caudate, right parietal lobe (BA 7 and 40), and right occipital lobe (BA 19). Subjects without PTSD had greater correlations of ACC with left superior frontal gyrus (BA 9), left anterior ACC (BA 32), left striatum (caudate), left parietal lobe (BA 40 and 43), and left insula (BA 13).(51) These findings are intriguing; however, our understanding of functional neural networks both in health and disease is still very limited. As methods for the analysis of functional connectivity continue to develop and the knowledge base regarding coordinated activation of brain regions grows these approaches will likely play an increasingly important role in delineating functional relationships between regions implicated in the pathophysiology of PTSD.

Summary of functional neuroimaging studies in PTSD

The studies reviewed above involve different cohorts (combat and CSA-related PTSD), different paradigms (symptom provocation vs. cognitive activation), and different modalities (fMRI,

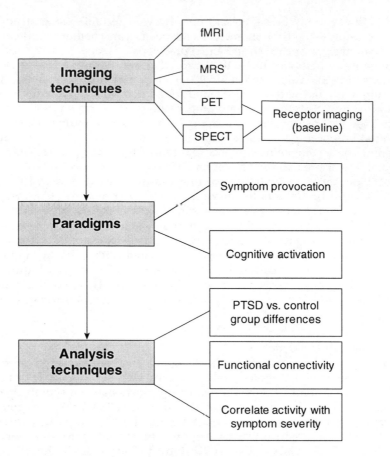

Figure 4.2   A summary of key imaging techniques, paradigms and analysis techniques discussed with in the chapter that are used to study the functional neuroanatomy associated with PTSD.

PET, and SPECT) [See Figure 4.2 for examples of imaging techniques]. Taken together, they lend tentative support to a neurocircuitry model that emphasizes the role of dysregulation in threat-related processing in PTSD. According to this model, trauma exposure sets off a cascade of neural changes that culminates in a state of amygdala hyperresponsivity to trauma-reminiscent and other threat-related stimuli that mediates symptoms of hyperarousal and vigilance associated with PTSD. The model also proposes associated inadequate top-down control by the mPFC that maintains and perpetuates the state of amygdala hyperresponsivity and also helps mediates the failure to suppress attention to trauma-related stimuli. Consistent with this model, several studies have demonstrated reduced activation of the mPFC (BA 10 and 11) and ACC (BA 32) in PTSD subjects compared to traumatized controls.(8–10, 21, 52) Other studies have reported increased responsivity of the amygdaloid region (4, 24, 29), though some have not (8, 10, 52). While the conceptualization of PTSD-related pathophysiology that emphasizes the role of threat-related processing has some empirical support, there is clearly a need for a broader conceptualization of the processes implicated in the disorder. This is because deficits in threat-related processing explain only some aspects of PTSD, and other significant manifestations of PTSD remain unexplained by this model. These include intrusive thoughts and memories, emotional numbing, vulnerability and resilience factors, and generalization of vigilance and avoidance from the initial traumatic event to other less closely related events. Thus to understand these complex phenomena, additional relevant mechanisms that may assist in understanding the complex phenomenology of PTSD need to be explored. The following section includes a selective review of emerging neuroimaging research that focuses on a number of mechanisms that are potentially relevant to the pathophysiology of PTSD, including fear conditioning and cognitive–emotional interactions.

PART II: PROCESSES IMPLICATED IN PTSD AND NEUROIMAGING

Studies of threat-related processing (fear conditioning, habituation, extinction, and extinction recall)

Studies using the fear-conditioning paradigm in rats over the past two decades have helped outline a specialized threat-related neurocircuitry with a number of functionally connected regions, including subregions of the PFC, the amygdala, and the hippocampus. A conceptual framework amalgamating their findings has been put forward, proposing the existence of two broad pathways in the processing of threat-related signals—a subcortical "fast" pathway that transmits features of the stimulus rapidly, but with poor specificity, and a cortical "slow" pathway that involves more integrated and detailed cognitive processing of stimulus characteristics.(53) Animal studies have identified the amygdaloid complex (central, lateral, and basolateral nuclei) as a crucial substrate in the formation of stimulus response associations involved in fear conditioning and aversive learning. Functional neuroimaging studies have used PET and fMRI to examine fear conditioning in humans, confirming that similar regions identified in animal research subserve fear conditioning in humans.(54) These usually examined classical conditioning to aversive stimuli, typically aversive tones, or mild electrical shocks. For example, Buchel and colleagues used event-related fMRI to study the classical conditioning of faces paired with aversive tones in nine healthy right-handed volunteers.(55) Comparison of the CS (+) condition to the CS (−) condition revealed greater activation of the ACC and greater activation in the amygdala in only early trials, suggesting a rapid habituation of the amygdala response in healthy volunteers.

There is also empirical work in healthy individuals indicating that the time course of amygdala activation during aversive conditioning is modulated by attention. Straube et al. (2007) demonstrated this empirically using stimulus processing to modulate attention. When attention was directed toward differences between CS (+) and CS (−), increased responses of the left amygdala to CS (+) versus CS (−) were rapidly established but absent at the end of conditioning trials, while directing attention to similarities between the CS (+) and CS (−) resulted in amygdala activation during the late but not early phase of conditioning.(56) This is significant, as it demonstrates that attention allocation can affect amygdala activation and potentially fear responding, implying that populations with aberrant patterns of attention allocation, such as attentional biases, may exhibit different patterns of amygdala activation and fear responses during conditioning.

Interestingly, studies designed to investigate the time course for amygdala response demonstrated that individuals with PTSD fail to show the same patterns of habituation of amygdala responding to negative stimuli, suggesting a possible longer maintenance of fear responses in PTSD.(18) In general, habituation and extinction are two processes that involve a time component that modulate conditioning and aversive learning and might be highly relevant to PTSD. Habituation refers to the process by which repeated presentation of the same CS–US pairing leads to a decreasing conditioned response (CR), while extinction refers to a reduction and disappearance of a CR on account of learning about a new stimulus–response association (i.e., the CS is no longer associated with the US). These are adaptive processes for organisms as they provide the organism with flexibility to reallocate critical resources to threat-related stimuli in a constantly changing environment. The failure of habituation to trauma-related stimuli and/ or the failure of extinction have been hypothesized to contribute to the development or maintenance of PTSD (i.e., trauma plays the role of the conditioning event). These phenomena have been extensively studied in animals and behaviorally in humans, but these processes have only recently been the subject of neuroimaging investigations.

A number of neuroimaging studies have found that presentation of emotionally expressive faces, presented both overtly as well as in a masked manner (fearful or happy faces masked with a neutral face such that subjects consciously perceive only the neutral face) activates the amygdala, a response that rapidly habituates with repeated presentation regardless of the mode of presentation (overt or masked).(57, 58) Several studies reviewed above, in which a CS is repeatedly paired with an aversive US, also found rapid habituation of the amygdala response.(55, 59, 60) One recent fMRI study suggests that repeated presentation of emotionally expressive faces may generate habituation in a regionally specific manner based on the valence of the facial stimulus. In this study fearful and happy faces were repeatedly presented in two 2-min runs to eight right-handed healthy men. Habituation was observed in the left dorsolateral prefrontal cortex (dlPFC) and premotor cortex and the right amygdala. The left dlPFC showed increased habituation to happy rather than fearful faces, the right amygdala exhibited greater habituation to emotionally valenced stimuli, and the left amygdala responded significantly more to negatively versus positively valenced stimuli (relative to the right).(61) Our laboratory has also demonstrated rACC habituation with repeated emotional picture (aversive minus neutral/ blank) presentation.(62) These studies provide evidence for habituation in the dlPFC, ACC, and the amygdala, with potentially differential habituation in prefrontal versus subcortical regions, or lateralized specialization. Interestingly, the only study that has specifically addressed the time course of amygdala responses to trauma cues (trauma-relevant words) in PP and healthy controls found an increased left amygdala response to trauma-relevant negative versus neutral stimuli in the first two but not last two runs. This response correlated with the symptom severity (CAPS total score). However, while sensitization to nontrauma negative words was seen in the PTSD group, failure of habituation to trauma-related words was not seen.(18)

The process of extinction has also been the subject of recent neuroimaging studies and it has been suggested that a failure to adequately extinguish fear responses is the mechanism underlying the maintenance of pathological fear in PTSD.(63) Phelps et al. (2004) used a simple discrimination, partial reinforcement, fear-conditioning paradigm with an event-related fMRI design. Colored squares were used for conditioned Stimulus (CS) (+) and conditioned Stimulus (CS) (–) (blue and yellow) and unconditioned stimulus (US) was a mild wrist shock. The study was conducted in three phases, an acquisition phase in which subjects were exposed to reinforced presentations of the CS, followed by Day 1 extinction and Day 2 extinction, in which subjects were exposed to unreinforced presentations of the CS. The authors reported that right amygdala activation predicted the CR in the early acquisition (positive correlation) and Day 1 extinction phase (negative correlation). The vmPFC (the subgenual anterior cingulate region of interest) response positively correlated with the CR magnitude during Day 2 extinction.(64) Milad et al. (2007) studied recall of fear extinction in healthy adults ($N = 17$). Context was manipulated, separating acquisition and extinction context, and extinction recall took place the next day, in the extinction context. Significant bilateral activations in the vmPFC and left amygdala were identified during fear extinction and two distinct loci within the vmPFC and bilateral hippocampi during extinction recall.(65)

Together, these findings appear to be consistent with those of animal research that implicate the amygdala in acquisition and extinction and the vmPFC in the retention and recall of the extinction learning process.(25, 64, 66–68) They are also intriguing in light of evidence reviewed earlier from human neuroimaging studies of altered connectivity between medial frontal regions and amygdala in PTSD. Thus, the evidence from human neuroimaging studies implicates subregions of the mPFC and OFC; subdivisions of the ACC; the extended amygdala; the hippocampus; and nuclei of the thalamus in the processes of fear conditioning, habituation, and extinction. The neuroimaging studies of these processes in healthy humans and also extending these studies to patients with PTSD are needed to better understand the roles of fear conditioning, habituation, and extinction in PTSD pathophysiology and symptom generation.

COGNITIVE–EMOTIONAL INTERACTIONS: APPRAISAL, REAPPRAISAL, AND EMOTIONAL REGULATION

Emotion regulation refers to the set of mental processes by which people amplify, attenuate, or otherwise modulate emotion states.(69) Key features of PTSD include emotional numbing and heightened and prolonged experience of fear, anxiety, and other negative affective states. While it is possible that abnormal threat-processing drives some of these symptoms, it is also possible that poor emotion regulation plays a key or complimentary role in this disorder and contributes significantly to behavioral dysfunction. If threat detection is a "bottom-up" process cognitive–emotional interaction can be seen as "top-down" regulation. Abnormalities in either one or in both of these processing streams can lead to similar outcomes, and in the case of PTSD, to similar psychopathology. For the purposes of this discussion, emotion regulation is understood in terms of a number of component processes that operate over different time scales. Appraisal refers to the cognitive interpretation of emotion-relevant stimuli by higher cortical centers. An increasing number of neuroimaging studies are providing evidence that cognitive appraisal can modulate emotional responses, which is reflected in changes in the activity of emotion processing areas. Cognitive reappraisal is a form of emotion regulation that involves volitionally reinterpreting the meaning of a stimulus to change one's emotional response to it.

A number of studies have manipulated the extent to which subjects cognitively attend to aspects of emotion-relevant stimuli. These studies suggest that even the simple process of appraising an emotion via labeling or rating can reduce the activity in structures that are responsive when the emotional stimulus is passively viewed or experienced. Hariri and colleagues examined the cognitive modulation of emotions by comparing the BOLD response in healthy subjects as they performed three different tasks (match, label, and control). In the match task, subjects were asked to match the affect of one of two faces to that of a simultaneously presented target face (angry or fearful) whereas in the label task, they were asked to assign one of two simultaneously presented linguistic labels (angry or afraid) to a target face. Matching was associated with increased activation in both the right and left amygdale, whereas linguistically labeling the expression was associated with a decreased activation in the amygdala. In addition, right PFC activity was inversely correlated with left amygdala activity, interpreted as it being the neural substrate for the cognitive modulation of emotion.(70) This finding has been replicated using threatening and fearful pictures as well.(71)

In our laboratory, we examined rCBF response in healthy subjects comparing a rating to a passive viewing condition.(72) Subjects saw aversive and neutral pictures while they performed a passive viewing and rating task. During passive viewing, subjects activated right amygdala / insula and left insula, and rating was associated with increased activation of the dorsomedial prefrontal cortex (dmPFC) and the ACC, and with reduced sadness and reduced activation of the right amygdala/insula and left insula. These findings demonstrate the involvement of the dmPFC and ACC in the cognitive rating task and suggest modulating effects of these structures on emotion-related structures, such as the amygdala and insula. These results extend findings from animal studies that have demonstrated the inhibitory influence of the mPFC over the amygdale.(73) If indeed dmPFC/ACC dysfunction is present in PTSD, these findings could suggest one explanation for exaggerated emotional responses of PTSD patients, as they are less effectively modulated by cognitive appraisal.

The ability to cognitively modulate emotions refers to the efficacy of individuals to effortfully change their emotional reaction to a stimulus. Recently, several groups of researchers have begun to investigate this empirically using imaging, adopting different strategies to induce cognitive modulation. Cognitive reappraisal is one strategy, and this refers to volitional reinterpretation of the meaning of a stimulus to modify one's emotional response. This line of work is likely very relevant to PTSD, where an inability to reinterpret the meaning of ambiguous stimuli might contribute to emotional dysregulation. It is also of much interest in the investigation of brain mechanisms of cognitive behavioral therapy, an effective treatment for some patients with PTSD. Ochsner and colleagues used an event-related fMRI design and aversive pictures to study cognitive reappraisal in healthy women. These women were asked to attend (be aware of feelings elicited by the picture) or to reappraise (reinterpret the picture so that it no longer elicits a negative emotional response) while being scanned.(74) Reappraising (vs. attending) was associated with increased activation of the dorsal and ventral left lateral prefronal cortex, dmPFC, left temporal pole, right supramarginal gyrus (SMG), and left lateral occipital cortex. Greater activation in the right ACC and SMG correlated with greater decreases in negative affect (greater reappraisal success); left ventral PFC activation during reappraisal was inversely correlated with activity in the amygdala. Effective reappraisal resulted in increased activation in lateral PFC and mPFC regions and in decreased activation of medial OFC and amygdala. Using a similar paradigm, Phan et al. (2005) showed highly aversive and arousing pictures to healthy subjects, who were instructed to either "maintain" (feel naturally) or "suppress" (by positive reframing or rationalizing) negative affect. Successful reduction of negative affect was associated with increasing activation of dmPFC, dorsal ACC, dlPFC, lateral OFC, and ventrolateral PFC/inferior frontal gyrus, and with decreasing activity in the left nucleus accumbens, left lateral PFC, and left extended amygdala. In addition, right dorsal ACC, right anterior insula, bilateral dlPFC, and bilateral ventrolateral PFC activity inversely correlated with the intensity of negative affect.(75)

These studies provide evidence for the emotion regulatory role of lateral PFC, dmPFC, SMG, and ACC.(75) The observed difficulty among patients with PTSD to cognitively regulate their emotions can be hypothesized to be a result of dysfunctional cognitive–emotional processes (such as cognitive appraisal and reappraisal) subserved by some of these regions. The therapeutic mechanisms of cognitive behavioral therapy in PTSD may also be related to these processes and structures. There is, therefore, a need to extend these innovative paradigms to the study of PTSD.

RECEPTOR IMAGING

Insight into which regions differ in activity as a function of PTSD can be gauged with fMRI, as the BOLD signal, a measure of the ratio of oxygenated to deoxygenated hemoglobin in the blood across regions of the brain, is likely to reflect changes in neuronal firing or postsynaptic activity. In contrast, differences that may exist in functional neurochemistry between those with and without PTSD can be directly gauged with receptor imaging. To date, only a few studies have used receptor imaging to investigate neurotransmitter abnormalities associated with PTSD. Previous research in both animals and humans has implicated gamma-Aminobutyric acid (GABA), the principle inhibitory neurotransmitter within the brain, to be involved in both the pathogenesis and pathophysiology of PTSD.(76, 77) In a recent study, Geuze et al. (2008) used [^{11}C]flumazenil and PET to assess differences in the benzodiazepine–GABA$_A$ receptor complex in veterans with and without PTSD.(78) They found reduced binding potential of [^{11}C]flumazenil in veterans with PTSD relative to control veterans without PTSD, specifically in the hippocampus, thalamus, and throughout the cortex, including the frontal, temporal, parietal, and occipital cortex.(78) This suggests that these specific regions may be associated with premorbid differences in the composition/expression of GABA$_A$ –benzodiazepines receptors in PTSD patients or a disease-induced modulation and/or downregulation of the GABA$_A$ receptor complex. Consistent with this study is a previous [^{123}I]iomazenil SPECT study in Vietnam veterans that also found decreased volume of distribution of [^{123}I]iomazenil in the medial prefrontal cortex in Vietnam veterans with PTSD relative to healthy controls.(79) It should be noted, however, that another study also using [^{123}I] iomazenil and SPECT was unable to find any differences in volume distribution of [^{123}I]iomazenil between Gulf War veterans with and without PTSD.(80)

In a recent study, our group investigated μ-opioid receptor binding in PTSD, using PET and the selective μ-opioid radiotracer [^{11}C] carfentanil.(81) We had previously demonstrated endogenous opioids to be involved in inhibiting and modulating emotional responses in healthy humans (82), and this was the first study to provide direct evidence of alterations in μ-opioid receptor in vivo availability in PTSD. We demonstrated significant regional differences in the binding of μ-opioid receptor between both the trauma-exposed groups and normal controls, as well as between PTSD patients and trauma-exposed individuals who did not develop PTSD. These differences between the groups indicate μ-opioid receptor alterations arising from trauma that can be differentiated from those specifically associated with PTSD. Changes were principally located in limbic forebrain and cortical regions known to be involved in emotion regulation, which likely reflect adaptive changes resulting from trauma exposure or stress, as well as maladaptive alterations associated with PTSD pathophysiology.(81)

Despite both receptor imaging and fMRI approaches implicating similar brain regions in the pathophysiology of PTSD (e.g., prefrontal cortex and hippocampus), reconciling the findings of these two methodologies poses a challenge. The receptor imaging data suggest decreased GABA$_A$ receptor binding potential in prefrontal regions in PTSD, suggesting potentially lower inhibitory tone, and therefore, enhanced reactivity. In contrast, the fMRI data indicate hypoactivation of cortical regions (specifically mPFC) associated with PTSD. However, if the decreased GABA binding potential reflects a decreased number of GABA$_A$ receptors on the inhibitory interneurons, this could explain overall higher inhibitory tone in the mPFC. Furthermore, while BOLD activity likely reflects overall neuronal activity within a particular region, changes both in inhibitory and excitatory neurotransmission can contribute to the overall BOLD output. Thus, the changes in one particular neurotransmitter system should not be interpreted as defining the overall changes in BOLD signal. Moreover, given the complex interconnectivity of the PFC, its heterogeneity, and its broad functionality, it is possible that PTSD is associated with both increased and decreased activity within distinct regions of the PFC. To date, receptor imaging in PTSD has focused on inhibitory systems (GABA and Opioids) and a focus for future research on glutamatergic (excitatory) systems, as well as other neurotransmitters/neuromodulators implicated in PTSD, such as serotonin (83), central catecholamines (84), and corticotrophin-releasing hormone (85), will further help elucidate the molecular basis of altered brain function associated with PTSD.

SUMMARY AND FUTURE DIRECTIONS

Neuroimaging studies of PTSD over the past decade have been based on a model that conceptualizes the disorder as a state of heightened responsivity to threatening stimuli and/or a state of insufficient inhibitory control over exaggerated threat-sensitivity. Consistent with this model, several studies have demonstrated reduced activation of the mPFC (BA 10 and 11) and ACC (BA 32) in PTSD subjects compared to traumatized controls. Other studies have reported increased responsivity of the amygdaloid region, although these findings are not always consistent. Results may be influenced by several methodological issues, such as small samples, heterogeneous populations, presence or absence of comorbidities, and varying imaging methods that limit broad generalization. More importantly, it is still not known what are acquired signs of the disorder and what are its predisposing factors. Innovative imaging work in twins discordant for PTSD is beginning to elucidate this issue, suggesting that reduced hippocampus size and function may be a predisposing factor. Prospective neuroimaging studies are costly and challenging to employ, though they are essential for the identification of endophenotypes indicative of PTSD vulnerability, as well as to effectively delineate what are the causes and consequence of PTSD in terms of brain morphology and function. PTSD is a complex disorder, and despite the progress made, existing models and findings are unable to fully capture the complexity of PTSD. Innovative paradigms being developed in cognitive and social neuroscience suggest novel directions for future work that can broaden our understanding of a range of pathophysiological processes in PTSD.

Future directions of research include neuroimaging studies of fear conditioning, habituation, extinction, and extinction recall, as well as studies investigating emotion regulation processes in PTSD. Complicated emotional and cognitive processes rely not only on the activation of discrete brain regions but also upon the strength and nature of distributed brain networks. Consequently, increased use of connectivity analyses will help illuminate how the relationship between different neuronal regions is also impaired in PTSD. There is also a need for prospective studies, as well as studies that integrate different lines of inquiry, including genetic, neuroendocrine (HPA axis, catecholamines, etc.) and neurochemical receptor studies, and blood flow parameters in PTSD. This research holds the exciting promise of helping to identify neurobiological factors that may confer vulnerability or resilience to PTSD and offer meaningful clues to the pathophysiology of PTSD. This progress will be essential for the future development of effective prevention and treatment strategies for this disorder.

REFERENCES

1. Liberzon I, Phan KL. Brain-imaging studies of posttraumatic stress disorder. CNS Spectr 2003; 8(9): 641–50.
2. Pitman RK, Shin LM, Rauch SL. Investigating the pathogenesis of posttraumatic stress disorder with neuroimaging. J Clin Psychiatry 2001; 62(Suppl 17): 47–54.
3. Rauch SL, Shin LM. Functional neuroimaging studies in posttraumatic stress disorder. Ann N Y Acad Sci. 1997; 821: 83–98.
4. Rauch SL, van der Kolk BA, Fisler RE et al. A symptom provocation study of posttraumatic stress disorder using positron emission tomography and script-driven imagery. Arch Gen Psychiatry 1996; 53(5): 380–7.
5. Shin LM, Kosslyn SM, McNally RJ et al. Visual imagery and perception in posttraumatic stress disorder. A positron emission tomographic investigation. Arch Gen Psychiatry 1997; 54(3): 233–41.
6. Liberzon I, Britton JC, Phan KL. Neural correlates of traumatic recall in posttraumatic stress disorder. Stress 2003; 6(3): 151–6.
7. Bremner JD, Narayan M, Staib LH et al. Neural correlates of memories of childhood sexual abuse in women with and without posttraumatic stress disorder. Am J Psychiatry 1999; 156(11): 1787–95.
8. Shin LM, McNally RJ, Kosslyn SM et al. Regional cerebral blood flow during script-driven imagery in childhood sexual abuse-related PTSD: A PET investigation. Am J Psychiatry 1999; 156(4): 575–84.
9. Lanius RA, Hopper JW, Menon RS. Individual differences in a husband and wife who developed PTSD after a motor vehicle accident: a functional MRI case study. Am J Psychiatry 2003; 160(4): 667–9.
10. Lanius RA, Williamson PC, Densmore M et al. Neural correlates of traumatic memories in posttraumatic stress disorder: a functional MRI investigation. Am J Psychiatry 2001; 158(11): 1920–2.
11. Hendler T, Rotshtein P, Hadar U. Emotion-perception interplay in the visual cortex: "the eyes follow the heart". Cell Mol Neurobiol 2001; 21(6): 733–52.

12. Shin LM, Orr SP, Carson MA et al. Regional cerebral blood flow in the amygdala and medial prefrontal cortex during traumatic imagery in male and female Vietnam veterans with PTSD. Arch Gen Psychiatry 2004; 61(2): 168–76.

13. Britton JC, Phan KL, Taylor SF, Fig LM, Liberzon I. Corticolimbic blood flow in posttraumatic stress disorder during script-driven imagery. Biol Psychiatry 2005; 57(8): 832–40.

14. Lanius RA, Frewen PA, Girotti M et al. Neural correlates of trauma script-imagery in posttraumatic stress disorder with and without comorbid major depression: a functional MRI investigation. Psychiatry Res 2007; 155(1): 45–56.

15. Hsu CC, Chong MY, Yang P, Yen CF. Posttraumatic stress disorder among adolescent earthquake victims in Taiwan. J Am Acad Child Adolesc Psychiatry 2002; 41(7): 875–81.

16. Osuch EA, Benson B, Geraci M et al. Regional cerebral blood flow correlated with flashback intensity in patients with posttraumatic stress disorder. Biol Psychiatry 2001; 50(4): 246–53.

17. Lanius RA, Williamson PC, Boksman K et al. Brain activation during script-driven imagery induced dissociative responses in PTSD: a functional magnetic resonance imaging investigation. Biol Psychiatry 2002; 52(4): 305–11.

18. Protopopescu X, Pan H, Tuescher O et al. Differential time courses and specificity of amygdala activity in posttraumatic stress disorder subjects and normal control subjects. Biol Psychiatry 2005; 57(5): 464–73.

19. Bush G, Luu P, Posner MI. Cognitive and emotional influences in anterior cingulate cortex. Trends Cogn Sci 2000; 4(6): 215–22.

20. Bremner JD, Vermetten E, Vythilingam M et al. Neural correlates of the classic color and emotional stroop in women with abuse-related posttraumatic stress disorder. Biol Psychiatry 2004; 55(6): 612–20.

21. Shin LM, Whalen PJ, Pitman RK et al. An fMRI study of anterior cingulate function in posttraumatic stress disorder. Biol Psychiatry 2001; 50(12): 932–42.

22. Shin LM, Bush G, Whalen PJ et al. Dorsal anterior cingulate function in posttraumatic stress disorder. J Trauma Stress 2007; 20(5): 701–12.

23. Davis M. The role of the amygdala in fear and anxiety. Annu Rev Neurosci 1992; 151: 353–75.

24. Liberzon I, Taylor SF, Amdur R et al. Brain activation in PTSD in response to trauma-related stimuli. Biol Psychiatry 1999; 45(7): 817–26.

25. Morgan MA, LeDoux JE. Differential contribution of dorsal and ventral medial prefrontal cortex to the acquisition and extinction of conditioned fear in rats. Behav Neurosci 1995; 109(4): 681–8.

26. Davis M, Whalen PJ. The amygdala: vigilance and emotion. Mol Psychiatry 2001; 6(1): 13–34.

27. Armony JL, Corbo V, Clement MH, Brunet A. Amygdala response in patients with acute PTSD to masked and unmasked emotional facial expressions. Am J Psychiatry 2005; 162(10): 1961–3.

28. Bryant RA, Kemp AH, Felmingham KL et al. Enhanced amygdala and medial prefrontal activation during nonconscious processing of fear in posttraumatic stress disorder: an fMRI study. Hum Brain Mapp 2008; 29(5): 517–23.

29. Rauch SL, Whalen PJ, Shin LM et al. Exaggerated amygdala response to masked facial stimuli in posttraumatic stress disorder: a functional MRI study. Biol Psychiatry 2000; 47(9): 769–76.

30. Bryant RA, Kemp AH, Felmingham KL et al. Enhanced amygdala and medial prefrontal activation during nonconscious processing of fear in posttraumatic stress disorder: an fMRI study. Hum Brain Mapp 2008; 29(5): 517–23.

31. Shin LM, Wright CI, Cannistraro PA et al. A functional magnetic resonance imaging study of amygdala and medial prefrontal cortex responses to overtly presented fearful faces in posttraumatic stress disorder. Arch Gen Psychiatry 2005; 62(3): 273–81.

32. Corcoran KA, Maren S. Hippocampal inactivation disrupts contextual retrieval of fear memory after extinction. J Neurosci 2001; 21(5): 1720–6.

33. Eichenbaum H. A cortical-hippocampal system for declarative memory. Nat Rev Neurosci 2000; 1(1): 41–50.

34. Bremner JD, Randall P, Scott TM et al. MRI-based measurement of hippocampal volume in patients with combat-related posttraumatic stress disorder. Am J Psychiatry 1995; 152(7): 973–81.

35. Bremner JD, Scott TM, Delaney RC et al. Deficits in short-term memory in posttraumatic stress disorder. Am J Psychiatry 1993; 150(7): 1015–9.

36. Bremner JD, Randall P, Vermetten E et al. Magnetic resonance imaging-based measurement of hippocampal volume in posttraumatic stress disorder related to childhood physical and sexual abuse--a preliminary report. Biol Psychiatry 1997; 41(1): 23–32.

37. Gurvits TV, Shenton ME, Hokama H et al. Magnetic resonance imaging study of hippocampal volume in chronic, combat-related posttraumatic stress disorder. Biol Psychiatry 1996; 40(11): 1091–9.

38. Stein MB, Koverola C, Hanna C, Torchia MG, McClarty B. Hippocampal volume in women victimized by childhood sexual abuse. Psychol Med 1997; 27(4): 951–9.

39. Villarreal G, Hamilton DA, Petropoulos H et al. Reduced hippocampal volume and total white matter volume in posttraumatic stress disorder. Biol Psychiatry 2002; 52(2): 119–25.

40. Schuff N, Neylan TC, Lenoci MA et al. Decreased hippocampal N-acetylaspartate in the absence of atrophy in posttraumatic stress disorder. Biol Psychiatry 2001; 50(12): 952–9.

41. Villarreal G, Petropoulos H, Hamilton DA et al. Proton magnetic resonance spectroscopy of the hippocampus and occipital white matter in PTSD: preliminary results. Can J Psychiatry 2002; 47(7): 666–70.

42. Shin LM, Shin PS, Heckers S et al. Hippocampal function in posttraumatic stress disorder. Hippocampus 2004; 14(3): 292–300.

43. Bonne O, Brandes D, Gilboa A et al. Longitudinal MRI study of hippocampal volume in trauma survivors with PTSD. Am J Psychiatry 2001; 158(8): 1248–51.

44. Carrion VG, Weems CF, Eliez S et al. Attenuation of frontal asymmetry in pediatric posttraumatic stress disorder. Biol Psychiatry 2001; 50(12): 943–51.

45. De Bellis MD, Keshavan MS, Clark DB et al. A.E. Bennett Research Award. Developmental traumatology. Part II: Brain development. Biol Psychiatry 1999; 45(10): 1271–84.

46. Gilbertson MW, Shenton ME, Ciszewski A et al. Smaller hippocampal volume predicts pathologic vulnerability to psychological trauma. Nat Neurosci 2002; 5(11): 1242–7.

47. Gilbertson MW, Williston SK, Paulus LA et al. Configural cue performance in identical twins discordant for posttraumatic stress disorder: theoretical implications for the role of hippocampal function. Biol Psychiatry 2007; 62(5): 513–20.

48. Friston KJ, Frith CD, Fletcher P, Liddle PF, Frackowiak RS. Functional topography: multidimensional scaling and functional connectivity in the brain. Cereb Cortex 1996; 6(2): 156–64.

49. Friston KJ, Frith CD, Liddle PF, Frackowiak RS. Functional connectivity: the principal-component analysis of large (PET) data sets. J Cereb Blood Flow Metab 1993; 13(1): 5–14.

50. Gilboa A, Shalev AY, Laor L et al. Functional connectivity of the prefrontal cortex and the amygdala in posttraumatic stress disorder. Biol Psychiatry 2004; 55(3): 263–72.

51. Lanius RA, Williamson PC, Densmore M et al. The nature of traumatic memories: a 4-T FMRI functional connectivity analysis. Am J Psychiatry 2004; 161(1): 36–44.

52. Bremner JD, Staib LH, Kaloupek D et al. Neural correlates of exposure to traumatic pictures and sound in Vietnam combat veterans with and without posttraumatic stress disorder: a positron emission tomography study. Biol Psychiatry 1999; 45(7): 806–16.

53. LeDoux JE. Emotion Circuits in the Brain. Annu Rev Neurosci 2000; 23: 155–84.

54. Buchel C, Dolan RJ. Classical fear conditioning in functional neuroimaging. Curr Opin Neurobiol 2000; 10(2): 219–23.

55. Buchel C, Dolan RJ, Armony JL, Friston KJ. Amygdala-hippocampal involvement in human aversive trace conditioning revealed through event-related functional magnetic resonance imaging. J Neurosci 1999; 19(24): 10869–76.

56. Straube T, Weiss T, Mentzel HJ, Miltner WH. Time course of amygdala activation during aversive conditioning depends on attention. Neuroimage 2007; 34(1): 462–9.

57. Breiter HC, Etcoff NL, Whalen PJ et al. Response and habituation of the human amygdala during visual processing of facial expression. Neuron 1996; 17(5): 875–87.

58. Whalen PJ, Rauch SL, Etcoff NL et al. Masked presentations of emotional facial expressions amygdala activity without explicit knowledge. J Neurosci 1998; 18: 411–8.

59. Buchel C, Morris J, Dolan RJ, Friston KJ. Brain systems mediating aversive conditioning: an event-related fMRI study. Neuron 1998; 20(5): 947–57.

60. LaBar KS, Gatenby JC, Gore JC, LeDoux JE, Phelps EA. Human amygdala activation during conditioned fear acquisition and extinction: a mixed-trial fMRI study. Neuron 1998; 20(5): 937–45.

61. Wright CI, Fischer H, Whalen PJ et al. Differential prefrontal cortex and amygdala habituation to repeatedly presented emotional stimuli. Neuroreport 2001; 12(2): 379–83.

62. Phan KL, Liberzon I, Welsh RC, Britton JC, Taylor SF. Habituation of rostral anterior cingulate cortex to repeated emotionally salient pictures. Neuropsychopharmacology 2003; 28(7): 1344–50.

63. Charney DS, Deutch AY, Krystal JH, Southwick SM, Davis M. Psychobiologic mechanisms of posttraumatic stress disorder. Arch Gen Psychiatry 1993; 50(4): 295–305.

64. Phelps EA, Delgado MR, Nearing KI, LeDoux JE. Extinction learning in humans: role of the amygdala and vmPFC. Neuron 2004; 43(6): 897–905.

65. Milad MR, Wright CI, Orr SP et al. Recall of fear extinction in humans activates the ventromedial prefrontal cortex and hippocampus in concert. Biol Psychiatry 2007; 62(5): 446–54.

66. Falls WA, Miserendino MJ, Davis M. Extinction of fear-potentiated startle: blockade by infusion of an NMDA antagonist into the amygdala. J Neurosci 1992; 12(3): 854–63.

67. Morgan MA, Romanski LM, LeDoux JE. Extinction of emotional learning: contribution of medial prefrontal cortex. Neurosci Lett 1993; 163(1): 109–13.

68. Morgan MA, Schulkin J, LeDoux JE. Ventral medial prefrontal cortex and emotional perseveration: the memory for prior extinction training. Behav Brain Res 2003; 146(1–2): 121–30.

69. Gross JJ. Antecedent- and response-focused emotion regulation: divergent consequences for experience, expression, and physiology. J Pers Soc Psychol 1998; 74(1): 224–37.

70. Hariri AR, Bookheimer SY, Mazziotta JC. Modulating emotional responses: effects of a neocortical network on the limbic system. Neuroreport 2000; 11(1): 43–8.

71. Hariri AR, Mattay VS, Tessitore A, Fera F, Weinberger DR. Neocortical modulation of the amygdala response to fearful stimuli. Biol Psychiatry 2003; 53(6): 494–501.

72. Taylor SF, Phan KL, Decker LR, Liberzon I. Subjective rating of emotionally salient stimuli modulates neural activity. Neuroimage 2003; 18(3): 650–9.

73. Rosenkranz JA, Grace AA. Cellular mechanisms of infralimbic and prelimbic prefrontal cortical inhibition and dopaminergic modulation of basolateral amygdala neurons in vivo. J Neurosci 2002; 22(1): 324–37.

74. Ochsner KN, Bunge SA, Gross JJ, Gabrieli JD. Rethinking feelings: an FMRI study of the cognitive regulation of emotion. J Cogn Neurosci 2002; 14(8): 1215–29.

75. Phan KL, Fitzgerald DA, Nathan PJ et al. Neural substrates for voluntary suppression of negative affect: a functional magnetic resonance imaging study. Biol Psychiatry 2005; 57(3): 210–9.

76. Harvey BH, Oosthuizen F, Brand L, Wegener G, Stein DJ. Stress-restress evokes sustained iNOS activity and altered GABA levels and NMDA receptors in rat hippocampus. Psychopharmacology 2004; 175: 494–502.

77. Vaiva G, Thomas P, Ducrocq F et al. Low posttrauma GABA plasma levels as a predictive factor in the development of acute posttraumatic stress disorder. Biol Psychiatry 2004; 55(3): 250–4.

78. Geuze E, van Berckel BNM, Lammertsma AA et al. Reduced GABAA benzodiazepine receptor binding in veterans with post-traumatic stress disorder. Mol Psychiatry 2008; 13: 74–83.

79. Bremner JD, Innis RB, Southwick SM et al. Decreased benzodiazepine receptor binding in prefrontal cortex in combat-related posttraumatic stress disorder. Am J Psychiatry 2000; 157(7): 1120–6.

80. Fujita M, Southwick SM, Denucci CC et al. Central type benzodiazepine receptors in Gulf War veterans with posttaumatic stress disorder. Biol Psychiatry 2004; 56: 95–100.

81. Liberzon I, Taylor SF, Phan KL et al. Altered central mu-opiod binding after psychological trauma. Biol Psychiatry 2007; 61(9): 1030–8.

82. Liberzon I, Zubieta JK, Fig LM et al. mu-Opioid receptors and limbic responses to aversive emotional stimuli. Proc Natl Acad Sci U S A 2002; 99: 7084–9.

83. Southwick SM, Krystal JH, Bremner JD et al. Noradrenergic and serotonergic function in posttraumatic stress disorder. Arch Gen Psychiatry 1997; 54(8): 749–58.

84. Yehuda R, Southwick SM, Giller EL, Ma XW, Mason JW. Urinary catecholamine excretion adn severity of PTSD symptoms in vietnam combat veterans. J Nerv Ment Dis 1992; 180(5): 321–5.

85. Bremner JD, Licinio J, Darnell A et al. Elevated CSF corticotropin-releasing factor concentrations in posttraumatic stress disorder. Am J Psychiatry 1997; 154(5): 624–9.

5 | Brain circuits in posttraumatic stress disorder

Eric Vermetten and Ruth Lanius

INTRODUCTION

With the notion that the primary goal in research in the clinical neuroscience of stress-related disorders is to apply findings related to the effects of stress on the brain in animals to patients with stress-related disorders (e.g., posttraumatic stress disorder [PTSD]), a variety of different methods have contributed to the working model of the neural circuitry of PTSD that is presented here. In addition to preclinical studies that look at brain tissue specificity to stress, in human studies the neural circuitry can be studied by measuring volumes of key brain structures with structural neuroimaging; the brain metabolic response to provocation of disease-specific symptoms in conjunction with functional neuroimaging, using neuroimaging to measure neuroreceptors; or neurotransmitters and hormone levels in blood, urine, and saliva, as well as assessing behavioral and biochemical responses to pharmacological challenge to specific neurochemical systems. The composite of these methods enables a definition of the circuitry that is involved in the pathophysiology of PTSD. As such the circuitry is mediating symptoms of the wider trauma-related disorders (e.g., acute stress disorders, dissociative disorders, pathological grief) [see also Liberman chapter].

Only since the last 10 years a model of PTSD could start to be validated with the newer neuroimaging methods. The imaging facilities and also the studies that have contributed to the model have improved over the past decade, mostly due to technical and software enhancements. Spatial and temporal resolution of neuroimaging methods have improved much (Dickerson, 2007) that promise to reveal novel insights into the function of fine-scale neural circuitry of the stress response. However, the findings of the various studies, research designs, methodologies, and techniques that will be discussed in this chapter vary to a great extent, show incoherence, or sometimes opposite results. Repeated studies across centers are an important prerequisite to generate consensus for a model. The lack of coherency of findings between studies may be accounted for by a large variety of parameters, among which standardization of the study protocol, and imaging parameters are of key importance. This review first focuses on the basic structures involved in the stress response and then moves on to discussing the compromised neural circuits in PTSD that were revealed through functional neuroimaging research. It covers various techniques (single positron emitted tomography (SPECT), positron emission tomography (PET), and functional neuroimaging (fMRI) that use different paradigms (resting, active tasks, stimulus presentation) and provides a global overview of the current findings of these studies. New developments in the field are also discussed briefly in the last section.

A WORKING MODEL FOR A NEURAL CIRCUITRY IN PTSD

Based on studies of the effects of stress on animals and emerging work in clinical neuroscience of PTSD, a working model for a neural circuitry of fear that is also applicable to PTSD can be described (see Vermetten and Bremner, 2002). This model is based on work of Charney and Bremner (Bremner et al. 1995, Charney et al. 1993). This work is ongoing and the models proposed may be subject to modification and revision as our knowledge base in this area continues to expand.

The brain structures that constitute a neurological working model for traumatic stress should have several features:

1 Sufficient afferent input should be provided to permit assessment of the fear-producing nature of the event;

2 The neuronal interactions between the brain structures must be capable of incorporation of a person's prior experience into the cognitive appraisal of stimuli;

3   The ability to effectively lay down memory traces related to a potential threat;
4   Efferent projections from the brain that are able to mediate an individual's neuroendo-
     crine, autonomic, and motor responses.

Critical brain structures involved in mediating fear behavior resulting from traumatic stress are locus coeruleus (LC), hippocampus, amygdala, prefrontal cortex, thalamus and hypothalamus, and periaqueductal grey (PAG), which contribute to neural mechanisms of fear conditioning, extinction, and behavioral sensitization in case of persistent symptoms of traumatic stress.

The model provides the neural circuitry that plays a role in describing how information related to a threatening stimulus (e.g., being threatened by someone at gunpoint or witnessing a deadly car accident) enters the primary senses (smell, sight, touch, hearing); is integrated into a coherent image that is grounded in space and time; activates memory traces of prior similar experiences with the appropriate emotional valence (necessary in order to evaluate the true threat potential of the stimulus); triggers a stress response and subsequently triggers appropriate and adaptive behavioral response, like defending yourself, running away, or calling for help.

Afferent sensory input enters through the eyes, ears, smell, touch, the body's own visceral information, or any combination of these. These sensory inputs are relayed through the dorsal thalamus to cortical brain areas, such as primary visual (occipital), auditory (temporal), or tactile (post-central gyrus) cortical areas. Olfactory sensory input, however, has direct inputs to the amygdala and entorhinal cortex (Turner et al. 1978). Input from peripheral visceral organs is relayed in the brainstem to the LC, site of the majority of the brain's noradrenergic neurons (see companion paper), and from here to central brain areas. These brain areas have projections to multiple areas, including amygdala, hippocampus, entorhinal cortex, orbitofrontal cortex, and cingulate, which are involved in mediating memory and emotion (Van Hoesen et al. 1972) (Vogt & Miller 1983).

Cognitive appraisal of potential threat, which involves placing the threatening object in space and time, is an important aspect of the stress response. Specific brain areas are involved in these functions (like localizing objects in space, visuospatial processing, memory, cognition, action, and planning). The anterior cingulate gyrus (Brodmann Area 32) is involved in selection of responses for action as well as emotion (Devinsky et al. 1995). This area and other medial portions of the prefrontal cortex, including Brodman's Area 25 and orbitofrontal cortex (OFC), modulate emotional and physiological responses to stress. If one is approached in a potentially threatening situation, it will be important to determine whether the face of the person you see is someone known to you or is a stranger who may be more threatening. Also, it is important to place the situation in time and place. Entering a dark alleyway may trigger prior memories of being robbed, with associated negative emotions and physiological arousal. These memories may have survival value in that the individual will avoid the situation where the previous negative event took place, with arousal stimulated and eventual flight prepared. Retrieval of prior memories of traumatic events has survival value for a true threatening situation; however, if retrieval occurs repeatedly in nonthreatening situations situation it can be maladaptive and so lead to symptoms of PTSD.

It is critical to effectively lay down memory traces related to a potential threat in order to prevent, defend against, or avoid types of threat in the future. The hippocampus and adjacent cortex mediate declarative memory function (e.g., recall of facts and lists) and play an important role in integration of memory elements at the time of retrieval and in assigning significance for events within space and time (Squire & Zola-Morgan 1991). The hippocampus also regulates the neuroendocrine response to the stress by its role in glucocorticoid negative feedback. The function of the amygdala in the processing of fear involves conditioning and addition of an emotional valence to the situation. The amygdala also has direct connections that initiate motor responses to fear (Sarter & Markowitsch 1985). It is most likely that fearful experiences will be stored in long-term memory. However, (dissociative) amnesia for traumatic events, a widely debated issue regarding memories for childhood abuse, is not an uncommon phenomenon in patients with trauma-related disorders (Bremner et al. 1996) (Chu et al. 1999) (van der Hart et al. 2005) (Vermetten and Bremner, 2000). With long-term storage, memories are felt to be shifted through hippocampal synaptic plasticity by protein synthesis, from hippocampus to the neocortical areas where also the sensory impressions are stored (Neves et al. 2008) (Bekinschtein et al. 2007).

In situations of extreme fear, a special category of memory is involved, which entails the implicit (probably unconscious) learning and storage of information about the emotional significance of events. The neural system underlying emotional memory involves the amygdala and structures with which it is connected. Afferent inputs from sensory processing areas of the thalamus and cortex mediate emotional learning in situations involving specific sensory cues, whereas learning about the emotional significance of more general, contextual cues involves projections to the amygdala from the hippocampal formation (LeDoux 1993). Associative processes can occur during the process of fear conditioning, and these may underlie the long-term associative plasticity that constitutes memory of the conditioning experience (Rogan et al. 1997). Fear conditioning to explicit and contextual cues has been proposed as a model for intrusive memories that in a kindling-like process, are reactivated by trauma-related stimuli and hyperarousal, respectively (Grillon et al. 1996). Clinicians often report that 'traumatic cues' such as a particular sight or sound reminiscent of the original traumatic event can trigger a cascade of anxiety- and fear-related symptoms in a patient, not uncommonly without conscious recall of the original traumatic event (Vermetten & Bremner 2003).

Frontal cortical areas modulate emotional responsiveness through inhibition of amygdala function, and it has been hypothesized that dysfunction in these regions may underlie pathological emotional responses in patients with PTSD, and possibly other anxiety disorders. Medial prefrontal cortex (mPFC) (area 24, 25 and 32) (incl. subcallosal gyrus) has projections to the amygdala (Buchanan et al. 1994), which are involved in the suppression of amygdala responsiveness to fearful cues. Dysfunction of this area may be responsible for the failure of extinction to fearful cues, which is an important part of the anxiety response (Morgan et al. 1993) (Anderson & Insel 2006). In animal models of extinction, the aversive association in the amygdala seems to be inhibited rather than removed; fear can be rapidly reinstated even long after extinction either by the presentation of the conditioned stimulus in a different context or by a single stimulus-shock pairing (Myers & Davis 2007). medial prefrontal cortex (MPF) is involved in regulation of peripheral responses to stress, including heart rate, blood pressure, and cortisol response (Roth et al. 1988). Finally, case studies of humans with brain lesions (e.g., the famous case of Phineas Gage) have implicated mPFC (including orbitofrontal cortex, Area 25, and anterior cingulate, Area 32) in "emotion" and socially appropriate interactions (Damasio et al. 1994). Auditory association areas (temporal lobe) have also been implicated in animal studies as mediating extinction to fear responses (Quirk et al. 1997). As reviewed later, in PTSD patients, dysfunction of medial prefrontal cortex and auditory cortex during exposure to traumatic reminders has been reported in several studies (Bremner et al. 1999, Bremner et al. 1999, Liberzon & Sripada 2008, Shin et al. 1997b).

A final component of the traumatic stress response involves preparation for a response to potential threat. Preparation for responding to threat requires integration between brain areas involved in assessing and interpreting the potentially threatening stimulus, and brain areas involved in response. For instance, prefrontal cortex and anterior cingulate play an important role in the planning of action and in holding multiple pieces of information in 'working memory' during the execution of a response (Goldman-Rakic 1988). Parietal cortex and posterior cingulate cortex are involved in visuospatial processing that is an important component of the stress response. Motor cortex may represent the neural substrate of planning for action. The cerebellum has a well-known role in motor movement, which would suggest that this region is involved in planning for action; however, recent imaging studies are consistent with a role in cognition as well (Katz & Steinmetz 2002). Connections between parietal and prefrontal cortex are required in order to permit the organism to rapidly and efficiently execute motor responses to threat. It is, therefore, not surprising that these areas have important innervations to precentral (motor) cortex, which is responsible for skeletal motor responses to threat, which facilitate survival. The striatum (caudate and putamen) modulates motor responses to stress. The dense innervation of the striatum and prefrontal cortex by the amygdala indicates that the amygdala can regulate both of these systems. These interactions between the amygdala and the extrapyramidal motor system may be very important for generating motor responses to threatening stimuli, especially those related to prior adverse experiences (Berretta 2005) (Charney & Deutch 1996).

The organism must also rapidly effect peripheral responses to threat, which are mediated by the stress hormones, cortisol, and arganine vasopressine (AVP), and the sympathetic and parasympathetic systems. Stimulation of the lateral hypothalamus results in sympathetic system activation producing increases in blood pressure and heart rate, sweating, piloerection, and pupil dilatation. Stress stimulates the release of corticotropin reseasing factor (CRF) from the hypothalamic periventricular nucleus (PVN), which in turn increases peripheral adrenocorticotrophic hormone (ACTH) and cortisol levels. The medial prefrontal cortex, as mentioned above, also mediates increased blood pressure and pulse as well as elevations in cortisol in response to stress. Striatum, amygdala, and bed nucleus of the stria terminalis also affect peripheral responses to threat through inputs to the lateral nucleus of the hypothamalus (Walker et al. 2003) (Grillon 2008). The vagus and splanchnic nerves are major projections of the parasympathetic nervous system. Afferents to the vagus include the lateral hypothalamus, PVN, LC, and the amygdala. Efferent connections to the splanchnic nerves have been described occurring from the LC (Clark & Proudfit 1991).

FORMATION OF TRAUMATIC MEMORIES

The molecular basis and brain locations of certain memories are also now becoming better understood. Storage of memories of stressful life events appears to involve changes in gene expression in response to a traumatic stimulus. Genes can be in a state of active transcription in open chromatin or kept in a silent state in condensed chromatin. Chromatin remodeling to allow gene transcription is a crucial early step in the memory encoding process. N methyl D aspartase (NMDA) receptor activation will lead to such chromatin modifications in a small subset of neurons in the dentate gyrus of the hippocampus (less than 10,000 neurons for each memory-inducing stress event) (see Chandramohan et al. 2008). These dentate neurons have a prominent role in the encoding of sensory information for the formation of memory and possibly also thus further downstream structures. This could explain why stress memories can stay so very prominent for an extended period, and at the same time it would open the possibility for intervention therapies, for example, NMDA antagonists or glutamate depressing drugs initiated soon after trauma (Reul and Nutt, 2008).

Thus, the pathophysiology of PTSD can be linked to several neurobiological mechanisms related to traumatic stress. Preclinical studies that investigated the effects of stress on neural processes such as learning and memory retention were initially used to model PTSD as humans experience it. These studies suggested that an altered fear response mechanism, behavioral sensitization, and failure of the extinction of fear play an important role in the pathophysiology of PTSD (Charney et al. 1993) (see Figure 5.1). These neuro- or psycho-biological mechanisms will be briefly described below:

Behavioral Sensitization (enhanced stress sensitivity)

Insomnia, poor concentration, hypervigilance, and exaggerated startle response are traits related to the increased susceptibility to stress of patients with PTSD (Vermetten & Bremner 2002). "Sensitization" may be defined as an increase in a certain response due to the presentation of a specific stimulus. In military veterans with PTSD, for example, a traumatic event, or series of events they witnessed, is thought to cause the onset of PTSD. Patients become more aroused and hypervigilant, among other characteristics, than do healthy individuals when presented with trauma-related stimuli. It is the experience or recurrent experience of traumas that facilitates or sensitizes this process. It is, therefore, possible to state that PTSD is a certain type of behavioral sensitization, in which trauma exposure causes the onset of increased stress sensitivity. Although few human subject studies have investigated these symptoms on a neurobiological level, more advances have been made in preclinical settings (Stam et al. 2000) (Stam 2007a, Stam 2007b).

The neural circuitry underlying the increased sensitivity to stress is not centralized to a specific anatomical or functional neurological component because sensitization is a very broad concept and even occurs at cellular levels throughout the body. In patients with PTSD, the (over) sensitization is more vivid in the structures and mechanisms involved in the stress response, as described earlier. An example of this, the glucocorticoid mechanism, is thought to be sensitized in patients with PTSD, (Yehuda et al. 2004, Yehuda et al. 1991, Rohleder et al. 1994), making them more susceptible to stress. However, some findings are in contrast with this model. De Kloet et al. (2007) measured the effect of dexamethasone on the mitogen-induced proliferative response and on pro- and anti-inflammatory cytokine secretion by PHA-stimulated phytohemagglutinin T cells. These results suggest that trauma exposure alone is sufficient to induce changes in GR binding characteristics, whereas resistance of T cell proliferation to dexamethasone only occurs in PTSD (de Kloet et al. 2007).

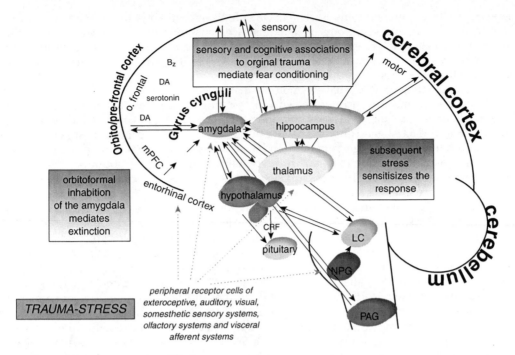

Figure 5.1   A schematic model for the neural circuits involved in the afferent input of fear and anxiety-inducing stimuli and the processing of the stimuli. The amygdala plays a pivotal role in the assessment of danger and the response. The LC is a critical component in both afferent and efferent systems, mainly through the NE release. The amygdala receives input from PAG, LC, thalamus, hippocampus, association cortices, entorhinal cortex, and visceral pathways. Input form mPFC is involved in determining the significance of fear producing sensory events, the choice and implementation and the type of behavior, and the extinction of conditioned fear responses. States of stress and fear result in a rapid increase in firing of neurons in the LC, with release of NE transmitter in different target sites in the brain. This results in an increase in attention and vigilance, as well as enhancement of memory recall, which can be life saving in threatening situations. Patients with anxiety disorder, however, develop long-term alterations in function of this system. The fear response is dependent on previous experience, sensitization, fear conditioning and extinction of previous fear responses. (from Vermetten and Bremner, 2002).

Fear Conditioning

Among the most characteristic feature of PTSD is that 'anxiogenic' memories (e.g., of the traumatic experience) can remain seemingly indelible for years or decades without causing problems and then can be reawakened by various sorts of stimuli and stressors. The strength of traumatic memories relates, in part, to the degree to which certain neuromodulatory systems, particularly catecholamines and glucocorticoids, are activated by the traumatic experience. Release of these stress hormones promotes the encoding of memories of the stressful event. Long-term alterations in these catecholaminergic and glucocorticoid systems may not only be responsible for symptoms of fragmentation of memories but also for hypermnesia, amnesia, deficits in declarative memory, delayed recall, and other aspects of the wide range of memory distortions in anxiety- and traumatic stress–related disorders. Experimental and clinical investigations provide evidence that memory processes remain susceptible to modulating influences after information has been acquired. The brain mechanisms by which sensory representations (such as colors, objects, or individuals) are selected for episodic encoding are not fully understood. It is thought that with long-term storage, memories are shifted from hippocampus to the neocortical areas, as the neocortex gradually comes to support stable, long-term storage (Murray et al. 2001; Wang et al. 2008). The shift in memory storage to the cortex may represent a shift from conscious representational memory to unconscious memory processes that indirectly affect behavior. "Traumatic cues" such as a particular sight or sound reminiscent of the original traumatic event will trigger a cascade of anxiety and fear-related symptoms will ensue, often without conscious recall of the original traumatic event. In patients with PTSD, however, the traumatic stimulus is always potentially identifiable. In contrast, in panic or phobic disorder patients, symptoms of anxiety may be related to fear responses to a traumatic cue (in individuals who are vulnerable to increased fear responsiveness, either through constitution or previous experience), where there is no possibility that the original fear-inducing stimulus will ever be identified.

Thus, patients with PTSD have symptoms that reflect a more or less continuous perception of threat with unconsciously processed fear responses (see Vermetten and Spiegel, 2007). The animal model of contextual fear-conditioning represents a good model for these symptoms. Preclinical data suggest that the hippocampus (as well as bed nucleus striae terminals (BNST) and periaquaeductal grey) plays an important role in the mediation of contextual fear and that increased responding to conditioned stimuli (CS) is due to hippocampal dysfunction. Hippocampal atrophy in PTSD, therefore, provides a possible neuroanatomical substrate for abnormal, contextual fear conditioning and chronic symptoms of feeling of threat and anxiety. Interestingly, in light of studies showing abnormal noradrenergic function in PTSD, the BNST has some of the densest noradrenergic innervation of any area in the brain (Yamada et al. 2006).

The startle reflex has been the subject of the few fear-conditioning-specific studies in PTSD that have been preformed in humans. Startle is a useful method for examining fear responding in experimental studies involving both animals and humans that is mediated by the amygdala and connected structures. Patients with combat-related PTSD were found to have elevated baseline startle compared with controls in some studies but not others. In the patients group these was asymmetry of baseline startle response (higher in patients) and increased heart rate responses during measurement of startle. From other studies, it becomes quite clear that unconscious emotional processes are involved in fear conditioning, for example, patients with anxiety disorders have demonstrated greater resistance to extinction of conditioned responses to angry facial expressions, but not to neutral facial expressions, compared with controls. In the neural circuitry, damage to the amygdala does not prevent patients from learning the relationship between the CS and the unconditioned stimulus (UCS), but it abolishes conditioned autonomic responses. In contrast, damage to the hippocampus does not affect conditioned autonomic responses, but does prevent learning of the conditioned stimulus (CS)–US unconditioned stimulus association. Further evidence for unconscious processes stems from backward masking techniques, which prevents conscious awareness of a stimulus. Using such a technique, fear conditioning to a certain class of stimuli called fear-relevant stimuli (e.g., spiders and snakes) proves to be mediated by preattentive, automatic information-processing mechanisms. These automatic mechanisms may be mediated in part by direct thalamic–amygdala connections. These thalamo–mygdala pathways that bypass the cerebral cortex may trigger conditioned responses before the stimulus reaches full awareness, providing an explanation for unconscious conditioned phobic responses to fear-relevant stimuli (Katkin et al. 2001).

Failure of Extinction

The process of fear extinction is closely linked to the conditioning of fear. When a person is exposed to a normally dangerous situation from which no aversive events result, this situation elicits a smaller fear response than before—a process which repeated leads to smaller and smaller responses called extinction. In patients with PTSD, this process does not occur efficiently, and fear of certain situations fails to extinguish. In military veterans this may be identified by persistent, fearful responses to large, noisy crowds, fireworks, and doors slamming, among other forms of traumatic recall. Therefore, some permanence in fear conditioning in patients is due to a dysfunction in the extinction of fear. Ultimately, this can be the cause of the persistence of the traumatic memories. The neural mechanisms involved in the extinction of fear greatly overlap with those involved in fear acquisition, as just described.

The main structures involved in the extinction of fear are the medial prefrontal cortex and the amygdalae (Quirk et al. 2006). NMDA receptors and voltage-gated calcium channels are essential to extinction processes (Charney 2004). Other systems include the neurotransmitters gamma-amino-butyric acid (GABA) (Berlau & McGaugh 2006), norepinephrine (Southwick et al. 1999), and dopamine (Pezze & Feldon 2004). During a fearful response of the amygdala, the mPFC is activated and attempts to regulate the initial response to the threat so that fear is contained and managed appropriately. If this prefrontal activation is absent or occurs to a lesser extent, the amygdala does not receive sufficient inhibitory feedback, resulting in higher autonomic arousal and exaggerated responses as we see in patients with PTSD. The amygdala–mPFC connection (feedback process) is thought to be mediated by GABA interneurons, which may be malfunctioning in PTSD (Berkowitz et al. 2007, Gilboa et al. 2004) as evidenced by a reduction in GABA-A receptor binding in mPFC (Bremner et al. 2000; Geuze et al. 2007).

MEMORY PERFORMANCE IN PTSD

A symptom that is common in PTSD patients that is negatively contributing to social and occupational function is forgetfulness (Geuze et al. 2008a). Patients with PTSD have showed significant deficits in hippocampal-mediated declarative memory (Bremner et al. 1995, Bremner et al. 1993) (Golier et al. 2002, Vasterling et al. 2002; see review Brewin et al. 2007). A large number of clinical studies have reported alterations in learning and memory in patients with PTSD, which are consistent with both deficits in encoding on explicit memory tasks, deficits in retrieval, as well as enhanced encoding or retrieval for specific trauma-related material (Pitman 1989; Wolfe and Schlesinger 1997; Vasterling et al. 1998; Bremner and Narayan 1998; Andrews et al. 2000; Buckley et al. 2000; Gilbertson et al. 2001; Roca and Freeman 2001). The majority of these studies found deficits in verbal memory, with a relative absence of deficits in tasks of attention or visuospatial memory. The alterations varied from self-reported difficulties in memory (Thygesen, 1970), to impairments of verbal declarative memory (Sutker et al. 1991; Uddo, 1993; Bremner et al. 1993a; Yehuda et al. 1995; Bremner et al. 1995; Jenkins et al. 1998; Moradi et al. 1999; Gilbertson et al. 2001). These studies, which involved heterogeneous groups of trauma populations and comorbidity status, all reported specific deficits in explicit memory function in PTSD (with no change in IQ). The memory impairments were not accounted for by attentional disturbances or intellectual functioning (Gilbertson et al. 2001; Vasterling et al. 2002). While attention and immediate memory is also associated with PTSD, some studies did not report verbal declarative memory deficits (Dalton et al. 1989; Zalewski et al. 1994).

Alterations in memory are correlated with specific brain structures and functional pathways that may be altered and are, therefore, possibly dysfunctional in patients with PTSD (Geuze et al. 2008c). Studies that look into the memory deficiencies in PTSD have found significant associations with reductions in hippocampal volume (Geuze et al. 2005b). The hippocampus has been linked to spatial and episodic memory, stress and emotional regulation, and novelty processing. Lesions of the hippocampus have been found to result in deficiencies of hippocampus-based learning and memory (Scoville & Milner 2000), 2000]. In conjunction with the clinical observation that patients with PTSD have been found to perform significantly more poorly on neuropsychological memory tasks, studies that have examined hippocampal structure in this population have found smaller hippocampal volumes in patients who have experienced combat trauma, physical and sexual abuse, and childhood sexual abuse. However, the findings for hippocampal reductions vary greatly (5–26%) and are found in different areas within this structure, depending on the methodology, (Geuze et al. 2005a) and are not specific for PTSD (Geuze et al. 2005b). Moreover, in some studies, trauma-exposed persons without PTSD also showed significantly smaller bilateral hippocampal compared to nonexposed controls. A recent meta-analyses also found significantly smaller left amygdala volumes in adults with PTSD compared with both healthy and trauma-exposed controls and significantly smaller anterior cingulate cortex compared with trauma-exposed controls (Karl et al. 2006).

Although changes in hippocampal volume have been attributed to PTSD, a causal relationship between a traumatic stressor and hippocampal volume reductions is difficult to prove. There are two current hypotheses about smaller hippocampal volume. One explanation for a reduced hippocampal volume in PTSD is the neurotoxicity caused by elevated glucocorticoids, reduced brain-derived neurotrophic factor (BDNF), and the inhibition of the regeneration of damaged brain tissue (Vermetten et al. 2003, who also found that treatment for 9 months with the selective serotonergic reuptake inhibitor (SSRI) paroxetine restored both the hippocampal volume and memory function). The second hypothesis is that people who have a smaller hippocampus by birth are (genetically) more at risk to develop PTSD. A twin study that provided some evidence for the latter hypothesis indicated that there is a negative correlation between PTSD severity and hippocampal volume in both the patients and their healthy, trauma-unexposed twin's hippocampi (Gilbertson et al. 2002). Furthermore, several studies suggested that childhood abuse may be a significant contributor to disturbances in hippocampal volume in patients with PTSD during a later stage in their lives. Ultimately, longitudinal studies in populations regularly exposed to traumatic events may provide evidence of whether hippocampal volume reduces over time or is initially lower in people who get PTSD.

FUNCTIONAL NEUROIMAGING STUDIES IN PTSD

The advent of modern, structural, and functional imaging techniques has opened a great window of opportunity for conducting neurological research in human patients. In the past years, such techniques have been used to reveal whether the hypotheses about changes in the brain in PTSD, made in the 1990s by Charney et al. (1993) and Bremner et al. (1995), were accurate. In more recent publications by the same authors, hypotheses supported by preclinical data are discussed in relation to research findings in human subjects (Bremner 2003, Charney 2004). These updates include neural structures, circuits, and functions that are altered in patients with PTSD. Although there is no definitive pathophysiology for PTSD and its biological cause, many theories that have been developed remain closely tied to the mechanisms from the preclinical findings.

Functional neuroimaging techniques are a relatively recent development in the field of neurological research. There are various ways to measure the activity that takes place in the brain, all based on different principles. Such techniques include SPECT, PET, and fMRI. These three techniques derive brain function indirectly from physiological measures such as cerebral blood flow, blood oxygen levels, and energy consumption. The assumption related to these techniques is that glucose metabolism and blood flow, among other parameters, alter when certain brain areas become activated or inhibited. When neural cells fire, their increase in activity requires a restoration of the energy they used. It is thought that the metabolic demands by such neurons result in an increased blood flow to these areas (Jueptner & Weiller 1995). Hence, these methods interpret physiological measures to deduce brain activity. Both SPECT and PET make use of regional cerebral blood flow (rCBF) and neuroreceptor concentration, whereas fMRI makes use of the blood oxygen level–dependent (BOLD) signal to show patterns of activity in the brain.

FUNCTIONAL NEUROIMAGING PARADIGMS

There are various types of strategies used in measuring functional activity of the brain. The most straightforward way of measuring brain activity is by observing a subject at rest. In PTSD, researchers have used both PET and SPECT to measure rCBF (Bonne et al. 2003) (Mirzaei et al. 2001) (Seedat et al. 2004), glucose metabolism (Bremner et al. 1997), and the binding potentials for both benzodiazepine (Bremner et al. 2000, Fujita et al. 2004, Geuze et al. 2008) and serotonin 1A (Bonne et al. 2005) receptors. Cerebral blood flow, and both receptor availability and affinity, are all indirect measures of activity, or potential activity, in the brain. Differences of these variables in persons with PTSD may be helpful in describing the pathophysiology of the disorder. Activity in the brain can also be observed by having subjects participate in an active task or by exposing them to certain stimuli. When a paradigm includes active tasks, subjects are asked to perform certain activities that elicit a predicted brain response. These tasks are usually designed so that they change neural activities in regions hypothesized to be dysfunctional in PTSD. Such tasks include emotional recall tasks (Pavic et al. 2003), memory recall tasks (Shin et al. 2004), memory encoding tasks (Bremner et al. 2003c), the counting Stroop task (Shin et al. 2001b), the emotional Stroop task (Bremner et al. 2004), and the auditory continuous performance task [auditory continuous performance task (ACPT); (Semple et al. 1996b, Semple et al. 2000a)]. Each of these methods measures variables of how well a subject performs a task and what actual neural activity is involved during these tasks. Ideally these two variables show some kind of correlation so the brain activity can explain the performance of a task (Vermetten & Bremner 2004). In the functional neuroimaging studies of PTSD, paradigms frequently consist of exposure to visual or auditory stimuli related to a specific type of trauma. In this way, neural activity can be studied when subjects are exposed to stimuli reminiscent of their traumatic past. Studies of Vietnam combat veterans have used combat sounds (Bremner et al. 1999, Liberzon et al. 1999, Pissiota et al. 2002, Zubieta et al. 1999) and combat slides (Bremner et al. 1999,

Hendler et al. 2003) as well as olfactory cues (Vermetten et al. 2007) to induce trauma-related stress by symptom provocation. Other studies that include victims of sexual assault or abuse have used personal traumatic scripts (Britton et al. 2005, Gilboa et al. 2004, Lanius et al. 2002, Lanius et al. 2003, Liberzon et al. 2003b, Rauch et al. 1996, Shin et al. 2004) to elicit an emotional response. Although it is interesting to observe these patients during a state of traumatic recall, it is important to have a baseline with which to compare this activity. This can be done intrapersonally by also measuring activity during a neutral activity or stimulus, or interpersonally, by having a healthy or trauma control group, or a combination of both.

SUMMARY OF CURRENT FINDINGS

MPFC and amygdala

The findings of the current studies indicate several trends in neural correlates of PTSD, permitting us to create a model of this disorder. Two of the most recurrent findings in patients with PTSD, using PET, fMRI, and SPECT are decreased medial prefrontal cortex and increased amygdalar activation. On the other hand, inconsistent findings have been tied to regions such as the hippocampus and the adjacent parahippocampal gyrus. These inconsistencies could be the result of a wide variation of parameters in different studies and of the complex nature of PTSD. Altered function in the amygdala is frequently discussed in the clinical presentation of PTSD. Studies using symptom provocation paradigms and active tasks have both found an increased amygdalar activation pattern in patients with PTSD compared to healthy controls. Symptom provocation studies target the fear response mechanism in which the amygdala is thought to play a pivotal role. Stimuli successfully used in these paradigms include combat sounds (e.g., Zubieta et al. 1999) and images (e.g., Hendler et al. 2003, Shin et al. 1997a), emotional faces (e.g., Britton et al. 2008, Rauch et al. 2000, Shin et al. 2005), emotional words (e.g., Protopopescu et al. 2005), and traumatic scripts (e.g., Lanius et al. 2001, Osuch et al. 2008). Furthermore, studies using active tasks found amygdala activation when subjects were instructed to perform an auditory continuous performance task (Semple et al. 2000b), explicit memory recall tasks (Shin et al. 2004), and active trauma recall (Driessen et al. 2004). On the whole, the amygdala appears to be more responsive in patients with PTSD. This hyperactivation is thought to be the reason for a failure of the extinction to fearful stimuli, a common component of the clinical presentation of PTSD (Vermetten & Bremner 2002). Another common finding in studies measuring neural activity in PTSD is a hypoactivation of the mPFC, which includes the OFC (Brodmann's Area 11), the anterior cyngulated gyrus (ACC) (Brodmann's Area 32), and mPFC proper (Brodmann's Areas 9 and 25). Symptom provocation paradigms that found this trend for the latter two regions in patients with PTSD made use of traumatic sounds and images (Bremner et al. 1999; Yang et al. 2004a), emotional faces (Britton et al. 2008, Shin et al. 2005), and traumatic scripts (Bremner et al. 1999; Britton et al. 2005; Lanius et al. 2001; Lanius et al. 2003, Liberson et al. 2003a, Lindauer et al. 2004, Shin et al. 1999, Shin et al. 2004) (Bremner et al. 1999, Britton et al. 2005, Lanius et al. 2001, Lanius et al. 2003, Liberzon et al. 2003a, Lindauer et al. 2004, Shin et al. 1999, Shin et al. 2004, Osuch et al. 2008). Furthermore, studies using active tasks found relative mPFC deactivation when subjects were instructed to perform an auditory continuous performance task (Semple et al. 2000b), memory tasks (Bremner et al. 2003b, Lanius et al. 2003), or a counting Stroop task using combat words (Shin et al. 2001b). Similarly, studies using resting paradigms (Bremner et al. 1997), symptom provocation (Driessen et al. 2004, Lanius et al. 2001), and active memory tasks also found OFC dysfunction. Studies using SPECT to measure benzodiazepine receptor-binding affinity have found both reductions (Bremner et al. 2000, Geuze et al. 2008) and unchanged (Fujita et al. 2004) binding in the mPFC of war veterans. The latter finding was related to Gulf War veterans, whereas the former included veterans from the Vietnam era. Several studies have suggested a relationship or direct functional link between the amygdala and the mPFC regions discussed here. In fact, four functional imaging studies (Driessen et al. 2004, Semple et al. 2000b, Shin et al. 2004, Shin et al. 2005) have found a decrease in mPFC activity and a simultaneous hyperactivation of the amygdala in patients with PTSD. It is thought that the mPFC provides a system of negative feedback to the amygdala, regulating its activation during emotional and fearful conditions: An increase in mPFC activity inhibits activation of the amygdala, whereas a decrease in mPFC activity, as found in numerous imaging studies in PTSD, seems to be connected to increased, or unchecked, amygdalar activity.

Although there is significant agreement about the connection of mPFC and amygdalar activity among the functional imaging studies, some findings point in different directions. Gilboa et al. (Gilboa et al. 2004) reported a parallel increase in mPFC and amygdalar activity, for example. Conversely, another study reported parallel hypoactivation of these structures in a group of combat veterans with PTSD (Liberzon et al. 2003a). Other PTSD studies report no changes in amygdalar (Bremner et al. 1999, Bremner et al. 1999, Britton et al. 2005, Lanius et al. 2007, Lanius et al. 2003a, Lanius et al. 2002, Lanius et al. 2001, Yang et al. 2004b) or mPFC (Bonne et al. 2005, Semple et al. 1996b) activity. One possible explanation for the lack of amygdalar activation in two of these studies (Britton et al. 2005, Lanius et al. 2001) is the use of traumatic scripts (internally generated stimuli as opposed to externally generated sounds or images). Yang et al. (Yang et al. 2004a) attributed their lack of amygdalar activation to paradigm design and small sample size (n = 11). The fact that Rauch et al. (2000) did not observe any mPFC changes is difficult to explain. In a more recent symptom provocation study using the presentation of emotional faces, activity in the mPFC was significantly reduced in patients with PTSD (Shin et al. 2005). Furthermore, studies using combat pictures (Bremner et al. 1999) and slides related to natural disaster (Yang et al. 2004a) found significantly reduced activation of the mPFC. One possibility for the lack of results in the study by Rauch et al. (Rauch et al. 2000) could be the presentation of masked emotional faces, a practice not employed by studies showing reduced mPFC activity. Semple et al. (Semple et al. 1996a) also failed to find a difference in mPFC activity, yet they did manage to do so in a more recent study using a similar auditory continuous performance task paradigm. Finally, Lanius et al. (Lanius et al. 2002) found an increase in mPFC/ACC region, as opposed to the decreased activation trend. A possible explanation for this is the exclusive participation of subjects with dissociative responses to fearful stimuli, as we discuss further on. In a SPECT study, Zubieta et al. (Zubieta et al. 1999) also reported an increased mPFC activity and hypothesized hyperactive dysfunction of the mPFC.

Hippocampus and parahippocampus

Inconsistencies are not uncommon in neuroimaging studies of PTSD. For instance, findings in the hippocampus and parahippocampus are highly inconsistent when considered both individually and compared to each other. The parahippocampal gyrus, a region anatomically adjacent to the hippocampus, is liaison for many neocortical projections from the hippocampus and also the source of most afferents to the hippocampus. Activity in these structures is, therefore, related and can be compared to a certain extent. Despite their functional relationship in one of the limbic pathways, results in functional imaging studies of PTSD appear to be altered regarding these regions, because the majority of findings suggest a decrease in hippocampal functioning alongside increased parahippocampal activity. When we look at these results more closely, however, it is possible to find trends of neural activity disruption in PTSD.

The hippocampus plays a critical role in the consolidation of novel memories of facts and events. Several studies have shown that patients with chronic PTSD perform significantly more poorly on hippocampal-based memory and learning tasks (Bremner et al. 1995, Bremner et al. 1993). Starting from this premise, a multitude of studies have explored the hippocampal structure of patients with PTSD. A recent review summarized the MRI-based hippocampal volume reduction studies in PTSD as being inconsistent because both reductions and insignificant differences were observed (Geuze et al. 2005b). Studies reporting differences in the functional properties of the hippocampus have similarly presented consistency issues. Altered hippocampal function was reported mostly in paradigms that employ memory to elicit hippocampal activity. PET studies by Bremner et al. using declarative memory tasks (Bremner et al. 2003a, Bremner et al. 2003c) and script-driven imagery (Bremner et al. 1999) have shown a failure or reduced activation of the hippocampus. In addition, Shin et al. (2004) demonstrated reduced hippocampal activation, using PET during a word-stem completion task. On the contrary, in the few fMRI studies to report hippocampal dysfunction, Shin et al. (Shin et al. 2001a) found increased hippocampal activity during a counting Stroop task that used emotionally valenced words. Some years earlier, using a resting paradigm, Bremner et al. (Bremner et al. 1997) observed reduced hippocampal functioning when administering the a2 receptor antagonist yohimbine. In conclusion, reduced activation of the hippocampus is found in patients with PTSD during memory-related tasks, whereas studies using tasks with emotional content report inconsistent findings.

The parahippocampal gyrus is to a great extent functionally related to the hippocampus. The majority of findings related to this structure show a trend of increased activity, which could contradict the theory of memory deficits in PTSD. The parahippocampus is an extensive neural structure with a large functional diversity. In analyzing the studies that specified the precise location of altered parahippocampal functioning, we can attempt to derive several interesting conclusions. The studies that suggest decreased parahippocampal functioning (Lanius et al. 2003b, Lanius et al. 2002) refer to more specific regions such as the entorhinal and perirhinal cortices (Brodmann's Areas 28 and 35, respectively). The entorhinal cortex has been found to be one of the major afferents to the hippocampus. Results for these specific regions reported a decrease in activity in patients with PTSD. Both regions are found to be functionally related to emotion, memory, and association of these memories. Another region, anatomically different but functionally similar to these areas, is the retrosplenial cortex, which is situated in the posterior cingulate cortex (Brodmann's Area 30). This region is also involved as an intermediary between the hippocampus and more cortical areas, and findings from the same studies show reduced activation in patients with PTSD. On the other hand, three studies that reported increases in parahippocampal activity referred more specifically to the more posterior-oriented lingual gyrus (Brodmann's Area 19; Bremner et al. 1999, Bremner et al. 1999, Shin et al. 2001a, Yang et al. 2004b). This specific region has previously been linked to visuospatial processing and visual association (Geuze et al. 2008b). A possible explanation for the increased activity of this area, and perhaps other regions of the parahippocampus, is that it may facilitate or trigger flashbacks and intrusive thoughts. The fact that some studies report the specific areas within a region of interest enables us to make the distinctions found above. Other studies unfortunately did not report their results in great detail, making it difficult to trace the trend within the parahippocampus. It is therefore important to note that a future direction in the field of neuroimaging should be a common way of reporting results, paying close attention to the level of detail. This includes a more specific categorization of parahippocampal structures and a better understanding of the role these play in various networks.

Thalamus

A less documented finding in functional neuroimaging studies is the involvement of the thalamus in patients with PTSD even though thalamic dysfunction in PTSD has previously been shown by several groups (Bremner et al. 1999; Liberzon et al. (1996/7); Lanius et al. 2001; 2003). The thalamus has also been suggested to be involved in mediating the interaction between attention and arousal (Portas et al. 1998), both of which are clearly relevant to the phenomenology of traumatic stress syndromes. Moreover, the thalamus is an important relay station for the transmission of external sensory information to different areas of the cerebral cortex and limbic system where this information is processed. Target regions include the frontal cortex, cingulated gyrus, amygdala, and hippocampus, all of which are closely related to the neural networks hypothesized to be active in PTSD. Two studies by Lanius et al. (Lanius et al. 2001, Lanius et al. 2004) using traumatic script-driven imagery and another using traumatic memory recall (Lanius et al. 2003a) reported decreased thalamic activity. The disruption in thalamic activity could lead to several of the traits displayed by the clinical presentation of PTSD. Due to its functional nature, a disruption in activity of the thalamus could lead to the misinterpretation of external stimuli. It is important to note, however, that the only research group that found altered activity in PTSD with regard to the thalamus, used MRI as opposed to SPECT or PET. Furthermore, this particular group uses a 4 Tesla MRI scanner as proposed to the more conventional (and lower resolution) 1.5 and 3 Tesla scanners. Due to the importance of the thalamus in relaying sensory information to higher cortical regions, it is a region of interest in PTSD research that deserves and requires further investigation.

Precuneus

The role of the precuneus has been neglected in PTSD research. When male veterans with and without PTSD (*n* = 12 per group) were subjected to fMRI during encoding of 12 neutral, non–trauma-related word pairs, the precuneus was less activated in veterans with PTSD, which correlated significantly with the severity of PTSD. Like frontotemporal regions the precuneus is differentially activated during memory formation in veterans with PTSD (Geuze et al. 2008b).

DEFAULT NETWORK

The notion that the brain has an intrinsic mode of functioning has received increasing attention over the past years, an idea that stems from observations that even when no explicit task is performed a consistent network of brain areas shows high levels of activity—the "default" network (Bruckner et al. 2008). In these studies the default network appeared to be more active at rest than in a range of explicit tasks. Two opposing brain systems have been identified with opposing functions, dorsal attention, and hippocampal-cortical memory systems, which are positioned anatomically to integrate information from the external world versus internally directed mentation that involves long-term memory (Vincent et al. 2008). Bluhm et al. have recently reported that at rest, spontaneous low-frequency activity in the posterior cingulate/precuneus was more strongly correlated with activity in other areas of the default network in healthy comparison subjects than in subjects with PTSD related to chronic childhood abuse. Direct comparison of the two groups showed that posterior cingulate/precuneus connectivity was also greater in healthy comparison subjects than in patients with PTSD in a number of areas previously associated with PTSD, including the right amygdala and the hippocampus/parahippocampal gyrus. In this patient population, the observed alterations may be associated with the disturbances in self-referential processing often observed in PTSD (Bluhm et al. 2008).

HETEROGENEITY OF RESPONSES IN PTSD

An emerging literature in PTSD has begun to examine the heterogeneity of response to traumatic reminders. Due to the different type of traumas that cause the onset of PTSD, the clinical presentation of symptoms can vary between patients. Recently, it has been hypothesized that there are two main categories of PTSD symptoms closely related to the criteria that make up the disorder. Whereas some patients tend to be hyperaroused, others show numbing in response to fearful situations. This latter often have moments of dissociation, as opposed to the former, who tend to be hypervigilant and experience flashbacks of their trauma (Bremner, 1996). In a study performed by Lanius et al. (Lanius et al. 2005), functional connectivity was measured using fMRI in both dissociated and flashback PTSD groups. The findings indicate a different neural connectivity between the two groups, with the dissociated group showing greater connectivity in the left inferior frontal gyrus, an area previously found to be related to the determination of self-relevance of emotional statements (Lanius et al. 2006). Moreover, in a case report of a married couple involved in a motor vehicle accident, Lanius et al. (Lanius et al. 2003a) clearly presented a case for different types of PTSD. The husband responded to a traumatic script about the accident in a state of hyperarousal, whereas his wife became numb and frozen. Because there is a possible difference in brain activation patterns between the flashback and dissociated PTSD groups, comparing these two groups of patients may lead to distortions in the outcome of a study. We recently reviewed evidence that dissociation reflects frontal inhibition of limbic and other temporal lobe structures. Moreover, these dissociative response states have been shown to be triggered by several classes of neurochemicals, including serotonergic hallucinogens, NMDA antagonists, and opioid agonists, acting through the hippocampus and other brain areas involved in memory and emotion.

The model of PTSD has focused on a model of hyperactivation of the noradrenergic system, for example, the locus coeruleus. Irritability; increased heart rate; and blood pressure associated with trauma reminders, flashbacks, and nightmares have been key symptoms targeted for treatments such as exposure, cognitive restructuring, and coping skills training. However, the neurobiology of these dissociative responses is a rapidly developing field as well. Different types of dissociation, involving somatoform, cognitive, and affective cognitive components have been identified, and brain mechanisms linking frontal cortical inhibition to amygdala and other limbic hypoactivation have been identified (see Vermetten et al. 2008; Lanius et al. in review; Vermetten, Dorahy, & Spiegel, 2007, Felmingham et al. 2008) as well. Thus, there is also potential to recognize in *DSM-V* the dissociative component of trauma response in peritraumatic, acute, and posttraumatic periods and symptomatology. A better integration of related disciplines may help to provide a more coherent nosology regarding trauma response and its treatment.

SUMMARY AND FUTURE DIRECTIONS

During the past decade, more than 60 studies were published that specifically used functional neuroimaging techniques in PTSD research. These studies make use of a wide range of methodologies: measuring resting brain activity, presenting a wide range of stimuli, and using active tasks performed by a subject. Within these main groupings, there are further distinctions to be made, such as the type of stimulus (auditory, visual, trauma script, personal script), type of task (active recall, counting Stroop task, auditory continuous performance task), and type of tracer used in PET or SPECT studies. Due to this variation, difficulties arise when comparing data across different studies. Another issue that confounds comparison is a wide array of subjects in specific studies and when comparing different studies, including patients with a broad trauma spectrum and of different sexes. It is important to distinguish between trauma types, such as trauma caused by motor vehicle accident (MVAs), sexual assault, combat situations, natural disasters, and so on. This could be one reason behind the inconsistency in hippocampal activation. Furthermore, studies have shown significant differences in properties between the male and female brain (Goldstein et al. 2001). PTSD is a complex disorder with foundations in an extensive neural circuitry (Rauch et al. 2006). By examining patients with a common traumatic history and sex, it is possible to analyze neural activity with higher precision, and potential differences between the groups can be brought to light.

An interesting observation can also be drawn from the discrepancy in abnormalities between functional versus structural neuroimaging. Although functional neuroimaging demonstrates abnormalities in the mPFC (including ACC) and amygdalar circuit, structural MRI studies have almost exclusively focused on the hippocampus and have only recently started to examine the amygdale factor. Functional neuroimaging studies suggest that there are clear differences in metabolic acticity in the mPFC–amygdale circuit; therefore, it would be interesting to investigate further whether patients with PTSD show structural differences with respect to their amygdalae (Karl et al. 2006) (Vermetten et al. 2006). As reported before, an important issue that needs to be raised is that one may wonder whether the abnormalities found in structural and functional neuroimaging studies are specific to PTSD. Similar findings have also been reported in other studies, targeting other anxiety disorders, such as obsessive–compulsive disorder (Nakao et al. 2005), panic disorder (van den Heuvel et al. 2005), and generalized social phobia (Phan et al. 2006). We must be careful, however, in assuming similarity with these other anxiety disorders due to the specificity of the experimental designs. Studies that target patients with PTSD use different experimental designs, with content specific to the disorder. For example, script-driven imagery for patients with PTSD differs from that used for patients with other anxiety disorders. In turn, this may elicit different, disease-specific brain activation patterns.

In conclusion, functional neuroimaging studies that use SPECT, PET, and fMRI have opened up a new window to uncover the biobehavioral mechanisms in PTSD. The most consistent finding in many research studies to date is a relative decrease in mPFC activity, in conjunction with an increased amygdalar activation. Although no conclusive evidence exists, a functional relationship between the two regions is hypothesized, which is altered in PTSD. The role of the hippocampus and parahippocampal gyrus in PTSD is ambiguous, despite several studies that support the involvement both in structural and functional studies. The numerous variations between the studies discussed and the complexity of PTSD symptomatology are potential causes for the inconsistent findings to date. More comprehensive meta-analyses of the findings across functional imaging studies in PTSD could be benefited by paradigm conformation. With a standard set of guidelines for subject inclusion, scanning procedures, stimulus presentation, tasks and other variables, results may become more comparable. Correspondingly, setting guidelines risks limiting novel methods and ultimately novel results, potentially impeding progress in uncovering the neural mechanisms underlying PTSD. As the research base deepens, the number of studies increases, facilitating comparison. Ultimately this may lead to more consistent trends. Even though the increase in the number of neuroimaging studies has contributed much to the insight in the neural circuits of PTSD, further research is imperative to fine-tune this model to better understand this complex and diverse disorder.

LIST OF ABBREVIATIONS

BNST - bed nucleus striae terminals
CS - conditioned stimulus

DSM - diagnostic statistical manual
UCS - unconditioned stimulus
mPFC - medial prefrontal cortex
ACC - anterior cyngulated gyrus
NMDA - N methyl D aspartase
GABA – gamma amino butyric acid
BDNF – brain derived neurotrophic factor
SPECT - single positron emitted tomography
PET - positron emission tomography
MRI - magnetic resonance imaging
BOLD - blood oxygen level dependent
rCBF – regional cerebral blood flow
Tc-99m HMPAO - technetium-99m hexamethyl propylenamine oxime
ACPT - auditory continuous performance task
^{18}F-FCWAY - ^{18}F-trans-4-Fluoro-N-2-[4-(2-methoxyphenyl)piperazin-1-yllethyl]-N-(2-pyridyl) cyclohexanecarboxamide
5HT1AR - Serotonin type 1A receptors
FDG - 18F-fluorodeoxyglucose
OFC – orbitofrontal gyrus
MVA – motor vehicle accident

REFERENCES

1. Anderson KC, Insel TR. The promise of extinction research for the prevention and treatment of anxiety disorders. Biol Psychiatry 2006; 60(4): 319–21.
2. Bekinschtein P, Cammarota M, Igaz LM et al. Persistence of long-term memory storage requires a late protein synthesis- and BDNF- dependent phase in the hippocampus. Neuron 2007; 53(2): 261–77.
3. Berkowitz RL, Coplan JD, Reddy DP, Gorman JM. The human dimension: how the prefrontal cortex modulates the subcortical fear response. Rev Neurosci 2007; 18(3–4): 191–207.
4. Berlau DJ, McGaugh JL. Enhancement of extinction memory consolidation: the role of the noradrenergic and GABAergic systems within the basolateral amygdala. Neurobiol Learn Mem 2006; 86(2): 123–32.
5. Berretta S. Cortico-amygdala circuits: role in the conditioned stress response. Stress 2005; 8(4): 221–32.
6. Bluhm RL, Osuch EA, Lanius RA et al. Default mode network connectivity: effects of age, sex, and analytic approach. Neuroreport 2008; 19(8): 887–91.
7. Bonne O, Bain E, Neumeister A et al. No change in serotonin type 1A receptor binding in patients with posttraumatic stress disorder. Am J Psychiatry 2005; 162(2): 383–5.
8. Bonne O, Gilboa A, Louzoun Y et al. Resting regional cerebral perfusion in recent posttraumatic stress disorder. Biol Psychiatry 2003; 54(10): 1077–86.
9. Bremner JD. Functional neuroanatomical correlates of traumatic stress revisited 7 years later, this time with data. Psychopharmacol Bull 2003; 37(2): 6–25.
10. Bremner JD. Stress and brain atrophy. CNS Neurol Disord Drug Targets 2006; 5(5): 503–12.
11. Bremner JD, Innis RB, Ng CK et al. Positron emission tomography measurement of cerebral metabolic correlates of yohimbine administration in combat-related posttraumatic stress disorder. Arch Gen Psychiatry 1997; 54(3): 246–54.
12. Bremner JD, Innis RB, Southwick SM et al. Decreased benzodiazepine receptor binding in prefrontal cortex in combat-related posttraumatic stress disorder. Am J Psychiatry 2000; 157(7): 1120–6.
13. Bremner JD, Krystal JH, Charney DS, Southwick SM. Neural mechanisms in dissociative amnesia for childhood abuse: relevance to the current controversy surrounding the "false memory syndrome". Am J Psychiatry 1996; 153(7): 71–82.
14. Bremner JD, Krystal JH, Southwick SM, Charney DS. Functional neuroanatomical correlates of the effects of stress on memory. J Trauma Stress 1995; 8(4): 527–53.
15. Bremner JD, Narayan M, Staib LH et al. Neural correlates of memories of childhood sexual abuse in women with and without posttraumatic stress disorder. Am J Psychiatry 1999; 156(11): 1787–95.
16. Bremner JD, Randall P, Scott TM et al. Deficits in short-term memory in adult survivors of childhood abuse. Psychiatry Res 1995; 59(1–2): 97–107.
17. Bremner JD, Scott TM, Delaney RC et al. Deficits in short-term memory in posttraumatic stress disorder. Am J Psychiatry 1995; 150(7): 1015–9.
18. Bremner JD, Staib LH, Kaloupek D et al. Neural correlates of exposure to traumatic pictures and sound in Vietnam combat veterans with and without posttraumatic stress disorder: a positron emission tomography study. Biol Psychiatry 1999; 45(7): 806–16.

19. Bremner JD, Vermetten E, Vythilingam M et al. Neural correlates of the classic color and emotional stroop in women with abuse-related posttraumatic stress disorder. Biol Psychiatry 2004; 55(6): 612–20.

20. Bremner JD, Vythilingam M, Vermetten E et al. MRI and PET study of deficits in hippocampal structure and function in women with childhood sexual abuse and posttraumatic stress disorder. Am J Psychiatry 2003a; 160(5): 924–32.

21. Bremner JD, Vythilingam M, Vermetten E et al. Neural correlates of declarative memory for emotionally valenced words in women with posttraumatic stress disorder related to early childhood sexual abuse. Biol Psychiatry 2003b; 53(10): 879–89.

22. Bremner JD, Vythilingam M, Vermetten E et al. Neural correlates of declarative memory for emotionally valenced words in women with posttraumatic stress disorder related to early childhood sexual abuse. Biol Psychiatry 2003c; 53(10): 879–89.

23. Brewin CR, Kleiner JS, Vasterling JJ, Field AP. Memory for emotionally neutral information in posttraumatic stress disorder: A meta-analytic investigation. J Abnorm Psychol 2007; 116(3): 448–63.

24. Britton JC, Phan KL, Taylor SF, Fig LM, Liberzon I. Corticolimbic blood flow in posttraumatic stress disorder during script-driven imagery. Biol Psychiatry 2005; 57(8): 832–40.

25. Britton JC, Shin LM, Barrett LF, Rauch SL, Wright CI. Amygdala and fusiform gyrus temporal dynamics: responses to negative facial expressions. BMC Neurosci 2008; 9: 44.

26. Buchanan SL, Thompson RH, Maxwell BL, Powell DA. Efferent connections of the medial prefrontal cortex in the rabbit. Exp Brain Res 1994; 100(3): 469–83.

27. Chandramohan Y, Droste SK, Arthur JS, Reul JM. The forced swimming-induced behavioural immobility response involves histone H3 phospho-acetylation and c-Fos induction in dentate gyrus granule neurons via activation of the N-methyl-D-aspartate/extracellular signal-regulated kinase/ mitogen- and stress-activated kinase signalling pathway. Eur J Neurosci 2008; 27(10): 2701–13.

28. Charney DS. Psychobiological mechanisms of resilience and vulnerability: implications for successful adaptation to extreme stress. Am J Psychiatry 2004; 161(2): 195–216.

29. Charney DS, Deutch A. A functional neuroanatomy of anxiety and fear: implications for the pathophysiology and treatment of anxiety disorders. Crit Rev Neurobiol 1996; 10(3–4): 419–46.

30. Charney DS, Deutch AY, Krystal JH, Southwick SM, Davis M. Psychobiologic mechanisms of posttraumatic stress disorder. Arch Gen Psychiatry 1993; 50(4): 295–305.

31. Chu JA, Frey LM, Ganzel BL, Matthews JA. Memories of childhood abuse: dissociation, amnesia, and corroboration. Am J Psychiatry 1999; 156(5): 749–55.

32. Clark FM, Proudfit HK. The projection of locus coeruleus neurons to the spinal cord in the rat determined by anterograde tracing combined with immunocytochemistry. Brain Res 1991; 538(2): 231–45.

33. Damasio H, Grabowski T, Frank R, Galaburda AM, Damasio AR. The return of Phineas Gage: clues about the brain from the skull of a famous patient. Science 1994; 264(5162): 1102–5.

34. de Kloet CS, Vermetten E, Bikker A et al. Leukocyte glucocorticoid receptor expression and immunoregulation in veterans with and without post-traumatic stress disorder. Mol Psychiatry 2007; 12(5): 443–53.

35. Devinsky O, Morrell MJ, Vogt BA. Contributions of anterior cingulate cortex to behaviour. Brain 1995; 118: 279–306.

36. Dickerson BC. Advances in functional magnetic resonance imaging: technology and clinical applications. Neurotherapeutics 2007; 4(3): 360–70.

37. Driessen M, Beblo T, Mertens M et al. Posttraumatic stress disorder and fMRI activation patterns of traumatic memory in patients with borderline personality disorder. Biol Psychiatry 2004; 55(6): 603–11.

38. Felmingham K, Kemp AH, Williams L et al. Dissociative responses to conscious and non-conscious fear impact underlying brain function in post-traumatic stress disorder. Psychol Med 2008; 38(12): 1771–80.

39. Fujita M, Southwick SM, Denucci CC et al. Central type benzodiazepine receptors in Gulf War veterans with posttraumatic stress disorder. Biol Psychiatry 2004; 56(2): 95–100.

40. Geuze E, van Berckel BN, Lammertsma AA et al. Reduced GABAA benzodiazepine receptor binding in veterans with post-traumatic stress disorder. Mol Psychiatry 2008; 13(1): 74–83, 3.

41. Geuze E, Vermetten E, Bremner JD. MR-based in vivo hippocampal volumetrics: 1. Review of methodologies currently employed. Mol Psychiatry 2005a; 10(2): 147–59.

42. Geuze E, Vermetten E, Bremner JD. MR-based in vivo hippocampal volumetrics: 2. Findings in neuropsychiatric disorders. Mol Psychiatry 2005b; 10(2): 160–84.

43. Geuze E, Vermetten E, de Kloet CS, Hijman R, Westenberg HG. Neuropsychological performance is related to current social and occupational functioning in veterans with posttraumatic stress disorder. Depress Anxiety 2009; 26(1): 7–15.

44. Geuze E, Vermetten E, de Kloet CS, Westenberg HG. Precuneal activity during encoding in veterans with posttraumatic stress disorder. Prog Brain Res 2008b; 167: 293–7.

45. Geuze E, Vermetten E, Ruf M, de Kloet CS, Westenberg HG. Neural correlates of associative learning and memory in veterans with posttraumatic stress disorder. J Psychiatr Res 2008c; 42(8): 659–69.

46. Gilbertson MW, Shenton ME, Ciszewski A et al. Smaller hippocampal volume predicts pathologic vulnerability to psychological trauma. Nat Neurosci 2002; 5(11): 1242–7.
47. Gilboa A, Shalev AY, Laor L et al. Functional connectivity of the prefrontal cortex and the amygdala in posttraumatic stress disorder. Biol Psychiatry 2004; 55(3): 263–72.
48. Goldman-Rakic PS. Topography of cognition: parallel distributed networks in primate association cortex. Annu Rev Neurosci 1988; 11:137–56.
49. Golier JA, Yehuda R, Lupien SJ et al. Memory performance in Holocaust survivors with posttraumatic stress disorder. Am J Psychiatry 2002; 159(10): 1682–8.
50. Grillon C. Models and mechanisms of anxiety: evidence from startle studies. Psychopharmacology (Berl) 2008; 199(3): 421–37.
51. Grillon C, Southwick SM, Charney DS. The psychobiological basis of posttraumatic stress disorder. Mol Psychiatry 1996; 1(4): 278–97.
52. Hendler T, Rotshtein P, Yeshurun Y et al. Sensing the invisible: differential sensitivity of visual cortex and amygdala to traumatic context. Neuroimage 2003; 19(3): 587–600.
53. Jueptner M, Weiller C. Review: does measurement of regional cerebral blood flow reflect synaptic activity? Implications for PET and fMRI. Neuroimage 1995; 2(2): 148–56.
54. Karl A, Schaefer M, Malta LS et al. A meta-analysis of structural brain abnormalities in PTSD. Neurosci Biobehav Rev 2006; 30(7): 1004–31.
55. Katz DB, Steinmetz JE. Psychological functions of the cerebellum. Behav Cogn Neurosci Rev 2002; 1(3): 229–41.
56. Katkin ES, Wiens S, Ohman A. Nonconscious fear conditioning, visceral perception, and the development of gut feelings. Psychol Sci 2001; 12(5): 366–70.
57. Lanius RA, Bluhm R, Lanius U, Pain C. A review of neuroimaging studies in PTSD: heterogeneity of response to symptom provocation. J Psychiatr Res 2006; 40(8): 709–29.
58. Lanius RA, Frewen PA, Girotti M et al. Neural correlates of trauma script-imagery in posttraumatic stress disorder with and without comorbid major depression: a functional MRI investigation. Psychiatry Res 2007; 155(1): 45–56.
59. Lanius RA, Hopper JW, Menon RS. Individual differences in a husband and wife who developed PTSD after a motor vehicle accident: a functional MRI case study. Am J Psychiatry 2003a; 160(4): 667–9.
60. Lanius RA, Hopper JW, Menon RS. Individual differences in a husband and wife who developed PTSD after a motor vehicle accident: a functional MRI case study. Am J Psychiatry 2003b; 160(4): 667–9.
61. Lanius RA, Williamson PC, Bluhm RL et al. Functional connectivity of dissociative responses in posttraumatic stress disorder: a functional magnetic resonance imaging investigation. Biol Psychiatry 2005; 57(8): 873–84.
62. Lanius RA, Williamson PC, Boksman K et al. Brain activation during script-driven imagery induced dissociative responses in PTSD: a functional magnetic resonance imaging investigation. Biol Psychiatry 2002; 52(4): 305–11.
63. Lanius RA, Williamson PC, Densmore M et al. Neural correlates of traumatic memories in posttraumatic stress disorder: a functional MRI investigation. Am J Psychiatry 2001; 158(11): 1920–2.
64. Lanius RA, Williamson PC, Densmore M et al. The nature of traumatic memories: a 4-T FMRI functional connectivity analysis. Am J Psychiatry 2004; 161(1): 36–44.
65. Lanius RA, Williamson PC, Hopper J et al. Recall of emotional states in posttraumatic stress disorder: an fMRI investigation. Biol Psychiatry 2003; 53(3): 204–10.
66. Lanius RA, Vermetten E, Loewenstein RJ et al. Neural and Endocrine Systems in Dissociation, Am J Psychiatry, submitted.
67. LeDoux JE. Emotional memory: in search of systems and synapses. Ann N Y Acad Sci 1993; 702: 149–57.
68. Liberzon I, Britton JC, Phan KL. Neural correlates of traumatic recall in posttraumatic stress disorder. Stress 2003a; 6(3): 151–6.
69. Liberzon I, Britton JC, Phan KL. Neural correlates of traumatic recall in posttraumatic stress disorder. Stress 2003b; 6(3): 151–6.
70. Liberzon I, Sripada CS. The functional neuroanatomy of PTSD: a critical review. Prog Brain Res 2008; 167: 151–69.
71. Liberzon I, Taylor SF, Amdur R et al. Brain activation in PTSD in response to trauma-related stimuli. Biol Psychiatry 1999; 45(7): 817–26.
72. Lindauer RJ, Booij J, Habraken JB et al. Cerebral blood flow changes during script-driven imagery in police officers with posttraumatic stress disorder. Biol Psychiatry 2004; 56(11): 853–61.
73. Mirzaei S, Knoll P, Keck A et al. Regional cerebral blood flow in patients suffering from post-traumatic stress disorder. Neuropsychobiology 2001; 43(4): 260–4.
74. Morgan MA, Romanski LM, LeDoux JE. Extinction of emotional learning: contribution of medial prefrontal cortex. Neurosci Lett 1993; 163(1): 109–13.

75. Murray EA, Bussey TJ. Consolidation and the medial temporal lobe revisited: methodological considerations. Hippocampus 2001; 11(1): 1–7.

76. Myers KM, Davis M. Mechanisms of fear extinction. Mol Psychiatry 2007; 12(2): 120–50.

77. Nakao T, Nakagawa A, Yoshiura T et al. Brain activation of patients with obsessive-compulsive disorder during neuropsychological and symptom provocation tasks before and after symptom improvement: a functional magnetic resonance imaging study. Biol Psychiatry 2005; 57(8): 901–10.

78. Neves G, Cooke SF, Bliss TV. Synaptic plasticity, memory and the hippocampus: a neural network approach to causality. Nat Rev Neurosci 2008; 9(1): 65–75.

79. Osuch EA, Willis MW, Bluhm R, Ursano RJ, Drevets WC. Neurophysiological responses to traumatic reminders in the acute aftermath of serious motor vehicle collisions using. Biol Psychiatry 2008; 64(4): 327–35.

80. Pavic L, Gregurek R, Petrovic R et al. Alterations in brain activation in posttraumatic stress disorder patients with severe hyperarousal symptoms and impulsive aggressiveness. Eur Arch Psychiatry Clin Neurosci 2003; 253(2): 80–3.

81. Pezze MA, Feldon J. Mesolimbic dopaminergic pathways in fear conditioning. Prog Neurobiol 2004; 74(5): 301–20.

82. Phan KL, Fitzgerald DA, Nathan PJ, Tancer ME. Association between amygdala hyperactivity to harsh faces and severity of social anxiety in generalized social phobia. Biol Psychiatry 2006; 59(5): 424–9.

83. Pissiota A, Frans O, Fernandez M et al. Neurofunctional correlates of posttraumatic stress disorder: a PET symptom provocation study. Eur Arch Psychiatry Clin Neurosci 2002; 252(2): 68–75.

84. Protopopescu X, Pan H, Tuescher O et al. Differential time courses and specificity of amygdala activity in posttraumatic stress disorder subjects and normal control subjects. Biol Psychiatry 2005; 57(5): 464–73.

84. Quirk GJ, Armony JL, LeDoux JE. Fear conditioning enhances different temporal components of tone-evoked spike trains in auditory cortex and lateral amygdala. Neuron 1997; 19(3): 613–24.

85. Quirk GJ, Garcia R, Gonzalez-Lima F. Prefrontal mechanisms in extinction of conditioned fear. Biol Psychiatry 2006; 60(4): 337–43.

86. Rauch SL, Shin LM, Phelps EA. Neurocircuitry models of posttraumatic stress disorder and extinction: human neuroimaging research--past, present, and future. Biol Psychiatry 2006; 60(4): 376–82.

87. Rauch SL, van der Kolk BA, Fisler RE et al. A symptom provocation study of posttraumatic stress disorder using positron emission tomography and script-driven imagery. Arch Gen Psychiatry 1996; 53(5): 380–7.

88. Rauch SL, Whalen PJ, Shin LM et al. Exaggerated amygdala response to masked facial stimuli in posttraumatic stress disorder: a functional MRI study. Biol Psychiatry 2000; 47(9): 769–76.

89. Rogan MT, Staubli UV, LeDoux JE. Fear conditioning induces associative long-term potentiation in the amygdala. Nature 1997; 390(6660): 604–7.

90. Rohleder N, Joksimovic L, Wolf JM, Kirschbaum C. Hypocortisolism and increased glucocorticoid sensitivity of pro-Inflammatory cytokine production in Bosnian war refugees with posttraumatic stress disorder. Biol Psychiatry 2004; 55: 745–51.

91. Reul JM, Nutt DJ. Glutamate and cortisol--a critical confluence in PTSD? J Psychopharmacol 2008; 22(5): 469–72.

92. Roth RH, Tam SY, Ida Y, Yang JX, Deutch AY. Stress and the mesocorticolimbic dopamine systems. Ann N Y Acad Sci 1988; 537: 138–47.

93. Sarter M, Markowitsch HJ. Involvement of the amygdala in learning and memory: a critical review, with emphasis on anatomical relations. Behav Neurosci 1985; 99(2): 342–80.

94. Scoville WB, Milner B. Loss of recent memory after bilateral hippocampal lesions. 1957. J Neuropsychiatry Clin Neurosci 2000; 12(1): 103–13.

95. Seedat S, Warwick J, van Heerden B et al. Single photon emission computed tomography in posttraumatic stress disorder before and after treatment with a selective serotonin reuptake inhibitor. J Affect Disord 2004; 80(1): 45–53.

96. Semple WE, Goyer PF, McCormick R et al. Attention and regional cerebral blood flow in posttraumatic stress disorder patients with substance abuse histories. Psychiatry Res 1996a; 67(1): 17–28.

97. Semple WE, Goyer PF, McCormick R et al. Attention and regional cerebral blood flow in posttraumatic stress disorder patients with substance abuse histories. Psychiatry Res 1996b; 67(1): 17–28.

98. Semple WE, Goyer PF, McCormick R et al. Higher brain blood flow at amygdala and lower frontal cortex blood flow in PTSD patients with comorbid cocaine and alcohol abuse compared with normals. Psychiatry 2000a; 63(1): 65–74.

99. Semple WE, Goyer PF, McCormick R et al. Higher brain blood flow at amygdala and lower frontal cortex blood flow in PTSD patients with comorbid cocaine and alcohol abuse compared with normals. Psychiatry 2000b; 63(1): 65–74.

100. Shin LM, Kosslyn SM, McNally RJ et al. Visual imagery and perception in posttraumatic stress disorder. A positron emission tomographic investigation. Arch Gen Psychiatry 1997a; 54(3): 233–41.

101. Shin LM, McNally RJ, Kosslyn SM et al. A positron emission tomographic study of symptom provocation in PTSD. Ann N Y Acad Sci 1997b; 821: 521–3.

102. Shin LM, McNally RJ, Kosslyn SM et al. Regional cerebral blood flow during script-driven imagery in childhood sexual abuse-related PTSD: a PET investigation. Am J Psychiatry 1999; 156(4): 575–84.

103. Shin LM, Orr SP, Carson MA et al. Regional cerebral blood flow in the amygdala and medial prefrontal cortex during traumatic imagery in male and female Vietnam veterans with PTSD. Arch Gen Psychiatry 2004; 61(2): 168–76.

104. Shin LM, Whalen PJ, Pitman RK et al. An fMRI study of anterior cingulate function in posttraumatic stress disorder. Biol Psychiatry 2001a; 50(12): 932–42.

105. Shin LM, Whalen PJ, Pitman RK et al. An fMRI study of anterior cingulate function in posttraumatic stress disorder. Biol Psychiatry 2001b; 50(12): 932–42.

106. Shin LM, Wright CI, Cannistraro PA et al. A functional magnetic resonance imaging study of amygdala and medial prefrontal cortex responses to overtly presented fearful faces in posttraumatic stress disorder. Arch Gen Psychiatry 2005; 62(3): 273–81.

107. Southwick SM, Bremner JD, Rasmusson A et al. Role of norepinephrine in the pathophysiology and treatment of posttraumatic stress disorder. Biol Psychiatry 1999; 46(9): 1192–204.

108. Squire LR, Zola-Morgan S. The medial temporal lobe memory system. Science 1991; 253(5026): 1380–6.

109. Stam R. PTSD and stress sensitisation: a tale of brain and body Part 1: human studies. Neurosci Biobehav Rev 2007a; 31(4): 530–57.

110. Stam R. PTSD and stress sensitisation: a tale of brain and body Part 2: animal models. Neurosci Biobehav Rev 2007b; 31(4): 558–84.

111. Stam R, Bruijnzeel AW, Wiegant VM. Long-lasting stress sensitisation. Eur J Pharmacol 2000; 405(1–3): 217–24.

112. Turner BH, Gupta KC, Mishkin M. The locus and cytoarchitecture of the projection areas of the olfactory bulb in Macaca mulatta. J Comp Neurol 1978; 177(3): 381–96.

113. van den Heuvel OA, Veltman DJ, Groenewegen HJ et al. Disorder-specific neuroanatomical correlates of attentional bias in obsessive-compulsive disorder, panic disorder, and hypochondriasis. Arch Gen Psychiatry 2005; 62(8): 922–33.

114. van der Hart O, Bolt H, van der Kolk BA. Memory fragmentation in dissociative identity disorder. J Trauma Dissociation 2005; 6(1): 55–70.

115. Van Hoesen GW, Pandya DN, Butters N. Cortical afferents to the entorhinal cortex of the Rhesus monkey. Science 1972; 175(29): 1471–3.

116. Vasterling JJ, Duke LM, Brailey K et al. Attention, learning, and memory performances and intellectual resources in Vietnam veterans: PTSD and no disorder comparisons. Neuropsychology 2002; 16(1): 5–14.

117. Vermetten E, Bremner JD. Dissociative Amnesia: Re-remembering traumatic memories. In: Memory disorders in psychiatric practice. Berrios GE, Hodges J, eds. Cambridge University Press: Cambridge, 2000: 400–32.

118. Vermetten E, Bremner JD. Circuits and systems in stress. II. Applications to neurobiology and treatment in posttraumatic stress disorder. Depress Anxiety 2002; 16(1): 14–38.

119. Vermetten E, Bremner JD. Olfaction as a traumatic reminder in posttraumatic stress disorder: case reports and review. J Clin Psychiatry 2003; 64(2): 202–7.

120. Vermetten E, Douglas Bremner J. Functional brain imaging and the induction of traumatic recall: a cross-correlational review between neuroimaging and hypnosis. Int J Clin Exp Hypn 2004; 52(3): 280–312.

121. Vermetten E, Schmahl C, Lindner S, Loewenstein RJ, Bremner JD. Hippocampal and amygdalar volumes in dissociative identity disorder. Am J Psychiatry 2006; 163(4): 630–6.

122. Vermetten E, Schmahl C, Southwick SM, Bremner JD. Positron tomographic emission study of olfactory induced emotional recall in veterans with and without combat-related posttraumatic stress disorder. Psychopharmacol Bull 2007; 40(1): 8–30.

123. Vermetten E, Spiegel D. Perceptual Processing and Traumatic Stress: Contributions from Hypnosis. In: Traumatic Dissociation: Neurobiology and Treatment, Vermetten, E, Dorahy, Spiegel D, eds. American Psychiatric Press 2007: 103–20.

124. Vermetten E, Dorahy M, Spiegel D. Traumatic Dissociation; Neurobiology and Treatment. Washington, American Psychiatric Press; 2007.

125. Vermetten E, Lanius R, Bremner JD. Contributions of traumatic stress studies to the neurobiology of dissociation and dissociative disorders: Implications for schizophrenia. In: Andrew M, Ingo S, Martin D, eds. Psychosis, Trauma and Dissociation; Emerging Perspectives on Severe Psychopathology. Wiley Blackwell: Oxford, 221–38.

126. Vincent JL, Kahn I, Snyder AZ, Raichle ME, Buckner RL. Evidence for a frontoparietal control system revealed by intrinsic functional connectivity. J Neurophysiol 2008; 100(6): 3328–42.

127. Vogt BA, Miller MW. Cortical connections between rat cingulate cortex and visual, motor, and postsubicular cortices. J Comp Neurol 1983; 216(2): 192–210.

128. Walker DL, Toufexis DJ, Davis M. Role of the bed nucleus of the stria terminalis versus the amygdala in fear, stress, and anxiety. Eur J Pharmacol 2003; 463(1–3): 199–216.

129. Wang JX, Poe G, Zochowski M. From network heterogeneities to familiarity detection and hippocampal memory management. Phys Rev E Stat Nonlin Soft Matter Phys 2008; 78: 041905.

130. Yamada S, Uenoyama Y, Maeda K, Tsukamura H. Role of noradrenergic receptors in the bed nucleus of the stria terminalis in regulating pulsatile luteinizing hormone secretion in female rats. J Reprod Dev 2006; 52(1): 115–21.

131. Yang P, Wu MT, Hsu CC, Ker JH. Evidence of early neurobiological alternations in adolescents with posttraumatic stress disorder: a functional MRI study. Neurosci Lett 2004a; 370(1): 13–8.

132. Yang P, Wu MT, Hsu CC, Ker JH. Evidence of early neurobiological alternations in adolescents with posttraumatic stress disorder: a functional MRI study. Neurosci Lett 2004b; 370(1): 13–8.

133. Yehuda R, Golier JA, Yang RK, Tischler L. Enhanced sensitivity to glucocorticoids in peripheral mononuclear leukocytes in posttraumatic stress disorder. Biol Psychiatry 2004; 55(11): 1110–6.

134. Yehuda R, Lowy MT, Southwick SM, Shaffer D, Giller EL Jr. Lymphocyte glucocorticoid receptor number in posttraumatic stress disorder. Am J Psychiatry 1991; 148(4): 499–504.

135. Zubieta JK, Chinitz JA, Lombardi U et al. Medial frontal cortex involvement in PTSD symptoms: a SPECT study. J Psychiatr Res 1999; 33(3): 259–64.

6 | The genetics of posttraumatic stress disorder

Eduard Maron and Jakov Shlik

The diagnostic definition of posttraumatic stress disorder (PTSD) postulates its onset in response to external terrifying events. While an exposure to traumatic conditions is likely to cause serious distress in almost any individual, only a proportion of them develop clinical features of PTSD (1). Epidemiological studies estimate that 40% to 90% of the general population may experience traumatic events during their life, but that only 15% to 24% develop PTSD (2-4). Thus, the exposure to a traumatic event is necessary, but not sufficient factor in the etiology of PTSD. Among various factors underlying the individual vulnerability to PTSD, the genetics may have an important role in the onset and course of this disease. The genetics of PTSD are often overlooked, with only few recent reviews drawing attention to this intriguing topic (5-8). Relatively scarce genetic research is in contrast with growing need to understand the predisposition and risks for PTSD. This chapter summarizes available studies and findings, which contribute to a better recognition of the genetic mechanisms of PTSD, keeping in mind limitations and problems accompanying this type of research. In addition, we discuss novel genetic approaches and directions to stimulate further investigations in this area.

FAMILIAL AGGREGATION STUDIES

Family studies explore the heritability of disease by estimation of its occurrence among first degree relatives of affected subjects. Generally these studies provide evidence of an increased rate of familial psychiatric morbidity among PTSD patients, whereas the stronger association was revealed for major depression with less consistent support for anxiety or PTSD. One family interview–based study involving 127 female probands and 639 first-degree relatives reported that PTSD following rape was associated with familial vulnerability to major depression that serves as a risk factor for developing PTSD (9). Several other studies demonstrated the two- to four-fold increased risk of developing PTSD in subjects with a family history of depression, anxiety disorders, psychosis, or personality disorders (2, 3, 10). Dierker and Merikangas (11) examined familial psychopathology in 263 probands and 1,206 adult first-degree relatives showing associations between PTSD in probands and affective disorders among female relatives or drug abuse among male relatives. However, no specific elevation in PTSD risk was detected in the relatives of probands with PTSD in their study. The familial relationship between PTSD and major depression was confirmed in a study by Sautter et al. (12), demonstrating that relatives of PTSD probands show higher levels of familial depression than the relatives of healthy comparison subjects. Although they found that the prevalence of both anxiety and PTSD appeared to be higher in the relatives of probands with PTSD, no statistically significant differences were shown when compared to controls. Their last finding was conflicting with a family study of Sack et al. (13), who reported that parental PTSD was associated with a five fold increased risk of PTSD in offspring of Cambodian refugees living in the Western United States.

Kozaric-Kovacic et al. (14) have found that familial psychopathology is reasonably stronger in case of comorbid PTSD. Specifically, the rate of family history of psychiatric illness was more frequent in Croatian combat veterans with comorbid depression and PTSD than in those with PTSD alone (35% vs. 6%, respectively). Previously Yehuda et al. (15) demonstrated a significantly higher prevalence of both current and lifetime PTSD and other psychiatric disorders in the offspring of Holocaust survivors than in the comparison subjects, even though these offspring as a group did not have greater exposure to life-threatening events. Several studies have shown that family history of affective disorders may predict exposure to traumatic stressors independently from the risk of developing PTSD (10, 16). The distinct hereditary aspects of exposure to trauma and PTSD may confound genetic research on traumatic stress. Furthermore, the PTSD symptoms in probands with familial PTSD could not be fully explained only by genetic transmission. It was found that children in close contact with traumatized first responders may develop posttraumatic symptoms through secondary traumatization. For example, one factor associated with probable emotional disturbance in children throughout New York City 6 months after the September 11, 2001 terrorist attack on the World Trade Center was having a family member exposed to the attack (17, 18). The examination of mental health problems in New York City public school children ($N = 8,236$) 6 months after the World Trade Center attack revealed that children with emergency medical technician in the family had nearly 19% prevalence of probable PTSD (19). The role of genetic factors in these findings is not known.

TWIN STUDIES

Twin studies compare resemblance for a condition between members of a twin pair, using the fact that identical (monozygotic, MZ) twins share 100% of their genes while nonidentical (dizygotic, DZ) twins share on average 50% of their genes. Interpretation of twin studies is limited by the fact that MZ twins tend to share similar environment more than DZ twins. In a small Norwegian sample of 81 adult twins with anxiety disorders, PTSD was only found in cotwins of anxiety probands and was twice as prevalent in MZ (20%) versus DZ (7%) twins (20). The most compelling evidence for a genetic predisposition to PTSD came from the Vietnam Era Twin (VET) Registry data, including 4,042 male veteran twin (2,224 MZ and 1,818 DZ) pairs. True et al. (21) explored in this sample the effects of heredity, shared environment, and unique environment on the liability for 15 self-reported symptoms of PTSD from symptom clusters of reexperiencing, avoidance, and hyperarousal. They found that the MZ twin correlations were higher than the DZ correlations for all of the symptoms and heritability estimates were in the range of 30% to 35% for most of the individual symptoms after controlling for the effects of trauma exposure. There was no evidence that environment shared by twin siblings have contributed to the development of PTSD symptoms. Their parallel VET Registry study examined the relationship of genetic influences on the extent of trauma exposure by analyzing specific events, like volunteering for service in Vietnam, time served in Southeast Asia, combat experiences, and combat decoration awards (22). In this study, the correlation within MZ and DZ twin pairs for volunteering for service in Vietnam were 0.40 and 0.22, respectively; for actual service in Southeast Asia, the MZ correlation was 0.41 and the DZ correlation was 0.24. Analysis of twin pairs in which both siblings served in Southeast Asia ($n = 820$) demonstrated a correlation for self-reported combat experiences within MZ and DZ pairs of 0.53 and 0.30, respectively. Genetic factors accounted for 36% of the variance in service in Southeast Asia, 47% of the variance in combat exposure, and 54% of the variance in the likelihood of receiving a combat medal. The family environment did not have a significant effect on any of these variables. Another smaller study by Stein et al. (1) in a sample of 291 female–female, 75 male–male, and 40 opposite-sex twin pairs from the Vancouver area in Canada showed that for pairs with both twins exposed to trauma, MZ pairs were more concordant for all clusters of PTSD than DZ pairs with heritability estimates similar to those in the VET Registry study.

MOLECULAR GENETIC STUDIES

In the research on the heritability of psychiatric disorders, linkage and association studies aim to clarify the molecular basis of epidemiological genetic findings. Linkage studies point to a chromosomal location of the gene or genes associated with a familial transmission of a phenotype of interest, estimating the likelihood of two gene loci to be inherited together. This model is difficult to apply to genetic research on PTSD because the essential condition for PTSD onset, exposure to trauma, is a variable that cannot be influenced (6). No linkage studies in

PTSD have been published. Main research efforts so far focus on candidate genes inferred from the knowledge on pathophysiology and drug action substrates in PTSD as well as relevant findings in other psychiatric disorders. This approach aims to link the illness to common variations in DNA sequence, such as sequence repeats or single nucleotide polymorphisms (SNPs) and patterns of their proximate occurrence (haplotypes). These studies employ the association method with case control design and/or family-based analyses. In contrast to other anxiety disorders, such as panic disorder or obsessive–compulsive disorder, fewer genetic association studies in PTSD have been published. All of them compared the allelic or genotype frequencies of candidate genes between cases and controls and only few explored haplotypes. Overall, these findings reviewed below are still preliminary to confirm the involvement of any specific genetic loci in the development of PTSD, but several of them deserve closer inspection (data summarized in Table 6.1).

DOPAMINE-RELATED GENES

Dopamine D2 receptor (DRD2) gene was the first candidate in PTSD association studies. Comings et al. (23, 24) implicated this gene in PTSD based on the association between this gene and alcohol abuse, the condition highly prevalent among individuals with PTSD. They reported significantly increased frequency of DRD2 TaqI "A1" alleles in the veterans who developed PTSD as compared to those who did not. Interpretation of these findings was limited by small sample size and comorbid drug or alcohol abuse. In attempt to replicate these findings, Gelernter et al. (25) studied DRD2 TaqI "A" allele frequencies in their sample of European–American Vietnam combat veterans with PTSD. Neither allelic nor haplotype frequencies significantly differed between the patient and control groups, excluding major role of genetic variation at the DRD2 locus in predisposition to PTSD. Their study was also restricted by small sample size and high comorbidity rates. A study of Young et al. (26) aimed to determine the effect of alcohol use on the possible association between PTSD and DRD2 A1 allele. In line with previous observations they found significantly higher frequency of the A1 allele in the Vietnam combat veterans of the Australian armed forces with PTSD than in the matched control group. However, further analysis revealed that A1 allelic frequency was about twice higher in PTSD subgroup of harmful drinkers then in nonharmful drinkers, whereas frequency of A1 allele in the latter subgroup did not significantly differ from control subjects. Moreover, daily amount and hourly rate of alcohol consumed were markedly higher in PTSD carriers of A1 allele than in those with A2 allele. In a subsequent study they extended the role of DRD2 locus on the four psychopathological factors, including somatic concerns, anxiety/insomnia, social dysfunction, and depression in untreated veterans with PTSD (27, 28). They found that the carriers of A1 allele were showing significantly higher anxiety, depression, and social dysfunction scores than A2 allele carriers. Interestingly, they also demonstrated that A1 allele is associated with greater improvements in social functioning in PTSD patients following 8-week treatment with paroxetine when compared to those without this allele. These findings indicate that DRD2 A1 allele may be implicated in expression of general psychopathological symptoms, such as depression, anxiety, or social dysfunction as well as alcohol use rather than associated with PTSD diagnosis. Pertinently, postmortem and positron emission tomography studies have demonstrated that A1 allele is associated with decreased density of DRD2 in human brain (29, 30). In another study, lower density of brain DRD2 was correlated with higher level of craving for alcohol (31). In the context of these findings, the nature of association between DRD2 A1 allele and PTSD remains unclear.

The gene of dopamine transporter (DAT), a key protein regulating synaptic reuptake of dopamine, is another marker recently associated with PTSD. Investigating a polymorphic variable number tandem repeats (VNTR) region in the SLC6A3 3' untranslated region, Segman et al. (32) found a significant association between nine repeat allele and nine repeat homozygous genotype, and the susceptibility to chronic PTSD. Notably, the PTSD association studies may be at risk for false negative results because of including potential unexposed cases as controls. More important, Segman et al. (32) diminished this risk by limiting their control group only to subjects who were exposed to similar traumatic events as patients, but

Table 6.1 Association studies in Posttraumatic Stress Disorder.

Genes	Polymorphisms	Sample (males)	Ethnicity	Comorbidity	Main findings [reference]
DRD2	TaqI "A1"	37 cases 19 controls	non-Hispanic Whites	Alcohol or drug dependence	Significantly more "A1" allele carriers among PTSD subjects as compared to non-PTSD (59% versus 5% p=0.0001) [Comings et al. 1996]
	TaqI "A1"	52 cases 87 controls	European-American	Alcohol or drug dependence	No difference in A1 allele frequencies between PTSD sample (0.15) and controls (0.19) [Gelernter et al. 1999]
	TaqI "A1"	57 cases	Caucasian	Excluded PSYH, BD, OCD, DEM	Significantly higher scores on GHQ 2 (anxiety/insomnia), GHQ 3 (social dysfunction) and GHQ 4 (depression) in A1 allele carriers [Lawford et al. 2006]
	TaqI "A1"	63 cases	Caucasian	Excluded PSYH, BD, OCD, DEM	Greater improvement in GHQ 3 (social dysfunction) in A1 allele carriers with paroxetine treatment [Lawford et al. 2003]
	TaqI "A1"	91 cases 51 (18) controls	Caucasian	Alcohol problems	Significantly higher frequency of A1 allele in PTSD harmful drinkers (28%) than in nonharmful drinkers (14%) or in controls (7%) [Young et al. 2002]
DAT	SLC6A3 3′ VNTR	102 (57) cases 104 (49) controls	Jewish	Anxiety disorders, depression	Association with 9 repeat allele (p=0.012, OR=1.72) and 9 repeat homozygous genotype (p=0.047) [Segman et al., 2002]
DBH	-1021C/T	133 cases 34 controls	Croatian Caucasian	Excluded	Significantly lower plasma DBH activity in PTSD combat veterans with CC genotype as compared to veterans without PTSD (p<0.001) [Mustapic et al., 2007]
5-HTT	5-HTTLPR	100 (43) cases 197 (76) controls	Korean	Mostly excluded	Higher frequency of S-allele in PTSD patients than in controls (0.87 versus 0.81; p=0.044, OR=1.65) [Lee et al. 2005]
	5-HTTLPR	19 (6) cases 570 (211) controls	American, mostly White	Depression	Significant association between low-expression variant and PTSD in adults with low social support and exposed to hurricane [Kilpatrick et al. 2007]
MAO-B	G/A substitution in intron 13	106 cases 242 controls	Croatian Caucasian	Depression, GAD, alcoholism	No significant difference in either the allelic (p=0.25-0.89) or genotype (p=0.24-1.00) frequencies [Pivac et al. 2007]

Table 6.1 (Continued)

genes	Investigated polymorphisms	Sample (males)	Ethnicity	Comorbidity	Main findings [reference]
APOE	€2, €3 and €4 isoforms	54 cases	Caucasian	Depression, PD, Alcohol problems	Significantly higher CAPS reexperiencing scores and poorer memory on the WMS-III in €2 allele carriers [Freeman et al. 2005]
BDNF	G-712A, C270T, Val66Met	96 (73) cases 250 (103) controls	European-American	Unspecified	No significant difference in either the allelic, genotype or haplotype frequencies (p=0.23-0.84) [Zhang et al. 2006]
	Val66Met	107 (45) cases 161 (52) controls	Korean	Mostly excluded	No significant difference in either the allelic (p=0.57) or genotype (p=0.81) frequencies [Lee et al. 2006]
GABRB3	CA repeat alleles (G1-G11)	86 cases	Caucasian	Not excluded	Higher total scores on GHQ in the G1 non-G1 hetero-zygotes than in homozygotes (p=0.002) [Feusner et al. 2001]
GCR	N363S, BclI	118 cases 42 controls	Unspecified	Excluded active comorbidity	No significant difference in either N363S allelic (p=0.46) or BclI genotype (p=0.40) frecuencies [Bachmann et al. 2005]
FKBP5	rs3800373 rs992105 rs9296158 rs737054 rs1360780 rs1334894 rs9470080 rs4713916	900 (384) nonpsychiatric clinic patients	> 95% Black-American		Significant interaction of 4 SNPs (rs9296158, rs3800373, rs1360780, and rs9470080; minimum p=0.0004) with the severity of child abuse to predict level of adult PTSD symptoms [Binder et al. 2008]
NPY	Leu7Pro	77 cases 202 controls	European-American	Alcohol dependence	No difference in Pro 7 allele frequencies between PTSD sample (3.9) and controls (2.0) [Lappalainen et al. 2002]

ApoE – apolipoprotein E, BDNF – brain-derived neurotrophic factor, DAT – dopamine transporter, DBN – dopamine beta-hydroxylase, DRD – dopamine receptor, FKBP5 – FK506 binding protein 5, GABA – gamma-amino-butyric acid, GABRB3 – gamma-amino-butyric acid type A receptor β3 subunit, GCR – gluccorticoid receptor, MAO-B – monoamine oxidases B, NPY – neuropeptide Y, 5-HTT – serotonin transporter, VNTR – variable number tandem repeat, CAPS – Clinician Administered PTSD Scale, GHQ – General Health Questionnaire-28 (comprises the somatic symptoms, depression, anxiety/insomnia and social dysfunction subscales), WMS-III – Weschler Memory Scale-Third Edition, BD – bipolar disorder, GAD – generalized anxiety disorder, DEM – dementia, OCD – obsessive-compulsive disorder, PD – panic disorder, PSYH – psychosis.

did not develop PTSD. Neuroimaging studies in various samples showed lack of a functional effect of SLC6A3 polymorphism on the availability of DAT in human brain (33-36). However, a recent study examining the effect of SLC6A3 genotype on brain DAT availability in a large sample of healthy subjects has revealed significantly higher striatal DAT density with mean increase about 9% in nine repeat allele carriers as compared to 10 repeat allele homozygotes (37). Whether increased removal of dopamine from synaptic cleft, as determined by nine repeat allele, is one of the pathogenetic factors in PTSD needs confirmation. Other disturbances in genetic regulation of catecholamine metabolism could be also related to PTSD. Similarly to patients with paranoid schizophrenia and psychotic depression (38), the war veterans with current and chronic PTSD have significantly lower plasma dopamine beta-hydroxylase (DBH) activity, in contrast to normal level of DBH activity in combat-exposed war veterans without PTSD (39). Furthermore, plasma DBH activity was significantly lower in veterans with PTSD carrying CC genotype of 1021C/T SNP in the five flanking region of DBH as compared to veterans without PTSD. However, neither genotypes nor allelic frequencies significantly differed between the two groups of war veterans. Notably, this polymorphism accounts for 35–52% of the interindividual variations in plasma DBH activity (40), whereas association between plasma DBH activity and CC genotype has been also reported in alcoholic subjects (41).

SEROTONIN TRANSPORTER GENE

Serotonin transporter (5-HTT), a key protein regulating serotonin neurotransmission, contains a functional polymorphism in the 5′ regulatory promoter region (5-HTTLPR), involving two alleles, corresponding to a 44-bp insertion (long or L-allele) or deletion (short or S-allele). This polymorphism became the usual suspect in genetic studies of psychiatric disorders after Lesch et al. (42) reported a decreased 5-HTT transcriptional activity and diminished serotonin uptake of S variant in comparison to LL genotype and a positive association of S allele with anxiety traits in humans. On the other hand, 5-HTT is the target for selective serotonin reuptake inhibitors—antidepressants commonly used in treatment of PTSD. There is only one published study reporting possible association between 5-HTTLPR and PTSD phenotype (43). This study was conducted in a Korean sample of PTSD patients, most of them with non–combat-related stressors, including serious accidents, fire, injury, or physical assault. The modest, but significant association was demonstrated in their sample with S allele been more frequent among patients. The interpretation of these results is limited by small sample size and a possibility that some of the control subjects may still develop PTSD upon exposure to a traumatic event. Moreover, the higher frequency of S allele in Korean and other Asian populations in comparison to Western populations may indicate the distinct role of 5-HTTLPR polymorphism in different ethnic groups. The finding of Lee et al. (43) is still of interest considering the findings in depression (44-47), where S allele of 5-HTTLPR contributed to development of depression via interaction with stressful life events. These data suggest that 5-HTTLPR may modify the risk of PTSD and other stress-related disorders. Supporting this view, a recent study of adults exposed to the 2004 Florida hurricanes conferred that 5-HTTLPR polymorphism may mediate risks of postdisaster PTSD and major depression, particularly in those with low social support (48). These relationships, are, however, not straightforward as other investigations, including a meta-analysis of 14 studies, found no clear influence of 5-HTTPLR polymorphism, or its interaction with life stressors, on the onset of affective disorders (49, 50).

MONOAMINE OXIDASE GENE

Monoamine oxidase (MAO), existing in two isoforms (MAO-A and MAO-B), catalyzes the oxidative deamination of several biogenic amines, including serotonin. Decreased platelet MAO-B activity was demonstrated in patients with PTSD in some studies, indicating possible involvement of this enzyme in PTSD (51-53). However, no difference in MAO-B enzymatic levels was found between patients and control subjects by Pivac et al. (54), who also evaluated the relationship between platelet MAO-B activity and G/A substitution polymorphism in intron 13 of MAO-B gene in combatrelated PTSD veterans with or without psychotic features, combat-exposed veterans without PTSD and healthy control male subjects. Higher platelet MAO-B activity was found only in PTSD patients with psychotic symptoms, whereas G/A polymorphism was unrelated to platelet MAO-B activity and was not associated with PTSD (55). The transcriptionally more active longer alleles or genotypes of the functional polymorphism of the MAO-A gene, uVNTR, were significantly associated with panic phenotypes in female but not male patients (56-58). Considering the high comorbidity rate between panic disorder and PTSD, this polymorphism deserves more attention in further association studies.

APOLIPOPROTEIN E GENE

Apolipoprotein E (APOE) is a mediator of lipoprotein binding to the low-density lipoprotein receptor, E4 isoform, which has been associated with memory impairment (59), smaller hippocampal volumes (60), and increased rates of hippocampal volume loss (61). The individuals with chronic PTSD exhibited more impaired memory, attentional, and executive function deficits (62) and smaller hippocampal volumes than comparison subjects (63). Based on these observations, Freeman et al. (64) have examined the possible effect of APOE4 allele on the specific cognitive symptoms in male veterans with combat-related PTSD. Their initial analysis did not reveal any associations with PTSD symptoms or memory functioning in APOE4 allele carriers as compared to those without this allele. However, they found that subjects with APOE2 allele had significantly worse symptoms of reexperiencing, but not avoidance or arousal clusters, and more impaired memory function than the remainder of the study sample. Despite the novelty of these findings, the study did not confirm the proposed hypothesis and do not allow to draw clear conclusions due to small sample size.

BRAIN-DERIVED NEUROTROPHIC FACTOR GENE

The possible involvement of brain-derived neurotrophic factor (BDNF) gene in the regulation of stress-related behaviors seems very intriguing due to its important role in the maintenance of neuronal plasticity (65). Rasmusson et al. (66) observed downregulated BDNF mRNA levels in the hippocampal dentate gyrus of rats exposed to footshock or reexposed to cues previously paired with footshock. Based on this finding, Zhang et al. (67) suggested that stress condition may inhibit hippocampal BDNF expression, which could be relevant to the pathogenesis of stress-related disorders, including PTSD. They screened a newly identified SNP, G-712A, and two previously reported SNPs—C270T and Val66Met—in the patients with Alzheimer's disease, affective disorders, schizophrenia, substance dependence, and PTSD. No significant differences in allele, genotype, or haplotype frequencies of the three BDNF SNPs were found between the patients with PTSD and normal controls. In addition, neither genotype nor allele frequencies of Val66Met polymorphism significantly differed between the patients with PTSD and unrelated healthy controls in Korean population (68). These studies have excluded a major role of BDNF gene in predisposition to PTSD what is in line with the findings on lack of associations between BDNF gene and panic disorder (69, 70).

GAMMA-AMINOBUTYRIC ACID GENE

The involvement of gamma-aminobutyric acid (GABA) system in the pathogenesis of PTSD is supported by peripheral measurements, animal models, and neuroimaging. The reduced benzodiazepine–GABA-A receptor binding was demonstrated in various brain regions in PTSD veterans in some but not all studies (71-73). To date, the role of GABA-related genes in PTSD has not been specifically examined in case-control association studies. Feusner et al. (74) had demonstrated an association between GABAA receptor α3 subunit gene locus and higher levels of General Health Questionnaire-28 (GHQ) cluster symptoms among Caucasian male PTSD veterans. In particular, total score of the GHQ subscale scores on the somatic symptoms, anxiety/insomnia, depression and social dysfunction were higher in PTSD subjects heterozygous for the G1 microsatellite polymorphism than in homozygous groups. Although the nature of this effect is not clear, these findings, similar to their above-mentioned consequent studies (27, 28) implicated the candidate genes in the expression of general psychopathology rather than in PTSD. The studies in other disorders frequently comorbid with PTSD have found that 485 G>A polymorphism in peripheral benzodiazepine receptor gene was significantly associated with panic disorder in Japanese sample (75); however, exonic sequence variants of the GABA-B receptor 1 gene were not implicated in susceptibility to panic disorder (76). Additionally, no associations were detected between depressive symptomatology and GABA-A receptor alpha-1 subunit gene in patients with mood disorders (77) or between two missense variations in peripheral benzodiazepine receptor gene and mood disturbances (78).

GLUCOCORTICOID RECEPTOR GENE

The possible involvement of glucocorticoid-related genes in predisposition to PTSD is suggested based on the apparent alterations in the hypothalamic–pituitary–adrenal (HPA) axis, resulting in neuroendocrine abnormalities, such as lowered cortisol levels, and increased sensitivity to glucocorticoids (79-82). A polymorphism in exon 2 of glucocorticoid receptor (GR) gene, N363S, which is known to alter the N terminal transactivation domain, was found to be associated with glucocorticoid hypersensitivity (83) and increased salivary cortisol response to psychosocial stress (84). The other polymorphism located in intron 2 of the same gene, defined as BclI, was associated with increased glucocorticoid sensitivity and greater cortisol suppression after lowdose dexamethasone (85, 86), but also with diminished cortisol response to stress (84). Bachmann et al. (87) examined the association between these polymorphisms and PTSD and their role in GR sensitivity in Vietnam veterans with PTSD and matched for combat exposure non-PTSD controls. In this study, the allelic and genotype frequencies of both polymorphisms did not differ between PTSD patients and controls or previously reported population. There was no clear relationship between the studied genotypes and glucocorticoid sensitivity as assessed by low-dose dexamethasone suppression test and the dermal vessel vasoconstrictor assay. Notably, in contrast to previous findings, the basal plasma cortisol levels did not significantly differ between PTSD veterans and combatexposed controls and the low-dose dexamethasone suppression test resulted in similar cortisol suppression in both groups. Only some trends were found in the subgroup of PTSD patients with BclI GG genotype, which were more responsive to dermal vessel vasoconstrictor assay and had higher clinician-administered PTSD scale scores that were significantly and negatively correlated with basal plasma cortisol levels.

FK506 BINDING PROTEIN 5 (FKBP5) GENE

FKBP5 is a cochaperone regulating GR signaling (88, 89). Several studies had served FKBP5 gene as an intriguing candidate gene for psychiatric disorders. The polymorphisms in FKBP5 were associated with recurrence or disease status of major depression and treatment response to antidepressants (90, 91). In addition, the positive association between FKBP5 variations and peritraumatic dissociation, which is considered to be a risk factor for PTSD, was demonstrated by Koenen et al. (92) in medically injured children. Binder et al. (93) have explored the interaction between genetic and environmental risk factors in the development of PTSD, including exposure to child abuse, non–child-abuse trauma, and genetic polymorphisms of the FKBP5 gene. In their cross-sectional study consisting of 762 genotyped, nonpsychiatric, mainly Black (>95%) male and female patients, several FKBP5 SNPs did not directly predict PTSD symptom outcome or interact with level of non–child-abuse trauma to predict PTSD symptom severity. However, four SNPs of the FKBP5 gene interacted with severity of child abuse as a predictor of adult PTSD symptoms, suggesting an interaction between this gene and childhood environment in the development of PTSD. They also observed significant interactions between FKBP5 risk allele carrier status, PTSD, and cortisol response to dexamethasone suppression test in a subgroup of this sample, demonstrating that the majority of patients with risk alleles and

PTSD showed enhanced cortisol suppression or enhanced GR sensitivity, which is a possible endocrine signature of PTSD. Notably, same SNPs were associated with higher FKBP5 protein levels or a stronger induction of FKBP5 mRNA by cortisol in healthy probands (90) and also as implicated by Koenen et al. (92) in psychological response to medical trauma in children. Interestingly, Segman et al. (94) detected upregualtion of FKBP5 mRNA expression in peripheral blood mononuclear cells immediately following trauma exposure in those subjects, who later developed chronic PTSD. These evidences strongly implicate FKBP5 gene in susceptibility to PTSD and its pathogenesis.

NEUROPEPTIDE Y GENE

Previously described functional Leu7Pro polymorphism in the neuropeptide Y (NPY) gene has been recently shown to affect intracellular processing and secretion of preproNPY peptide. Kallio et al. (95) demonstrated that healthy subjects with Pro7/Leu7 genotype have an average of 42% higher maximal increases in the plasma concentration of NPY during exercise-induced sympathetic activation as compared with Leu7/Leu7 carriers. This study has linked Leu7Pro polymorphism to magnitude of NPY release in response to physiological stressor. On the other hand, the lower baseline plasma NPY and blunted yohimbine-stimulated increases in plasma NPY were demonstrated in PTSD patients in comparison to healthy controls (96). In this study, baseline plasma NPY levels in patients correlated negatively with combat exposure scale scores, baseline PTSD, and panic symptoms. In a parallel study by the same group, a significant increase of plasma NPY was demonstrated in response to high-intensity military training in healthy soldiers and significant depletion of plasma NPY occurred when stress was extended (97). Consequently, Lappalainen et al. (98) had tested whether the Leu7Pro polymorphism of NPY gene is associated with a greater risk of alcohol dependence, secondarily investigating an independent sample of patients with PTSD. A significantly higher frequency of the Pro7 allele was observed in alcohol-dependent sample as compared to controls, but not in PTSD patients.

GENE EXPRESSION STUDIES

Investigation of gene expression patterns has a potential to expand the knowledge about genetic substrates of psychiatric disorders on transcriptional levels. Microarray studies of peripheral gene transcription signatures have suggested a shared expression of the majority of genes in brain and peripheral blood (99) and showed promising results in somatic and psychiatric disorders (100-104). To date, two studies exploring peripheral gene expression in PTSD have been published.

Segman et al. (94) were first to hypothesize that transcriptional response of peripheral blood mononuclear cell may correlate with the development of PTSD among trauma survivors. To examine this, the gene expression patterns of subjects exposed to traumatic event, mostly to motor vehicle accident, were screened using oligonucleotide microarrays, immediately following trauma at the emergency and four months later. This study provided initial evidence that peripheral transcriptional signatures at both time points distinguished survivors who had developed acute or chronic PTSD from those who were well at follow-up and correlated with the severity of PTSD symptom clusters. From the 4,512 active transcripts identified in their set, they found 656 transcripts that were differentially expressed between PTSD-affected and nonaffected subjects. A general reduction in expression of transcription activators in PTSD affected survivors was detected, whereas several differentiating genes were encoding for proteins that are known to be involved in stress response, transcriptional activation, cell cycle and proliferation, immune activation, signal transduction, and apoptosis. On the other hand, the subjects with PTSD demonstrated significantly increased representations of genes involved in RNA or nucleotide metabolism and processing as well as significantly enriched signatures for genes that encode for neural and endocrine proteins. More important, 533 from 656 differentially expressed transcripts were known to be expressed in pertinent brain and neuroendocrine regions. For example, gene transcripts expressed in the amygdala, hippocampus, and HPA axis were particularly abundant among the genes distinguishing the subjects with PTSD.

Another data set on peripheral gene expression signatures in PTSD was recently presented by Zieker et al. (105). Their study assessed the transcriptional activity of gene expression in whole blood of eight patients who developed PTSD after Ramstein air show catastrophe (1989) and eight control subjects. The authors hypothesized that PTSD results from a failure of the body to reverse the acute stress response; therefore, genes involved in stress and immune responses could be differentially transcribed in PTSD patients. Using customized "stress/immune chips" for selected genes related to inflammation, apoptosis, stress response, and related pathways, they found that four upregulated and 14 downregulated genes, with 5% of total valid transcripts compared, differentiated the patients from controls. Most downregulated transcripts were associated with immune functions or with reactive oxygen species. The additional polymerase chain reaction confirmed downregulation of the following genes: coding endothelial differentiation sphingolipid, interleukin-18 and 16, superoxide dismutase 1, and thioredoxin reductase 1. Notably, the assessment of peripheral gene expression profiles was conducted in patients 16 years after the traumatic event. Despite this long interval, authors argued that patients maintained the specific features of PTSD. However, patients did not differ from controls on metabolic level, where comparable levels of cortisol, adrenaline, noradrenaline, vanillylmandelic acid, homovanillic acid, and cytokines were detected in both groups. Taken together, the transcripts identified in this investigation indicate that a number of genes related to oxidative pathway and immune system could be good candidates for further genetic association studies and treatment targets in PTSD.

The studies above warrant replications in larger controlled and more homogenous samples. The indications of altered gene expression in PTSD challenge whole-genome association studies to explore novel polymorphisms in the genes demonstrating different transcriptional activity.

COMORBIDITY AND GENETICS

High comorbidity between PTSD and other psychiatric disorders indicate that PTSD and comorbid conditions may share genetic components. This is not surprising considering the universal pathogenic role of stress in mental illness. As mentioned above, the S allele of 5-HTTLPR polymorphism is probably one of the important genetic modifiers, which contributes to development of both major depression and PTSD via interaction with adverse life events or traumas. Unfortunately, no consistent confirmation from molecular studies exploring this aspect exists today; however, twin studies lend indirect support for shared or common genetic vulnerability.

Several recent studies have estimated the degree to which a common genetic vulnerability can explain the nature of associations between PTSD and various psychiatric conditions based on the data from 6,744 male veterans of VET Registry. Koenen et al. (106) found that common genetic liability explained 62.5% of PTSD and major depression comorbidity, whereas genetic influences common to major depression explained 15% of the total variance in risk for PTSD and 58% of the genetic variance in PTSD. In addition, they showed that individual-specific environmental influences common to major depression explained only 11% of the individual-specific environmental variance in PTSD, indicating that environmental influences on both disorders appear to be largely disorder specific. Subsequent analysis demonstrated that the magnitude of covariance (genetic plus individual-specific environmental) between major depression and PTSD was about twice as large as that of the covariance (shared plus individual-specific environmental) between conduct disorder and PTSD (107). This suggests that the etiology of PTSD is more closely related to major depression than to conduct disorder. In contrast, the shared genetic effects explained 63% of the association between PTSD and nicotine dependence, whereas the remaining covariance was explained by individual-specific environmental effects (108). These studies underscore a substantial genetic overlap between PTSD and major depression and nicotine dependence, making the genes implicated in the etiology of comorbid disorders strong candidates for PTSD and vice versa.

Earlier, Chantarujikapong et al. (109) estimated the magnitude of genetic and environmental contributions to the lifetime co-occurrence of generalized anxiety disorder, panic disorder, and PTSD using smaller sample from VET Registry consisting of 3,327 MZ and DZ male–male twin pair members. The liability for symptoms of generalized anxiety disorder was due to a 37.9% additive genetic contribution common to symptoms of panic disorder and PTSD. Liability for symptoms of panic disorder was due to a 20.7% additive genetic contribution common to symptoms of generalized anxiety disorder and PTSD, and a 20.1% additive genetic influence specific to panic symptoms. Additive genetic influences common to symptoms of generalized anxiety disorder and panic disorder accounted for 21.3% of the genetic variance in PTSD. Additive genetic influences specific to PTSD accounted for 13.6% of the genetic variance in PTSD. Remaining variance for all three disorders was due to unique environmental factors both common and specific to each phenotype. These results suggest that each of these disorders has etiologically distinct components as well as common genetic and unique environmental contributions.

Taken together, the high comorbidity between PTSD and other psychiatric disorders may represent the evidence of pleiotropy, where the same genes contribute to the development of several different disorders or endophenotypes.

ANIMAL GENETIC STUDIES

The animal studies applying stress models are largely used in exploring various PTSD- related aspects, including neuroendocrine status or reactivity of autonomic nervous system and behavioral changes in response to stress (reviewed in next chapter). These models are also useful in the genetic research. Two strategies are used to establish the nature of interactions between stress and genes. One direction is to study the effects of gene knockout or transgenic overexpression on stress-related behavior. Another approach investigates the effect of exposure to stress on changes in gene expression profiles or their transcriptional activity.

Despite the advantages of knockout models in research on anxiety, the relevance of these studies to PTSD remains uncertain. For example, several animal studies demonstrated that knockout mice lacking 5-HTT or 5-HT1A receptor exhibit increased anxiety-related behaviors in conflict tests, including the open-field, elevated-plus maze, elevated-zero maze, and novelty-suppressed feeding paradigms (110-116). The 5-HT1A receptor knockout mice also showed increased behavioral inhibition when faced with complex and ambiguous threatening cues (117). Although the generalization of fearful behavior to contextual fear conditioning may serve as a model of PTSD and thus implicate 5-HT1A receptor in this anxiety disorder, it should be noted that 5-HT1A density was not altered in the brain of patients with PTSD (118). Other knockout studies found a decrease in anxiety-like behavior associated with elevated baseline and poststress exposure levels of corticosterone in mice lacking the beta3 nicotinic receptor subunit (119) and less anxiety-related responses and less freezing to a tone after auditory fear conditioning and stress sensitization in transient receptor potential vanilloid type 1 channel knock-out mice (120). Moreover, significantly decreased anxiety response was observed after acute stress in mice with knockout of cellular prion protein (121), whereas anxiety- and stress-related responses were lowered in mice lacking melanin-concentrating hormone 1 receptor (122) or interleukin 6 (123). On the other hand, anxiety-like behaviors and/or sensitivity to stress responses increased in mice deficient in corticotropin-releasing hormone receptor type 1 and 2 (124-126) and in galanin GAL-R1 receptor subtype (127). However, anxious behavior and stress hormone levels remained unaffected during stress exposure in the mice deficient in both the GABAB(1) receptor isoforms (128) and neuromedin U central receptor (129) or were not clearly related to stress exposure in 5-HT3A receptor knockout mice (130).

The stress paradigms are also used in exploring the effect of behavioral and hormonal responses to stress exposure on the transcriptional levels of relevant genes. In particular, expression of mRNA for GR was significantly reduced across all hippocampal subfields in the animals after single prolonged stress, whereas mRNA level of mineralocorticoid receptor (MR), but not GR, remained persistently downregulated during following 2 weeks. Furthermore, the animals exhibited hypersensitive glucocorticoid fast feedback induced by the stress exposure, demonstrating a decreased MR/GR ratio; by contrast, chronically stressed animals with normal fast feedback demonstrated normalization in their glucocorticoid receptor mRNA levels (131). These findings may confirm that hypersensitive glucocorticoid fast feedback induced by specific stress paradigm may serve as an animal model of PTSD-specific neuroendocrine abnormality. Interestingly, the mice with transgenic overexpression of forebrain MR demonstrated diminished anxiety-like behavior accompanying by decrease in the hippocampal GR and increase in 5HT1A expressions, whereas female mice also exhibited moderate suppression of the corticosterone response to restraint stress (132). The rats exposed to restraint stress in the water demonstrated initial downregulation of mRNA for growth hormone receptor (GHR) in the dentate gyms, which level rapidly enhanced up to 4 hours after stress. This biphasic enhancement of GHR mRNA expression followed the elevation of plasma glucocorticoid levels and paralleled with biphasic expressions of mRNAs for MR and GR in the same region, suggesting that glucocorticoids may interact with GHR in modulation of hippocampal reactions to stress (134). The other recent study demonstrated that animals subjected to single prolonged stress exhibited increase in hippocampal levels of both glycine transporter 1 and vesicle-associated membrane protein 2 mRNA in response to contextual fear (135). In addition, animals with stronger changes of both behavior and corticosterone levels in response to predator-scent stress displayed a lack of upregulation in hippocampal mRNA expression for activity-regulated, cytoskeletal-associated protein (Arc), in contrast to those with the partial and minimal stress responses (136). On the other hand, the animals showing extreme behavioral response selectively displayed persistent downregulation of mRNA for BDNF and upregulation of mRNA for its intracellular kinaseactivating receptor, TrkB, in the CA1 subregion of the hippocampus, compared to animals with partial or minimal responses or to unexposed controls (137). Since both BDNF and Arc seem to be involved in the longer phases of long-term potentiation and consequently memory formation (138, 139), their persistently reduced expression in animals with extreme behavioral response might reflect or mediate changes in neural plasticity and synaptic functioning underlying chronic stress-induced psychopathologic processes (136). Earlier findings revealed that exposure to stress has lead to increased expression of messenger RNA encoding the early immediate transcription factor c-Fos (140), and those for acetylcholinesterase, but to decreased levels for the acetylcholine-synthesizing enzyme choline acetyltransferase and the vesicular acetylcholine transporter (141). These data may indicate that stress-induced changes in cholinergic gene expression could result in a reduction of available acetylcholine and decline in cholinergic neurotransmission. Preliminary microarray tests showed that the gene expression profiles in the hippocampus region in clusters of cell signaling, metabolism, cytoskeleton, and apoptosis, differentiated the stressed maladapted rats from stressed, well-adapted rats. In addition, the two pathways (mainly with immunoactivity), cell growth and cycle, and proliferation and apoptosis functionality, were upregulated, while one, namely, calcium-signaling pathway was downregulated in the amygdala of stressed rats (142). These findings are of particular interest considering above-mentioned human microarray findings in PTSD; however, direct parallels can not yet be drown.

Recently, the concept of epigenetic regulatory mechanisms, and specifically, modifications of chromatin remodelling has been applied in animal models investigating stress-related behaviors. Most attention has been given to the effects of stress on histone H3 phosphorylation, which modifies transcriptional activation of silent genes in distinct neuronal populations (143). Chandramohan et al. (144) have found that exposure to novelty enhanced phosphorylation and phosphoacetylation of histone H3 in the dentate gyrus throughout the rostrocaudal axis of the hippocampus, suggesting that selected population of mature dentate neurons is recruited to allow transcriptional induction of genes necessary for the cellular adaptation to stress. These studies indicate a high potential of epigenetic approach in advancing genetic research on PTSD.

CONCLUSIONS

Similar to other multifactorial and complex diseases, the genetic studies in PTSD face critical scrutiny and methodological challenges. To date, the genetic research on PTSD has made modest progress, whereas interpretation of available findings is often complicated and cannot clearly explain the vulnerability to PTSD. Most of the data are obtained from small samples and ethnically heterogeneous comorbid populations mainly consisting of males with combat PTSD, suggesting that the findings may not apply to females, children, or individuals exposed to other types of trauma. Possible impact of personality traits or individual characteristics on the vulnerability to traumatic experience has not been well delineated, and only few genetic studies recognized the necessity to compare PTSD patients to non-PTSD subjects exposed to the same or similar stressor. PTSD offers a unique opportunity to study interactions between the genes and the environment. The hypothesis-driven approach to association studies in PTSD, based on findings in other psychiatric disorders or animal studies, may be significantly augmented by genomewide association and gene expression studies using advanced biotechnology and informatics. The emerging research on imaging genomics (145) may further broaden the understanding of interplay between genetic and neurobiological bases of anxiety regulation, including PTSD. More transaltional research is warranted to link the findings on genetic basis of anxiety and stress response in animal and human subjects. The recognition of genetic factors influencing vulnerability to stressors and PTSD may help to develop more effective prevention and remediation efforts in this increasingly important area of public health.

REFERENCES

1. Stein MB, Jang KL, Taylor S, Vernon PA, Livesley WJ. Genetic and environmental influences on trauma exposure and posttraumatic stress disorder symptoms: a twin study. Am J Psychiatry 2002; 159(10): 1675–81.
2. Breslau N, Davis GC, Andreski P, Peterson E. Traumatic events and posttraumatic stress disorder in an urban population of young adults. Arch Gen Psychiatry 1991 48(3): 216–22.
3. Breslau N, Kessler RC, Chilcoat HD et al. Trauma and posttraumatic stress disorder in the community: the 1996 Detroit Area Survey of Trauma. Arch Gen Psychiatry 1998; 55(7): 626–32.
4. Kessler RC, Sonnega A, Bromet E, Hughes M, Nelson CB. Posttraumatic stress disorder in the National Comorbidity Survey. Arch Gen Psychiatry 1995; 52(12): 1048–60.
5. Segman RH, Shalev AY. Genetics of posttraumatic stress disorder. CNS Spectr 2003; 8(9): 693–8.
6. Broekman BF, Olff M, Boer F. The genetic background to PTSD. Neurosci Biobehav Rev 2007 31(3): 348–62.
7. Koenen KC. Genetics of posttraumatic stress disorder: Review and recommendations for future studies. J Trauma Stress 2007; 20(5): 737–50.
8. Maron E, Hettema JH, Shlik J. The genetics of human anxiety disorders. In: Huston JP, Robert J, Blanchard D. Caroline Blanchard, Guy Griebel, David Nutt, eds. Handbook of Anxiety and Fear 2008; 17: 475–510.
9. Davidson JR, Tupler LA, Wilson WH, Connor KM. A family study of chronic post-traumatic stress disorder following rape trauma. J Psychiatr Res 1998; 32(5): 301–9.
10. Reich J, Lyons M, Cai B. Familial vulnerability factors to post-traumatic stress disorder in male military veterans. Acta Psychiatr Scand 1996; 93(2): 105–12.
11. Dierker LC, Merikangas KR. Familial psychiatric illness and posttraumatic stress disorder: findings from a family study of substance abuse and anxiety disorders. J Clin Psychiatry 2001; 62(9): 715–20.
12. Sautter FJ, Cornwell J, Johnson JJ, Wiley J, Faraone SV. Family history study of posttraumatic stress disorder with secondary psychotic symptoms. Am J Psychiatry 2002; 159(10): 1775–7.
13. Sack WH, Clarke GN, Seeley J. Posttraumatic stress disorder across two generations of Cambodian refugees. J Am Acad Child Adolesc Psychiatry 1995; 34(9): 1160–6.
14. Kozaric´-Kovacic´ D, Hercigonja DK, Grubisic´-Ilic´ M. Posttraumatic stress disorder and depression in soldiers with combat experiences. Croat Med J 2001; 42(2): 165–70.
15. Yehuda R, Schmeidler J, Wainberg M, Binder-Brynes K, Duvdevani T. Vulnerability to posttraumatic stress disorder in adult offspring of Holocaust survivors. Am J Psychiatry 1998; 155(9): 1163–71.
16. Bromet E, Sonnega A, Kessler RC. Risk factors for DSM-III-R posttraumatic stress disorder: findings from the National Comorbidity Survey. Am J Epidemiol 1998; 147(4): 353–61.
17. Hoven CW, Duarte CS, Lucas CP et al. Psychopathology among New York city public school children 6 months after September 11. Arch Gen Psychiatry 2005 62(5): 545–52.
18. Hoven CW, Duarte CS, Mandell DJ. Children's mental health after disasters: the impact of the World Trade Center attack. Curr Psychiatry Rep 2003; 5(2): 101–7.

19. Duarte CS, Hoven CW, Wu P et al. Posttraumatic stress in children with first responders in their families. J Trauma Stress 2006; 19(2): 301–6.
20. Skre I, Onstad S, Torgersen S, Lygren S, Kringlen E. A twin study of DSM-III-R anxiety disorders. Acta Psychiatr Scand 1993; 88(2): 85–92.
21. True WR, Rice J, Eisen SA et al. A twin study of genetic and environmental contributions to liability for posttraumatic stress symptoms. Arch Gen Psychiatry 1993 50(4): 257–64.
22. Lyons MJ, Goldberg J, Eisen SA et al. Do genes influence exposure to trauma? A twin study of combat. Am J Med Genet 1993; 48(1): 22–7.
23. Comings DE, Comings BG, Muhleman D et al. The dopamine D2 receptor locus as a modifying gene in neuropsychiatric disorders. JAMA 1991; 266(13): 1793–800.
24. Comings DE, Muhleman D, Gysin R. Dopamine D2 receptor (DRD2) gene and susceptibility to posttraumatic stress disorder: a study and replication. Biol Psychiatry 1996; 40(5): 368–72.
25. Gelernter J, Southwick S, Goodson S et al. No association between D2 dopamine receptor (DRD2) "A" system alleles, or DRD2 haplotypes, and posttraumatic stress disorder. Biol Psychiatry 1999; 45(5): 620–5.
26. Young RM, Lawford BR, Noble EP et al. Harmful drinking in military veterans with post-traumatic stress disorder: association with the D2 dopamine receptor A1 allele. Alcohol Alcohol 2002; 37(5): 451–6.
27. Lawford BR, McD Young R, Noble EP et al. D2 dopamine receptor gene polymorphism: paroxetine and social functioning in posttraumatic stress disorder. Eur Neuropsychopharmacol 2003; 13(5): 313–20.
28. Lawford BR, Young R, Noble EP, Kann B, Ritchie T. The D2 dopamine receptor (DRD2) gene is associated with co-morbid depression, anxiety and social dysfunction in untreated veterans with post-traumatic stress disorder. Eur Psychiatry 2006; 21(3): 180–5.
29. Noble EP, Blum K, Ritchie T, Montgomery A, Sheridan PJ. Allelic association of the D2 dopamine receptor gene with receptor-binding characteristics in alcoholism. Arch Gen Psychiatry 1991; 48(7): 648–54.
30. Pohjalainen T, Rinne JO, Någren K et al. The A1 allele of the human D2 dopamine receptor gene predicts low D2 receptor availability in healthy volunteers. Mol Psychiatry 1998; 3(3): 256–60.
31. Heinz A, Siessmeier T, Wrase J et al. Correlation between dopamine D(2) receptors in the ventral striatum and central processing of alcohol cues and craving. Am J Psychiatry 2004; 161(10): 1783–9.
32. Segman RH, Cooper-Kazaz R, Macciardi F et al. Association between the dopamine transporter gene and posttraumatic stress disorder. Mol Psychiatry 2002; 7(8): 903–7.
33. Heinz A, Goldman D, Jones DW et al. Genotype influences in vivo dopamine transporter availability in human striatum. Neuropsychopharmacology 2000; 22(2): 133–9.
34. Jacobsen LK, Staley JK, Zoghbi SS et al. Prediction of dopamine transporter binding availability by genotype: a preliminary report. Am J Psychiatry 2000; 157(10): 1700–3.
35. Martinez D, Gelernter J, Abi-Dargham A et al. The variable number of tandem repeats polymorphism of the dopamine transporter gene is not associated with significant change in dopamine transporter phenotype in humans. Neuropsychopharmacology 2001; 24(5): 553–60.
36. Lynch DR, Mozley PD, Sokol S et al. Lack of effect of polymorphisms in dopamine metabolism related genes on imaging of TRODAT-1 in striatum of asymptomatic volunteers and patients with Parkinson's disease. Mov Disord 2003; 18(7): 804–12.
37. van Dyck CH, Malison RT, Jacobsen LK et al. Increased dopamine transporter availability associated with the 9-repeat allele of the SLC6A3 gene. J Nucl Med 2005; 46(5): 745–51.
38. Cubells JF, Zabetian CP. Human genetics of plasma dopamine beta-hydroxylase activity: applications to research in psychiatry and neurology. Psychopharmacology (Berl) 2004; 174(4): 463–76.
39. Mustapic´ M, Pivac N, Kozaric´-Kovacic´ D et al. Dopamine beta-hydroxylase (DBH) activity and -1021C/T polymorphism of DBH gene in combat-related post-traumatic stress disorder. Am J Med Genet B Neuropsychiatr Genet 2007; 144(8): 1087–9.
40. Zabetian CP, Anderson GM, Buxbaum SG et al. A quantitative-trait analysis of human plasma dopamine beta-hydroxylase activity: evidence for a major functional polymorphism at the DBH locus. Am J Hum Genet 2001; 68(2): 515–22.
41. Köhnke MD, Zabetian CP, Anderson GM et al. A genotype-controlled analysis of plasma dopamine beta-hydroxylase in healthy and alcoholic subjects: evidence for alcohol-related differences in noradrenergic function. Biol Psychiatry 2002; 52(12): 1151–8.
42. Lesch KP, Bengel D, Heils A et al. Association of anxiety-related traits with a polymorphism in the serotonin transporter gene regulatory region. Science 1996; 274(5292): 1527–31.
43. Lee HJ, Lee MS, Kang RH et al. Influence of the serotonin transporter promoter gene polymorphism on susceptibility to posttraumatic stress disorder. Depress Anxiety 2005; 21(3): 135–9.
44. Caspi A, Sugden K, Moffitt TE et al. Influence of life stress on depression: moderation by a polymorphism in the 5-HTT gene. Science 2003; 301(5631): 386–9.
45. Eley TC, Sugden K, Corsico A et al. Gene-environment interaction analysis of serotonin system markers with adolescent depression. Mol Psychiatry 2004; 9(10): 908–15.

46. Kendler KS, Kuhn JW, Vittum J, Prescott CA, Riley B. The interaction of stressful life events and a serotonin transporter polymorphism in the prediction of episodes of major depression: a replication. Arch Gen Psychiatry 2005; 62(5): 529–35.

47. Kim JM, Stewart R, Kim SW et al. Interactions between life stressors and susceptibility genes (5-HTTLPR and BDNF) on depression in Korean elders. Biol Psychiatry 2007; 62(5): 423–8.

48. Kilpatrick DG, Koenen KC, Ruggiero KJ et al. The serotonin transporter genotype and social support and moderation of posttraumatic stress disorder and depression in hurricane-exposed adults. Am J Psychiatry 2007; 164(11): 1693–9.

49. Gillespie NA, Whitfield JB, Williams B, Heath AC, Martin NG. The relationship between stressful life events, the serotonin transporter (5-HTTLPR) genotype and major depression. Psychol Med 2005; 35(1): 101–11.

50. Lasky-Su JA, Faraone SV, Glatt SJ, Tsuang MT. Meta-analysis of the association between two polymorphisms in the serotonin transporter gene and affective disorders. Am J Med Genet B Neuropsychiatr Genet 2005; 133(1): 110–5.

51. Davidson J, Lipper S, Kilts CD, Mahorney S, Hammett E. Platelet MAO activity in posttraumatic stress disorder. Am J Psychiatry 1985; 142(11): 1341–3.

52. Cicin-Sain L, Mimica N, Hranilovic D et al. Posttraumatic stress disorder and platelet serotonin measures. J Psychiatr Res 2000; 34(2): 155–61.

53. Kozaric´-Kovacic´ D, Ljubin T, Rutic´-Puz L et al. Platelet monoamine oxidase activity, ego strength, and neuroticism in soldiers with combat-related current posttraumatic stress disorder. Croat Med J 2000; 41(1): 76–80.

54. Pivac N, Mück-Seler D, Sagud M, Jakovljevic´ M. Platelet serotonergic markers in posttraumatic stress disorder. Prog Neuropsychopharmacol Biol Psychiatry 2002; 26(6): 1193–8.

55. Pivac N, Knezevic J, Kozaric-Kovacic D et al. Monoamine oxidase (MAO) intron 13 polymorphism and platelet MAO-B activity in combat-related posttraumatic stress disorder. J Affect Disord 2007; 103(1–3): 131–8.

56. Deckert J, Catalano M, Syagailo YV et al. Excess of high activity monoamine oxidase A gene promoter alleles in female patients with panic disorder. Hum Mol Genet 1999; 8(4): 621–4.

57. Maron E, Lang A, Tasa G et al. Associations between serotonin-related gene polymorphisms and panic disorder. Int J Neuropsychopharmacol 2005; 8(2): 261–6.

58. Samochowiec J, Hajduk A, Samochowiec A et al. Association studies of MAO-A, COMT, and 5-HTT genes polymorphisms in patients with anxiety disorders of the phobic spectrum. Psychiatry Res 2004; 128(1): 21–6.

59. Flory JD, Manuck SB, Ferrell RE, Ryan CM, Muldoon MF. Memory performance and the apolipoprotein E polymorphism in a community sample of middle-aged adults. Am J Med Genet 2000; 96(6): 707–11.

60. Kuller LH, Shemanski L, Manolio T et al. Relationship between ApoE, MRI findings, and cognitive function in the Cardiovascular Health Study. Stroke 1998; 29(2): 388–98.

61. Cohen RM, Small C, Lalonde F, Friz J, Sunderland T. Effect of apolipoprotein E genotype on hippocampal volume loss in aging healthy women. Neurology 2001; 57(12): 2223–8.

62. Golier J, Yehuda R. Neuropsychological processes in post-traumatic stress disorder. Psychiatr Clin North Am 2002; 25(2): 295–315.

63. Bremner JD, Randall P, Scott TM et al. MRI-based measurement of hippocampal volume in patients with combat-related posttraumatic stress disorder. Am J Psychiatry 1995; 152(7): 973–81.

64. Freeman T, Roca V, Guggenheim F, Kimbrell T, Griffin WS. Neuropsychiatric associations of apolipoprotein E alleles in subjects with combat-related posttraumatic stress disorder. J Neuropsychiatry Clin Neurosci 2005; 17(4): 541–3.

65. McAllister AK, Katz LC, Lo DC. Neurotrophins and synaptic plasticity. Annu Rev Neurosci 1999; 22: 295–318.

66. Rasmusson AM, Shi L, Duman R. Downregulation of BDNF mRNA in the hippocampal dentate gyrus after re-exposure to cues previously associated with footshock. Neuropsychopharmacology 2002; 27(2): 133–42.

67. Zhang H, Ozbay F, Lappalainen J et al. Brain derived neurotrophic factor (BDNF) gene variants and Alzheimer's disease, affective disorders, posttraumatic stress disorder, schizophrenia, and substance dependence. Am J Med Genet B Neuropsychiatr Genet 2006; 141(4): 387–93.

68. Lee HJ, Kang RH, Lim SW et al. Short Communication: No association between the brain-derived neurotrophic factor gene Val66Met polymorphism and posttraumatic stress disorder. Stress and Health 2006; 22: 115–9.

69. Lam P, Cheng CY, Hong CJ, Tsai SJ. Association study of a brain-derived neurotrophic factor (Val66Met) genetic polymorphism and panic disorder. Neuropsychobiology 2004; 49(4): 178–81.

70. Shimizu E, Hashimoto K, Koizumi H et al. No association of the brain-derived neurotrophic factor (BDNF) gene polymorphisms with panic disorder. Prog Neuropsychopharmacol Biol Psychiatry 2005; 29(5): 708–12.

71. Bremner JD, Innis RB, Southwick SM et al. Decreased benzodiazepine receptor binding in prefrontal cortex in combat-related posttraumatic stress disorder. Am J Psychiatry 2000; 157(7): 1120–6.

72. Fujita M, Southwick SM, Denucci CC et al. Central type benzodiazepine receptors in Gulf War veterans with posttraumatic stress disorder. Biol Psychiatry 2004; 56(2): 95–100.

73. Geuze E, van Berckel BN, Lammertsma AA et al. Reduced GABAA benzodiazepine receptor binding in veterans with post-traumatic stress disorder. Mol Psychiatry 2008; 13(1): 74–83.

74. Feusner J, Ritchie T, Lawford B et al. GABA(A) receptor beta 3 subunit gene and psychiatric morbidity in a post-traumatic stress disorder population. Psychiatry Res 2001; 104(2): 109–17.

75. Nakamura K, Yamada K, Iwayama Y et al. Evidence that variation in the peripheral benzodiazepine receptor (PBR) gene influences susceptibility to panic disorder. Am J Med Genet B Neuropsychiatr Genet 2006; 141(3): 222–6.

76. Sand PG, Godau C, Riederer P et al. Exonic variants of the GABA(B) receptor gene and panic disorder. Psychiatr Genet 2000; 10(4): 191–4.

77. Serretti A, Macciardi F, Cusin C et al. GABAA alpha-1 subunit gene not associated with depressive symptomatology in mood disorders. Psychiatr Genet 1998; 8(4): 251–4.

78. Kurumaji A, Nomoto H, Yamada K, Yoshikawa T, Toru M. No association of two missense variations of the benzodiazepine receptor (peripheral) gene and mood disorders in a Japanese sample. Am J Med Genet 2001; 105(2): 172–5.

79. Smith MA, Davidson J, Ritchie JC et al. The corticotropin-releasing hormone test in patients with posttraumatic stress disorder. Biol Psychiatry 1989; 26(4): 349–55.

80. Yehuda R, Kahana B, Binder-Brynes K et al. Low urinary cortisol excretion in Holocaust survivors with posttraumatic stress disorder. Am J Psychiatry 1995; 152(7): 982–6.

81. Yehuda R, Levengood RA, Schmeidler J et al. Increased pituitary activation following metyrapone administration in post-traumatic stress disorder. Psychoneuroendocrinology 1996; 21(1): 1–16.

82. Stein MB, Yehuda R, Koverola C, Hanna C. Enhanced dexamethasone suppression of plasma cortisol in adult women traumatized by childhood sexual abuse. Biol Psychiatry 1997; 42(8): 680–6.

83. Huizenga NA, Koper JW, De Lange P et al. A polymorphism in the glucocorticoid receptor gene may be associated with and increased sensitivity to glucocorticoids in vivo. J Clin Endocrinol Metab 1998; 83(1): 144–51.

84. Wüst S, Van Rossum EF, Federenko IS et al. Common polymorphisms in the glucocorticoid receptor gene are associated with adrenocortical responses to psychosocial stress. J Clin Endocrinol Metab 2004; 89(2): 565–73.

85. Panarelli M, Holloway CD, Fraser R et al. Glucocorticoid receptor polymorphism, skin vasoconstriction, and other metabolic intermediate phenotypes in normal human subjects. J Clin Endocrinol Metab 1998; 83(6): 1846–52.

86. van Rossum EF, Roks PH, de Jong FH et al. Characterization of a promoter polymorphism in the glucocorticoid receptor gene and its relationship to three other polymorphisms. Clin Endocrinol (Oxf) 2004; 61(5): 573–81.

87. Bachmann AW, Sedgley TL, Jackson RV et al. Glucocorticoid receptor polymorphisms and posttraumatic stress disorder. Psychoneuroendocrinology 2005; 30(3): 297–306.

88. Denny WB, Valentine DL, Reynolds PD, Smith DF, Scammell JG. Squirrel monkey immunophilin FKBP51 is a potent inhibitor of glucocorticoid receptor binding. Endocrinology 2000; 141(11): 4107–13.

89. Schiene-Fischer C, Yu C. Receptor accessory folding helper enzymes: the functional role of peptidyl prolyl cis/trans isomerases. FEBS Lett 2001; 495(1–2): 1–6.

90. Binder EB, Salyakina D, Lichtner P et al. Polymorphisms in FKBP5 are associated with increased recurrence of depressive episodes and rapid response to antidepressant treatment. Nat Genet 2004; 36(12): 1319–25.

91. Lekman M, Laje G, Charney D et al. The FKBP5-Gene in depression and treatment response-an association study in the sequenced treatment alternatives to relieve depression (STAR*D) cohort. Biol Psychiatry 2008; 63(12):1103-10.

92. Koenen KC, Saxe G, Purcell S et al. Polymorphisms in FKBP5 are associated with peritraumatic dissociation in medically injured children. Mol Psychiatry 2005; 10(12): 1058–9.

93. Binder EB, Bradley RG, Liu W et al. Association of FKBP5 polymorphisms and childhood abuse with risk of posttraumatic stress disorder symptoms in adults. JAMA 2008; 299(11): 1291–305.

94. Segman RH, Shefi N, Goltser-Dubner T et al. Peripheral blood mononuclear cell gene expression profiles identify emergent post-traumatic stress disorder among trauma survivors. Mol Psychiatry 2005; 10(5): 500–13.

95. Kallio J, Pesonen U, Karvonen MK et al. Enhanced exercise-induced GH secretion in subjects with Pro7 substitution in the prepro-NPY. J Clin Endocrinol Metab 2001; 86(11): 5348–52.

96. Rasmusson AM, Hauger RL, Morgan CA et al. Low baseline and yohimbine-stimulated plasma neuropeptide Y (NPY) levels in combat-related PTSD. Biol Psychiatry 2000; 47(6): 526–39.

97. Morgan CA 3rd, Wang S, Southwick SM et al. Plasma neuropeptide-Y concentrations in humans exposed to military survival training. Biol Psychiatry 2000 47(10): 902–9.

98. Lappalainen J, Kranzler HR, Malison R et al. A functional neuropeptide Y Leu7Pro polymorphism associated with alcohol dependence in a large population sample from the United States. Arch Gen Psychiatry 2002; 59(9): 825–31.

99. Liew CC, Ma J, Tang HC, Zheng R, Dempsey AA. The peripheral blood transcriptome dynamically reflects system wide biology: a potential diagnostic tool. J Lab Clin Med 2006; 147: 126–32.

100. Barnes MG, Aronow BJ, Luyrink LK et al. Gene expression in juvenile arthritis and spondyloarthropathy: pro-angiogenic ELR+ chemokine genes relate to course of arthritis. Rheumatology (Oxford) 2004; 43(8): 973–9.

101. Morello F, de Bruin TW, Rotter JI et al. Differential gene expression of blood-derived cell lines in familial combined hyperlipidemia. Arterioscler Thromb Vasc Biol 2004; 24(11): 2149–54.

102. Bull TM, Coldren CD, Moore M et al. Gene microarray analysis of peripheral blood cells in pulmonary arterial hypertension. Am J Respir Crit Care Med 2004 170(8): 911–9.

103. Philibert RA, Crowe R, Ryu GY et al. Transcriptional profiling of lymphoblast lines from subjects with panic disorder. Am J Med Genet B Neuropsychiatr Genet 2007; 144(5): 674–82.

104. Maron E, Kallassalu K, Tammiste A, et al. Peripheral gene expression profiling of CCK-4-induced panic in healthy subjects. Am J Med Genet B Neuropsychiatr Genet. 2008 Dec 2. [Epub ahead of print]

105. Zieker J, Zieker D, Jatzko A et al. Differential gene expression in peripheral blood of patients suffering from post-traumatic stress disorder. Mol Psychiatry 2007; 12(2): 116–8.

106. Koenen KC, Fu QJ, Ertel K et al. Common genetic liability to major depression and posttraumatic stress disorder in men. J Affect Disord 2008; 105(1–3): 109–15.

107. Fu Q, Koenen KC, Miller MW et al. Differential etiology of posttraumatic stress disorder with conduct disorder and major depression in male veterans. Biol Psychiatry 2007; 62(10): 1088–94.

108. Koenen KC, Hitsman B, Lyons MJ et al. A twin registry study of the relationship between posttraumatic stress disorder and nicotine dependence in men. Arch Gen Psychiatry 2005; 62(11): 1258–65.

109. Chantarujikapong SI, Scherrer JF, Xian H et al. A twin study of generalized anxiety disorder symptoms, panic disorder symptoms and post-traumatic stress disorder in men. Psychiatry Res 2001; 103(2–3): 133–45.

110. Gross C, Zhuang X, Stark K et al. Serotonin1A receptor acts during development to establish normal anxiety-like behaviour in the adult. Nature 2002; 416(6879): 396–400.

111. Heisler LK, Chu HM, Brennan TJ et al. Elevated anxiety and antidepressant-like responses in serotonin 5-HT1A receptor mutant mice. Proc Natl Acad Sci U S A 1998; 95(25): 15049–54.

112. Holmes A, Lit Q, Murphy DL, Gold E, Crawley JN. Abnormal anxiety-related behavior in serotonin transporter null mutant mice: the influence of genetic background. Genes Brain Behav 2003; 2(6): 365–80.

113. Parks CL, Robinson PS, Sibille E, Shenk T, Toth M. Increased anxiety of mice lacking the serotonin1A receptor. Proc Natl Acad Sci U S A 1998; 95(18): 10734–9.

114. Pattij T, Groenink L, Hijzen TH et al. Autonomic changes associated with enhanced anxiety in 5-HT(1A) receptor knockout mice. Neuropsychopharmacology 2002; 27(3): 380–90.

115. Ramboz S, Oosting R, Amara DA et al. Serotonin receptor 1A knockout: an animal model of anxietyrelated disorder. Proc Natl Acad Sci U S A 1998; 95(24): 14476–81.

116. Sibille E, Pavlides C, Benke D, Toth M. Genetic inactivation of the Serotonin(1A) receptor in mice results in downregulation of major GABA(A) receptor alpha subunits, reduction of GABA(A) receptor binding, and benzodiazepine-resistant anxiety. J Neurosci 2000; 20(8): 2758–65.

117. Klemenhagen KC, Gordon JA, David DJ, Hen R, Gross CT. Increased fear response to contextual cues in mice lacking the 5-HT1A receptor. Neuropsychopharmacology 2006; 31(1): 101–11.

118. Bonne O, Bain E, Neumeister A et al. No change in serotonin type 1A receptor binding in patients with posttraumatic stress disorder. Am J Psychiatry 2005; 162(2): 383–5.

119. Booker TK, Butt CM, Wehner JM, Heinemann SF, Collins AC. Decreased anxiety-like behavior in beta3 nicotinic receptor subunit knockout mice. Pharmacol Biochem Behav 2007; 87(1): 146–57.

120. Marsch R, Foeller E, Rammes G et al. Reduced anxiety, conditioned fear, and hippocampal long-term potentiation in transient receptor potential vanilloid type 1 receptor-deficient mice. J Neurosci 2007; 27(4): 832–9.

121. Nico PB, de-Paris F, Vinadé ER et al. Altered behavioural response to acute stress in mice lacking cellular prion protein. Behav Brain Res 2005; 162(2): 173–81.

122. Smith DG, Davis RJ, Rorick-Kehn L et al. Melanin-concentrating hormone-1 receptor modulates neuroendocrine, behavioral, and corticolimbic neurochemical stress responses in mice Neuropsychopharmacology 2006; 31(6): 1135–45.

123. Chourbaji S, Urani A, Inta I et al. IL-6 knockout mice exhibit resistance to stress-induced development of depression-like behaviors. Neurobiol Dis 2006; 23(3): 587–94.

124. Bale TL, Contarino A, Smith GW et al. Mice deficient for corticotropin-releasing hormone receptor-2 display anxiety-like behaviour and are hypersensitive to stress. Nat Genet 2000; 24(4): 410–4.

125. Gammie SC, Hasen NS, Stevenson SA, Bale TL, D'Anna KL. Elevated stress sensitivity in corticotropinreleasing factor receptor 2 deficient mice decreases maternal, but not intermale aggression. Behav Brain Res 2005; 160(1): 169–77.

126. Müller MB, Zimmermann S, Sillaber I et al. Limbic corticotropin-releasing hormone receptor 1 mediates anxiety-related behavior and hormonal adaptation to stress. Nat Neurosci 2003; 6(10): 1100–7.

127. Holmes A, Kinney JW, Wrenn CC et al. Galanin GAL-R1 receptor null mutant mice display increased anxiety-like behavior specific to the elevated plus-maze. Neuropsychopharmacology 2003; 28(6):1031–44.

128. Jacobson LH, Bettler B, Kaupmann K, Cryan JF. Behavioral evaluation of mice deficient in GABA(B(1)) receptor isoforms in tests of unconditioned anxiety. Psychopharmacology (Berl) 2007; 190(4):541–53.

129. Zeng H, Gragerov A, Hohmann JG et al. Neuromedin U receptor 2-deficient mice display differential responses in sensory perception, stress, and feeding. Mol Cell Biol 2006; 26(24): 9352–63.

130. Bhatnagar S, Sun LM, Raber J et al. Changes in anxiety-related behaviors and hypothalamicpituitary-adrenal activity in mice lacking the 5-HT-3A receptor. Physiol Behav 2004; 81(4): 545–55.

131. Liberzon I, López JF, Flagel SB, Vázquez DM, Young EA. Differential regulation of hippocampal glucocorticoid receptors mRNA and fast feedback: relevance to post-traumatic stress disorder. J Neuroendocrinol 1999; 11(1): 11–7.

132. Rozeboom AM, Akil H, Seasholtz AF. Mineralocorticoid receptor overexpression in forebrain decreases anxiety-like behavior and alters the stress response in mice. Proc Natl Acad Sci U S A 2007;104(11): 4688–93.

134. Fujikawa T, Soya H, Fukuoka H et al. A biphasic regulation of receptor mRNA expressions for growth hormone, glucocorticoid and mineralocorticoid in the rat dentate gyrus during acute stress. Brain Res 2000; 874(2): 186–93.

135. Iwamoto Y, Morinobu S, Takahashi T, Yamawaki S. Single prolonged stress increases contextual freezing and the expression of glycine transporter 1 and vesicle-associated membrane protein 2 mRNA in the hippocampus of rats. Prog Neuropsychopharmacol Biol Psychiatry 2007; 31(3): 642–51.

136. Kozlovsky N, Matar MA, Kaplan Z et al. The immediate early gene Arc is associated with behavioral resilience to stress exposure in an animal model of posttraumatic stress disorder. Eur Neuropsychopharmacol 2008; 18(2): 107–16.

137. Kozlovsky N, Matar MA, Kaplan Z et al. Long-term down-regulation of BDNF mRNA in rat hippocampal CA1 subregion correlates with PTSD-like behavioural stress response. Int J Neuropsychopharmacol 2007; 10(6): 741–58.

138. Guzowski JF, Lyford GL, Stevenson GD et al. Inhibition of activity-dependent arc protein expression in the rat hippocampus impairs the maintenance of long-term potentiation and the consolidation of long-term memory. J Neurosci 2000; 20(11): 3993–4001.

139. Plath N, Ohana O, Dammermann B et al. Arc/Arg3.1 is essential for the consolidation of synaptic plasticity and memories. Neuron 2006; 52(3): 437–44.

140. Friedman A, Kaufer D, Shemer J et al. Pyridostigmine brain penetration under stress enhances neuronal excitability and induces early immediate transcriptional response. Nat Med 1996; 2(12):1382–5.

141. Kaufer D, Friedman A, Seidman S, Soreq H. Acute stress facilitates long-lasting changes in cholinergic gene expression. Nature 1998; 393(6683): 373–7.

142. Zhang L, Zhou R, Xing G, et al. Identification of gene markers based on well validated and subcategorized stressed animals for potential clinical applications in PTSD. Med Hypotheses. 2006;66(2):309-14.

143. Bilang-Bleuel A, Ulbricht S, Chandramohan Y et al. Psychological stress increases histone H3 phosphorylation in adult dentate gyrus granule neurons: involvement in a glucocorticoid receptordependent behavioural response. Eur J Neurosci 2005 22(7): 1691–700.

144. Chandramohan Y, Droste SK, Reul JM. Novelty stress induces phospho-acetylation of histone H3 in rat dentate gyrus granule neurons through coincident signalling via the N-methyl-D-aspartate receptor and the glucocorticoid receptor: relevance for c-fos induction. J Neurochem 2007; 101(3):815–28.

145. Hariri AR, Weinberger DR. Functional neuroimaging of genetic variation in serotonergic neurotransmission. Genes Brain Behav 2003; 2(6): 341–9.

7 | Setting apart the affected—a novel animal model for posttraumatic stress disorder and its translational perspective

Joseph Zohar, Michael Matar, and Hagit Cohen

INTRODUCTION

Although animal models of psychiatric disorders are limited to the assessment of measurable and observable behavioral parameters and cannot assess complex psychological symptoms such as thought, meaning, and dreams, they are still useful. Valid and reliable animal models may provide a means for researching biomolecular, pathophysiological, and pharmacological features of the disorder in ways which are not feasible in human studies. They are not only relatively cheap but also enable an intervention with compounds and methods that would not be allowed in humans. Animal models also enable a prospective follow-up design, in which the disorder is triggered at a specified time and in a uniform manner, in controllable and statistically sound population samples (in terms of size and composition, including genetically manipulated and inbred strains), and enable the assessment of behavioral and gross physiological parameters. Moreover, and unlike studies in human subjects, they enable the assessment of concomitant biomolecular changes in dissected brain areas.

Certain criteria must be fulfilled in order to achieve a satisfactory degree of reliability and validity in modeling the complexities of psychiatric disorders. For example, the behavioral responses must be clearly observable and measurable, must reliably reflect clinical symptomatology, and pharmacological agents known to affect symptoms in human subjects should correct the parameters that model symptoms with equal efficacy.

However, many animal models for psychiatric disorders are from their onset subject to a hypothetical paradigm, for example, bulbectomy or inescapable shock for an animal model of depression, and so on. In posttraumatic stress disorder (PTSD) the situation is entirely different; the trigger is well-known and universal—exposure to a traumatic event, and hence the center of gravity shifts from how to induce it to how to "diagnose" those animals who develop PTSD vs. those who do not. The behavioral cutoff criteria were introduced, based on this concept—setting apart the affected—isolates and studies those animals who developed "PTSD-like behavior," comparing them to those who did not develop PTSD (although they were exposed to trauma) and to those who were not exposed.

Researchers who work with animals have long been aware that individual study subjects tend to display a varying range of responses to stimuli, certainly where stress paradigms are concerned. This heterogeneity in responses was accepted for many years, regarded as unavoidable, and mostly swept under the carpet. The hallmark of PTSD is the differential response to trauma, and the main issue is why the majority of those exposed to trauma do not develop PTSD (the resilience issue), and only a minority do. Hence, in an animal model of PTSD, the heterogeneity in animal responses might be regarded the heart of the model as it presents face validity rather than a problem. It stands to reason that an animal model that includes "diagnostic criteria" may augment the validity of the disorder studied. However, the criteria for classification should be clearly defined, reliably reproducible, and yield results that conform to findings in human subjects.

This chapter will present findings from a series of studies in an animal model of PTSD employing individual behavioral response classification. A brief introduction to the standard stress paradigm, the standard behavioral methods, and the definition of the cutoff behavioral criteria (CBC) employed for classification will precede this.

The Predator-Scent Stress Paradigm

Stress paradigms in animals studies aim to model criterion A of the *DSM-IV-TR* diagnostic criteria (1) They have thus consisted of extremely stressful experiences that create a sense of threat and helplessness in the study subjects. Many of the paradigms emphasize the ethological validity of the threatening or painful experience.

The standard stressor in the following studies consists of exposure of rodents to the scent of the urine of their prime predator—the cat. Blanchard et al. (2–7), Adamec et al. (8–13), and others (14–16) have established the validity of this paradigm, in which adult rodents are inescapably exposed to urine-soiled substrate (cat litter) for 5–10 minutes in a closed environment, where both "fight" and "flight" options are ineffective. Predator stress has ecological validity in that it mimics brief, intense threatening experiences inducing the expected range of behavioral and physiological responses. The potency of predator scent stress (PSS) is comparable to that of paradigms in which the threat is more tangible and immediate, as compared to paradigms based on induction of other stressors such as inescapable pain, electric shock, or direct (protected) proximity to a kitten or a cat. Exposure to unsoiled cat litter serves as the standard trauma-cue paradigm, and immediate response to the cue is assessed by freezing behavior recorded on an overhead camera.

Behavioral Assessments

A variety of mazes and open environments have been employed to assess changes in exploratory behavior resulting from stress exposure and to reflect the response amplitude. These test environments assess behaviors that indicate anxiety-like fearful behaviors and behaviors reflecting avoidance. Various learning and memory tasks are employed in which both exploration and learned task performance can be assessed. Some studies have investigated social behavior in home cages and in challenge situations. The startle response that characterizes many PTSD patients has also been employed as one of the more definitively measurable parameters for the hypervigilant/hyperalert component of the behavioral responses.(8, 15) In the following studies, exploratory behavior on the elevated plus maze (EPM) serves as the main platform for the assessment of overall behavior, and the acoustic startle response (ASR) paradigm provides a precise quantification of hyperalertness, in terms of magnitude of response and habituation to the stimulus. For details regarding these tests, see Cohen et al.(17–23)

As to the timing of behavioral assessments, a large number of studies performed in a range of research centers indicate quite clearly that behavioral changes that are observed in rodents at Day 7 after stress exposure are unlikely to change significantly over the next 30 days.(23) The average life expectancy for the domestic rat is between 2.5 and 3 years. Hence, behavioral patterns observed at Day 7 can reliably be taken to represent PTSD-like responses (i.e., "translating" a week for a rat to a month for a human).

Classification according to Cutoff Behavioral Criteria

Data from a series of studies had previously shown that 7 days after a single 10-minute predator-scent exposure, the overall exposed population displayed significantly decreased time spent in the open arms and increased time in the closed arms of the EPM (which is translated to "avoidant" and "anxiety-like behavior"), and higher mean startle responses as compared to control rats (Figure 7.1). It is important to note that the rats' behavior was not uniformly disturbed but rather demonstrated a broad range of variation in response severity. The pooled data were reexamined for definable behavioral criteria and revealed a group of animals whose behavioral response patterns clearly demonstrated no significant difference from unexposed control animals, and a second group whose responses to both test paradigms were equally significantly at the extreme end on all measures. Each of these groups was significantly distinct from animals whose behavior lay between the extremes.

The behavioral measures for each of these groups on the EPM and ASR tests were employed to define the basic cutoff behavioral criteria (CBC). As clinical diagnostic criteria require a sufficient number of symptoms from three symptom clusters in order to achieve satisfactory diagnostic specificity, the CBC response classification process would require that a given rat fulfill all criteria on *both* tests to be performed in series. The standard algorithm for the CBC classification model also requires that prior to classification, a significant overall effect be demonstrated. (Figure 7.2).

The CBCs enable us to clearly define a given rat as displaying extreme behavioral response (EBR) or minimal behavioral response (MBR; that is, extreme responses on *both* EPM and ASR tests led to classification as EBR, whereas minimal responses were defined as MBR)—both of which have been validated in a large series of studies. The remaining rats display clearly disrupted behavior patterns compared to controls, but the extent of the disruption does not

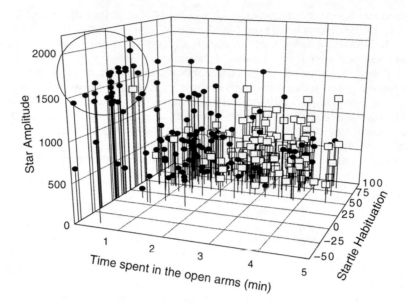

Figure 7.1 The effect of single PSS-exposure vs. unexposed control on rat anxiety-like behavior and acoustic startle response & habituation. The graphic representation of the data from both paradigms (EPM and ASR) reveals two obvious and rather distinct features. Firstly, it is clear that PSS-exposure alters the response of the majority of individuals to at least some degree. Secondly the cluster of individuals that forms in the upper left hand corner of the graph (i.e. more extreme responses to exposure) is quite distinct from the majority of individuals and could therefore be interpreted as representing "PTSD-like" behavior.

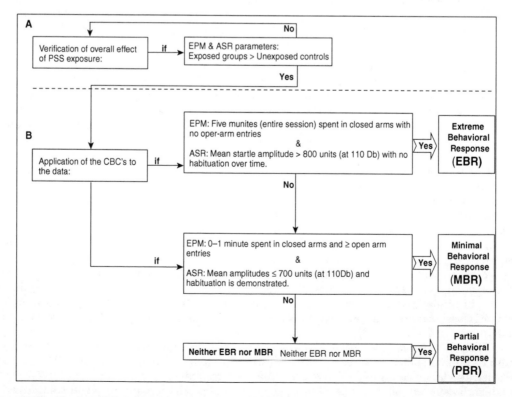

Figure 7.2 The Cut-off Behavioral Criteria (CBC) algorithm.

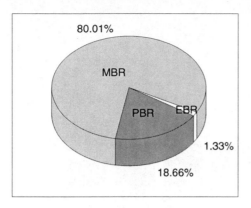
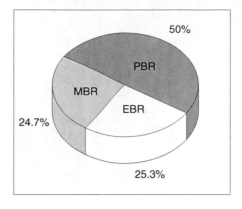

A: Unexposed populations   B: PSS-exposed animals

Figure 7.3   Re-analysis of data applying Cut-off Behavioral Criteria A) Unexposed populations B) PSS-exposed animals.

cross the threshold for EBR. These are labeled partial behavioral responders (PBR) and have as yet not been further subclassified.(19, 22, 23)

The pooled behavioral data for entire exposed populations were reexamined according to the CBCs, revealing that the overall prevalence rate for EBR rats was approximately 25% (Figure 7.3A), as compared to 1.3% in unexposed control populations (Figure 7.3B). The prevalence of MBR rats in the PSS-exposed groups was 24.7% (Figure 7.3A) as compared to 80.0% in the control groups (Figure 7.2B).

The implication of this initial finding was that all prior study analyses must have included a significant proportion of animals whose behavior had not been affected by the stressor (MBR) and many animals whose response was of uncertain significance (PBR), alongside those whose response was unequivocally one of severely disrupted behavioral patterns (EBR). Hence, the method offered a feasible means for classifying animal response patterns to trauma, thereby increasing the conceptual accuracy of the data.

It is interesting to note that the proportion of the entire exposed population fulfilling criteria for extreme responses (EBR) was also compatible with epidemiological data for PTSD among trauma-exposed human populations (24), which report that between 15% and 35% fulfill criteria for PTSD and that approximately 20% to 30% display partial or subsymptomatic clinical pictures.(24–26) This compatibility further supported the concept of criterion-based classification in terms of face validity.

SELECTED CBC-BASED STUDIES

Behavioral response patterns vs. time
Time is an integral factor in traumatic stress–induced disorders. The prevalence rates of EBR rats were assessed among PSS-exposed rats on Days 1, 3, 5, 7, 30, and 90 after exposure (Figure 7.4). Initially (Day 1) almost all animals displayed extreme disruptions of behavior (EBR = 90%). The proportion of EBR animals dropped rapidly over Days 3 and 5 to about 25% at Day 7. This proportion remained stable till Day 30, dropping to about 15% by Day 90. The resulting time curve of EBR prevalence rates parallels the rates of stress-related symptoms in humans, culminating in acute and chronic traumatic stress disorders.(23)

Physiological correlates
Physiological data were correlated with behavioral classification in a series of studies, including the HPA axis (circulating corticosterone, dehydroepiandrosterone (DHEA), and its sulphate derivative DHEA-S levels), autonomic nervous system (heart rate and heart rate variability) (19, 27), and immune system.(28) Although the gross population data had shown that the parameters

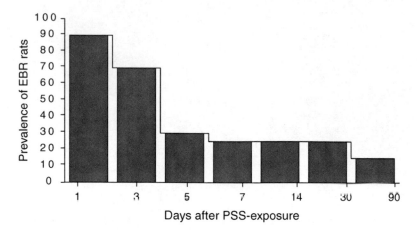

Figure 7.4   Prevalence of EBR rats after single PSS-exposure as a function of time.

in each study displayed significant responses to the stressor, CBC classification revealed that animals whose behavior conformed to EBR criteria were characterized by significantly more disturbances on all measures, whereas MBR rats displayed almost none.

Strain/genetic studies

The CBC classification model was applied to genetically manipulated rodent strains in order to examine two aspects of PTSD. One study assessed the HPA-axis response in rat strains inbred to have either deficient or excessive HPA-axis responsiveness, compared to outbred rats. The other examined the heritability of vulnerability vs. resilience factors using inbred (near-isogenic) mouse strains exposed to PSS and classified according to the CBC method.

a) HPA-axis response Lewis and Fischer rats: PTSD has been associated with disordered levels of circulating cortisol, an integral component of the stress response (increased levels according to some studies, and decreased in others).(29–45) Naturalistic clinical observations in intensive care units (46) and treatment of septic shock (47, 48) show that administration of cortisol reduces the incidence of cases of PTSD.(46–48)

The animal model provides an opportunity to address questions such as whether low basal cortisol levels represent a consequence of traumatic exposure (i.e., possible neurotoxic effects of trauma) or a predisposing trait for pathological stress reactions, by looking at populations of inbred Lewis and Fischer rats compared to outbred Sprague–Dawley rats. Lewis rats exhibit a reduced synthesis and secretion of corticotrophin-releasing factor (CRF), leading to reduced plasma ACTH and reduced CORT release from the adrenal cortex, whereas Fischer rats possess a hyperresponsive HPA axis. Prevalence rates of EBR individuals were significantly higher in Lewis (50%) than in Fischer rats (10%), or controls (25%) (49). Moreover, exogenous administration of cortisol to Lewis rats, before applying the stressor, decreased the prevalence of EBR significantly (8%).(49) These results suggest that a blunted HPA-axis response to stress may play a role in the susceptibility to experimentally induced PTSD-like behavioral changes, especially as these effects were reversed by preexposure administration of corticosterone.

b) Stress-induced behavioral responses in inbred mouse strains: Twin and family studies of PTSD patients raise questions as to a possible genetic predisposition to PTSD, although the relative contributions of the genotype and environment to endophenotypic expression are unclear.

Six inbred strains of mice frequently employed in transgenic research were assessed at baseline and 7 days after PSS exposure.(50) Inbred strains are expected to demonstrate ~97.5% homozygosity of loci as the result of at least 20 generations of sibling matings. The results, however, revealed an unexpectedly high degree of within-strain individual heterogeneity at baseline and in the degree of response to stress. This within-strain phenotypic heterogeneity might imply that environmental factors play a significant role in characterizing individual responses, in spite of the significant strain-related, that is, genetic, underpinnings.(51, 52)

Molecular Neurobiological Correlates

Selected brain areas, especially hippocampal substructures and frontal cortex, of rats classified according to the CBC procedure have been studied in correlation to both their behavioral and physiological response patterns. The studies have examined the expression of genes and gene products for key intracellular and intercellular biomolecules associated with neuromodulation, synaptic plasticity, and receptor systems. In some studies, these data have also been correlated to individual performance on memory-related tasks.

The development of an EBR response has been shown to be associated with a distinct pattern of long-term and persistent downregulation of mRNA for brain-derived neurotrophic factor (BDNF) and synaptophysin, and an upregulation of glucocorticoid receptor (GR) protein levels and tyrosine kinase receptor (TrkB) mRNA in the CA1 subregion of the hippocampus, compared to PBR and MBR animals and to unexposed controls.(53) The persistently higher levels of glucocorticoids are associated with the attenuation of BDNF, synaptophysin, and immediately early genes such as activity-regulated, cytoskeletal-associated protein (Arc) and zif/268 expression in the EBR rats, suggesting that they reflect or mediate the characteristic changes in neural plasticity and synaptic functioning underlying chronic stress-induced behavioral disruption. Neurotrophins, and particularly BDNF, are known to modulate many aspects of neuronal plasticity (54, 55) and the selection of functional neuronal connections in the CNS. (56–58) The decreased expression of BDNF (mRNA and protein) levels in EBR individuals may be associated with a decrease in synaptic plasticity and impairment of the stabilization of synaptic connectivity, which may be linked to vulnerability to psychopathology. Decreased hippocampal expression of synaptophysin, a major integral protein on synaptic vesicles, might also be associated with hippocampal damage that may occur during stress exposure.(59) Taken together, decreased hippocampal expression of these genes may have physiological consequences, for example, inducing damage to hippocampal neurons.

SSRIs and other antidepressant drugs were found to reinforce synaptic strength in mood-related brain regions in a manner akin to that achieved in experimental models of synaptic plasticity.(60, 61) Pei et al. (62) reported that repeated administration of the monoamine reuptake inhibitors— paroxetine, venlafaxine, or desipramine—induced region-specific increases in Arc mRNA (in the frontal and parietal cortex and hippocampal CA1 area). Thus, whereas downregulation of Arc mRNA has been shown to promote stress-induced psychopathology in synaptic networks, long-term administration of SSRIs and so on might either prevent or reverse this effect. Taken together, SSRIs might, therefore, be able to protect and/or to rescue the functional integrity of neuronal circuitry from the effects of stress.(53)

Drug studies

Acute-phase pharmacotherapeutic interventions that effectively alleviate symptoms and possess potential preventive effects on the development of PTSD founded on large-scale, double-blind, controlled, and prospective clinical trails are lacking. The CBC classification model affords distinct advantages in the prospective study of the therapeutic and preventive potential of medications. The model enables the prospective study of associations between the behavioral efficacy of the drug in question in a quantifiable manner over specific periods of time, and the biomolecular and physiological correlates of these behavioral effects. The CBC model was applied to the study of number of drugs—a selective serotonin reuptake inhibitor (sertraline), corticosteroids, and a benzodiazepine (alprazolam).

a) Early intervention with an SSRI (Sertraline): Based on the rationale that the acute phase in rodents is represented by the first 7 days following stress exposure (discussed in "Behavioral Assessments" in this chapter), rats were randomly allocated to 7 days of treatment either immediately following exposure or as of day 7, compared to saline treatment. Behavioral and biomolecular assessments performed at Day 7 (or Day 14) demonstrated the following: Brief, immediate postexposure intervention with sertraline had an observable short-term effect on stress-induced behavioral changes that was comparable to the later treatment regimen and compared to the saline-treated control group.(63) Seven days of treatment with sertraline immediately after PSS-exposure elicited a statistically significant reduction (14%) in prevalence rates of EBR and an increase of 5% in prevalence rates of minimal response (MBR) compared to the placebo-control group. The early treatment group displayed a reduced prevalence of extreme anxiety-like and avoidant behaviors on the EPM and an attenuation of the exaggerated

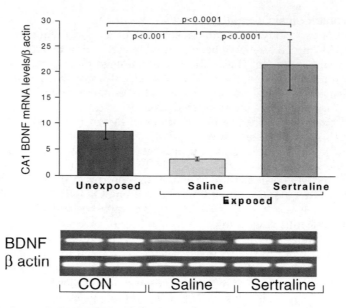

Figure 7.5 Quantitative analysis of BDNF mRNA expression. BDNF mRNA expression levels in the CA1 hippocampal subregion following saline or sertraline treatment.

hyperarousal responses, equivalent to the patterns of behavior of unexposed animals, and a significant degree of reversal of the deficit in habituation of the acoustic startle response observed in controls.(63) These finding suggest that SSRI drugs represent potential agents for secondary intervention in the acute aftermath of traumatic stress exposure and are thus worthy of further investigation. Moreover, 7 days of treatment with sertraline immediately after PSS-exposure normalized long-term changes of BDNF mRNA in PTSD-like animals in parallel with the improvement in their behavioral responses (Unpublished data - Figure 7.5).

b) Early intervention with corticosterone: As corticosteroid treatment is clinically indicated only in cases in which there is significant physical illness or polytrauma, recurrent clinical reports of a significant preventive effect in terms of the incidence of concomitant PTSD are difficult to interpret, despite their relative frequency and impressive results.(46–48, 64–66) The CBC model was employed to examine the effect of a single high-dose intervention with the adrenocorticoid stress hormone CORT given immediately after exposure. This regimen was compared to lower doses, later treatment, and saline. Stress-induced behavioral responses were assessed at Day 30 and trauma-cue triggered freezing-response was assessed on Day 31.

The results clearly showed that a single 25 mg/kg dose of CORT administered immediately after exposure to the scent of predator urine resulted in a statistically significant reduction of 13.2% in the prevalence rates of EBR individuals at 30 days, with a concomitant increase of 12.4% in the prevalence of MBR individuals, as compared to saline , that is, a significant shift toward less extreme behavioral disruption ensuing from traumatic stress.(67) Rats in the high-dose CORT group responded markedly less extremely to exposure to the trauma cue (24% of time freezing) than the saline-control group (80% of time freezing). This pattern of response suggests that the single high-dose CORT treatment had conferred some degree of resilience to future trauma-related stress exposure.(67) Lower doses of CORT (0.1–5.0 mg/kg) were ineffective in attenuating behavioral disruptions and significantly increased the prevalence of EBR (at Day 30) and the vulnerability to the trauma cue as compared to placebo.

The marked attenuation of the response of treated individuals to the trauma cue 31 days after exposure is of significance. The time frame in which CORT was administered (1 hour after stress exposure) conforms to the time frame within which the memory consolidation process takes place at the cellular level (3–6 hours after initiation of data acquisition). The time at which the effect was assessed was sufficiently distant from the initial exposure, which goes to show that the effect was mediated by memory-related processes. Furthermore, the same pattern was observed in another study, where the protein synthesis inhibitor Anisomycin was effective when administered within an hour after exposure, but not when administered later on (after reactivation of the trauma by a trauma cue).(68) This may suggest that the single high-dose CORT treatment interfered similarly, by disrupting consolidation of the short-term memory to long-term memory.(67)

    c) Early intervention with benzodiazepine (Alprazolam): Benzodiazepines are commonly used to relieve distress. Because it has been claimed that early administration of BNZ may be associated with a less favorable outcome (69) and because there is a possibility that BNZ may impede adequate processing of acute grief (70), their effects vis-à-vis exposure to stress were examined in the CBC model.

    In this placebo-controlled study, the short-term efficacy and the long-term sequelae of brief early postexposure administration of a commonly prescribed benzodiazepine (Alprazolam) for the prevention of subsequent PTSD-like behavioral changes were examined. The results demonstrated that rats treated immediately after the initial exposure were rendered significantly more vulnerable to the trauma cue and by far more vulnerable to reexposure to PSS than the placebo control groups. However, when the treatment was initiated after 1 week, it did not affect vulnerability.(71) It will be important to establish whether this finding is replicable and whether it is related to specific benzodiazepines and/or a certain time frame, both in animal and in clinical studies. How could this finding be explained? What might be the mechanism? One possible mechanism might be related to the effect of Alprazolam on cortisol secretion. The marked suppression of corticosterone activity during alprazolam treatment and the sharp rebound after its cessation may well be key factors in the pathogenesis of some behavioral responses observed in this study when BNZ treatment was initiated. As was mentioned above, the protective effect of cortisol secretion being entirely abolished by early administration of BNZ coupled with polarity of plasma corticosterone levels may be of great pathogenetic significance, especially in the consolidation phase.(71)

CONCLUSIONS

Animal models might complement clinical research and enable modalities that are difficult to attain in clinical studies. However, it is difficult to come up with an adequate animal model for psychiatric disorders. Because it is possible, in PTSD, to accurately mimic the main etiological factor, that is, exposure to trauma, an animal model of PTSD may be easier to defend. The animal model presented, which is a combination of an exposure to predator and a focus on setting apart the affected based on behavioral cutoff criteria, demonstrated high face validity, construct validity, and predictive validity. The cumulative results of our studies indicate that the validity of this contribution can be further enhanced by classifying individual animal study subjects according to their response patterns. This approach enables researchers to test interventions that might be impossible (i.e., Anisomycin) or difficult (e.g., BNZ, SSRI, Cortisol) to carry out in a clinical setting without any proper preclinical basis. The animal model also enables the researcher to go one step further and correlate specific anatomic biomolecular and physiological parameters with the degree and pattern of individual behavioral response.

REFERENCES

1. American Psychiatric Association. Diagnostic and Statistical Manual of Mental Disorders. 4 ed. Washington, DC. American Psychiatric Association; 2005.
2. Blanchard DC, Griebel G, Blanchard RJ. Conditioning and residual emotionality effects of predator stimuli: some reflections on stress and emotion. Prog Neuropsychopharmacol Biol Psychiatry 2003; 27(8): 1177–85.
3. Blanchard RJ, Blanchard DC. Anti-predator defense as models of fear and anxiety. In: Blanchard RJ and S. Parmigiani, ed. Brain. London: Harwood Academic Publishers, 1990.
4. Blanchard RJ, Blanchard DC, Rodgers J, Weiss SM. The characterization and modelling of antipredator defensive behavior. Neurosci Biobehav Rev 1990; 14(4): 463–72.
5. Blanchard RJ, Griebel G, Henrie JA, Blanchard DC. Differentiation of anxiolytic and panicolytic drugs by effects on rat and mouse defense test batteries. Neurosci Biobehav Rev 1997; 21(6): 783–9.

6.   Blanchard RJ, Nikulina JN, Sakai RR et al. Behavioral and endocrine change following chronic predatory stress. Physiol Behav 1998; 63(4): 561–9.

7.   Blanchard RJ, Yang M, Li CI, Gervacio A, Blanchard DC. Cue and context conditioning of defensive behaviors to cat odor stimuli. Neurosci Biobehav Rev 2001; 25(7–8): 587–95.

8.   Adamec R. Transmitter systems involved in neural plasticity underlying increased anxiety and defense--implications for understanding anxiety following traumatic stress. Neurosci Biobehav Rev 1997; 21(6): 755–65.

9.   Adamec R, Head D, Blundell J, Burton P, Berton O. Lasting anxiogenic effects of feline predator stress in mice: sex differences in vulnerability to stress and predicting severity of anxiogenic response from the stress experience. Physiol Behav 2006; 88(1–2): 12–29.

10. Adamec R, Muir C, Grimes M, Pearcey K. Involvement of noradrenergic and corticoid receptors in the consolidation of the lasting anxiogenic effects of predator stress. Behav Brain Res 2007; 179(2): 192–207.

11. Adamec R, Strasser K, Blundell J, Burton P, McKay DW. Protein synthesis and the mechanisms of lasting change in anxiety induced by severe stress. Behav Brain Res 2006; 167(2): 270–86.

12. Adamec RE, Blundell J, Burton P. Relationship of the predatory attack experience to neural plasticity, pCREB expression and neuroendocrine response. Neurosci Biobehav Rev 2006; 30(3): 356–75.

13. Adamec RE, Shallow T. Lasting effects on rodent anxiety of a single exposure to a cat. Physiol Behav 1993; 54(1): 101–9.

14. Diamond DM, Campbell AM, Park CR et al. Influence of predator stress on the consolidation vs. retrieval of long-term spatial memory and hippocampal spinogenesis. Hippocampus 2006; 16(7): 571–6.

15. File SE, Zangrossi Jr H, Sanders FL, Mabbutt PS. Dissociation between behavioral and corticosterone responses on repeated exposures to cat odor. Physiol Behav 1993; 54: 1109–11.

16. Griebel G, Blanchard DC, Jung A et al. Further evidence that the mouse defense test battery is useful for screening anxiolytic and panicolytic drugs: effects of acute and chronic treatment with alprazolam. Neuropharmacology 1995; 34(12): 1625–33.

17. Cohen H, Benjamin J, Kaplan Z, Kotler M. Administration of high-dose ketoconazole, an inhibitor of steroid synthesis, prevents posttraumatic anxiety in an animal model. Eur Neuropsychopharmacol 2000; 10: 429–35.

18. Cohen H, Friedberg S, Michael M, Kotler M, Zeev K. Interaction of CCK-4 induced anxiety and post-cat exposure anxiety in rats. Depress Anxiety 1996; 4(3): 144–5.

19. Cohen H, Zohar J, Matar M. The relevance of differential response to trauma in an animal model of post-traumatic stress disorder. Biol Psychiatry 2003; 53(6): 463–73.

20. Cohen H, Kaplan Z, Kotler M. CCK-antagonists in a rat exposed to acute stress: implication for anxiety associated with post-traumatic stress disorder. Depress Anxiety 1999; 10(1): 8–17.

21. Cohen H, Matar MA, Richter-Levin G, Zohar J. The contribution of an animal model toward uncovering biological risk factors for PTSD. Ann N Y Acad Sci 2006; 1071: 335–50.

22. Cohen H, Zohar J. Animal models of post traumatic stress disorder: the use of cut off behavioral criteria. Ann N Y Acad Sci 2004; 1032: 167–78.

23. Cohen H, Zohar J, Matar MA et al. Setting apart the affected: the use of behavioral criteria in animal models of post traumatic stress disorder. Neuropsychopharmacology 2004; 29(11): 1962–70.

24. Breslau N, Davis GC, Andreski P, Peterson E. Traumatic events and posttraumatic stress disorder in an urban population of young adults. Arch Gen Psychiatry 1991; 48(3): 216–22.

25. Breslau N, Kessler RC, Chilcoat HD et al. Trauma and posttraumatic stress disorder in the community: the 1996 Detroit Area Survey of Trauma. Arch Gen Psychiatry 1998; 55(7): 626–32.

26. Resnick HS, Kilpatrick DG, Dansky BS, Saunders BE, Best CL. Prevalence of civilian trauma and posttraumatic stress disorder in a representative national sample of women. J Consult Clin Psychol 1993; 61(6): 984–91.

27. Cohen H, Maayan R, Touati-Werner D et al. Decreased circulatory levels of neuroactive steroids in behaviorally more extremely affected rats subsequent to exposure to a potentially traumatic experience. Int J Neuropsychopharmacol 2007; 10(2): 203–9.

28. Cohen H, Ziv Y, Cardon M et al. Maladaptation to mental stress mitigated by the adaptive immune system via depletion of naturally occurring regulatory CD4+CD25+ cells. J Neurobiol 2006; 66(6): 552–63.

29. Mason JW, Giller EL, Kosten TR, Ostroff RB, Podd L. Urinary free-cortisol levels in posttraumatic stress disorder patients. J Nerv Ment Dis 1986; 174(3): 145–9.

30. Mason JW, Giller EL, Kosten TR, Harkness L. Elevation of urinary norepinephrine/cortisol ratio in posttraumatic stress disorder. J Nerv Ment Dis 1988; 176(8): 498–502.

31. Pitman RK, Orr SP. Twenty-four hour urinary cortisol and catecholamine excretion in combat-related posttraumatic stress disorder. Biol Psychiatry 1990; 27(2): 245–7.

32. Yehuda R, Lowy MT, Southwick SM, Shaffer D, Giller EL Jr. Lymphocyte glucocorticoid receptor number in posttraumatic stress disorder. Am J Psychiatry 1991a; 148(4): 499–504.

33. Yehuda R, Giller EL, Southwick SM, Lowy MT, Mason JW. Hypothalamic-pituitary-adrenal dysfunction in posttraumatic stress disorder. Biol Psychiatry 1991b; 30(10): 1031–48.

34. Yehuda R, Southwick S, Giller EL, Ma X, Mason JW. Urinary catecholamine excretion and severity of PTSD symptoms in Vietnam combat veterans. J Nerv Ment Dis 1992; 180(5): 321–5.

35. Resnick HS, Yehuda R, Pitman RK, Foy DW. Effect of previous trauma on acute plasma cortisol level following rape. Am J Psychiatry 1995; 152(11): 1675–7.

36. Yehuda R. Risk and resilience in posttraumatic stress disorder. J Clin Psychiatry 2004; 65(1): 29–36.

37. Bremner JD, Innis RB, Ng CK et al. Positron emission tomography measurement of cerebral metabolic correlates of yohimbine administration in combat-related posttraumatic stress disorder. Arch Gen Psychiatry 1997; 54(3): 246–54.

38. Foa EB, Stein DJ, McFarlane AC. Symptomatology and psychopathology of mental health problems after disaster. J Clin Psychiatry 2006; 67(2): 15–25.

39. Delahanty DL, Raimonde AJ, Spoonster E. Initial posttraumatic urinary cortisol levels predict subsequent PTSD symptoms in motor vehicle accident victims. Biol Psychiatry 2000; 48(9): 940–7.

40. Rasmusson AM, Lipschitz DS, Wang S et al. Increased pituitary and adrenal reactivity in premenopausal women with posttraumatic stress disorder. Biol Psychiatry 2001; 50(12): 965–77.

41. Elzinga BM, Schmahl CG, Vermetten E, van Dyck R, Bremner JD. Higher cortisol levels following exposure to traumatic reminders in abuse-related PTSD. Neuropsychopharmacology 2003; 28(9): 1656–65.

42. Yehuda R, McEwen BS. Protective and damaging effects of the biobehavioral stress response: cognitive, systemic and clinical aspects: ISPNE XXXIV meeting summary. Psychoneuroendocrinology 2004; 29(9): 1212–22.

43. Spivak B, Shohat B, Mester R et al. Elevated levels of serum interleukin-1 beta in combat-related posttraumatic stress disorder. Biol Psychiatry 1997; 42(5): 345–8.

44. Maes M, Lin AH, Delmeire L et al. Elevated serum interleukin-6 (IL-6) and IL-6 receptor concentrations in posttraumatic stress disorder following accidental man-made traumatic events. Biol Psychiatry 1999; 45(7): 833–9.

45. Baker DG, Ekhator NN, Kasckow JW et al. Plasma and cerebrospinal fluid interleukin-6 concentrations in posttraumatic stress disorder. Neuroimmunomodulation 2001; 9(4): 209–17.

46. Schelling G, Richter M, Roozendaal B et al. Exposure to high stress in the intensive care unit may have negative effects on health-related quality-of-life outcomes after cardiac surgery. Crit Care Med 2003; 31(7): 1971–80.

47. Schelling G, Stoll C, Kapfhammer HP et al. The effect of stress doses of hydrocortisone during septic shock on posttraumatic stress disorder and health-related quality of life in survivors. Crit Care Med 1999; 27(12): 2678–83.

48. Schelling G, Briegel J, Roozendaal B et al. The effect of stress doses of hydrocortisone during septic shock on posttraumatic stress disorder in survivors. Biol Psychiatry 2001; 50(12): 978–85.

49. Cohen H, Zohar J, Gidron Y et al. Blunted HPA axis response to stress influences susceptibility to posttraumatic stress response in rats. Biol Psychiatry 2006; 59(12): 1208–18.

50. Cohen H, Zohar J, Matar M, Loewenthal U, Kaplan Z. The impact of environment factors in determining post-exposure responses in isogenic strains of mice: can genetic predisposition explain phenotypic vulnerability? Int J Neuropsychopharmacol 2007; in press.

51. Caspi A, Moffitt T. Gene–environment interactions in psychiatry: joining forces with neuroscience. Nat Rev Neurosci 2006; 7: 583–90.

52. Moffitt T, Caspi A, Rutter M. Measured gene–environment interactions in psychopathology. Perspect Psychol Sci 2006; 1: 5–27.

53. Kozlovsky N, Matar MA, Kaplan Z et al. The immediate early gene Arc is associated with behavioral resilience to stress exposure in an animal model of posttraumatic stress disorder. Eur Neuropsychopharmacol 2007; 2: 2.

54. Shieh PB, Ghosh A. Molecular mechanisms underlying activity-dependent regulation of BDNF expression. J Neurobiol 1999; 41(1): 127–34.

55. Thoenen H. Neurotrophins and neuronal plasticity. Science 1995; 270(5236): 593–8.

56. Poo MM. Neurotrophins as synaptic modulators. Nat Rev Neurosci 2001; 2(1): 24–32.

57. Wang MJ, Huang HM, Chen HL, Kuo JS, Jeng KC. Dehydroepiandrosterone inhibits lipopolysaccharide-induced nitric oxide production in BV-2 microglia. J Neurochem 2001; 77(3): 830–8.

58. Mamounas LA, Altar CA, Blue ME et al. BDNF promotes the regenerative sprouting, but not survival, of injured serotonergic axons in the adult rat brain. J Neurosci 2000; 20(2): 771–82.

59. Thome J, Pesold B, Baader M et al. Stress differentially regulates synaptophysin and synaptotagmin expression in hippocampus. Biol Psychiatry 2001; 50(10): 809–12.

60. Duman RS. Synaptic plasticity and mood disorders. Mol Psychiatry 2002; 7: 29–34.

61. Manji HK, Drevets WC, Charney DS. The cellular neurobiology of depression. Nat Med 2001; 7: 541–7.

62. Pei Q, Zetterstrom TS, Sprakes M, Tordera R, Sharp T. Antidepressant drug treatment induces Arc gene expression in the rat brain. Neuroscience 2003; 121(4): 975–82.

63. Matar MA, Cohen H, Kaplan Z, Zohar J. The effect of early poststressor intervention with sertraline on behavioral responses in an animal model of post-traumatic stress disorder. Neuropsychopharmacology 2006; 31(12): 2610–8.

64. Schelling G. Effects of stress hormones on traumatic memory formation and the development of posttraumatic stress disorder in critically ill patients. Neurobiol Learn Mem 2002; 78(3): 596–609.

65. Schelling G, Kilger E, Roozendaal B et al. Stress doses of hydrocortisone, traumatic memories, and symptoms of posttraumatic stress disorder in patients after cardiac surgery: a randomized study. Biol Psychiatry 2004; 55(6): 627–33.

66. Weis F, Kilger E, Roozendaal B et al. Stress doses of hydrocortisone reduce chronic stress symptoms and improve health-related quality of life in high-risk patients after cardiac surgery: a randomized study. J Thorac Cardiovasc Surg 2006; 131(2): 277–82.

67. Cohen H, Matar MA, Buskila D, Kaplan Z, Zohar J. Early post-stressor intervention with high dose corticosterone attenuates post traumatic stress response in an animal model of PTSD. Biol Psychiatry 2008; 64(8):708–717.

68. Cohen H, Kaplan Z, Matar M et al. Anisomycin, a protein synthesis inhibitor, disrupts traumatic memory consolidation and attenuates post traumatic stress response in rats. Biol Psychiatry 2006; 60(7): 767–76.

69. Gelpin E, Bonne O, Peri T, Brandes D, Shalev AY. Treatment of recent trauma survivors with benzodiazepines: a prospective study. J Clin Psychiatry 1996; 57(9): 390–4.

70. British Medical Association & Royal Pharmaceutical Society of Great Britain. British National Formulary, London & Wallingford: BMJ Books and Pharmaceutical Press; 2000.

71. Matar M, Zohar J, Kaplan Z, Cohen H. Alprazolam treatment immediately after stress exposure interferes with the normal HPA-stress response and increases vulnerability to subsequent stress in an animal model of PTSD. Eur Neuropsychopharmacology 2009; 19(4):283–295.

8 | Psychosocial treatments of posttraumatic stress disorder

Kerry J Ressler and Barbara O Rothbaum

INTRODUCTION

Impressive advances in treating posttraumatic stress disorder (PTSD) have been made in the past decade with respect to group psychotherapy, individual psychodynamically oriented therapy, and cognitive–behavioral therapy. Notably the Institute of Medicine (1) has recently confirmed the efficacy for exposure-based psychotherapy treatment for PTSD while finding that the current data are inadequate to determine the efficacy of medication treatment for PTSD.(1)

During this same period of time, the neuroscience that underlies the psychotherapy for treating fear-based disorders is rapidly progressing and is being translated to the clinic in the form of pharmacological augmentation of emotional learning.

This chapter summarizes the literature on psychosocial interventions for PTSD, beginning with a brief review of traditional therapies. We then examine the larger literature on the efficacy of cognitive–behavioral procedures with PTSD, along with exciting experimental approaches such as virtual reality–based treatment for PTSD and pharmacological augmentation of emotional learning combined with psychotherapy.

TRADITIONAL INTERVENTIONS

Hypnotherapy

Hypnosis has been advocated in the treatment of trauma since it was introduced by Freud to attain the abreaction and catharsis he deemed necessary to resolve a psychic conflict (see (2) for a review) and continues to be used to treat trauma survivors. Spiegel noted that hypnosis may be useful in treating PTSD because hypnotic phenomena such as dissociation are common in coping with trauma as it occurs and in its sequelae, and hypnosis may facilitate the recall of traumatic events that were encoded in a dissociative state and that, therefore, are not available to conscious recollection.

A number of case studies have reported that hypnosis was useful in treating posttrauma disturbances following a variety of traumas, but most of these lack methodological rigor and thus cannot allow strong conclusions to be drawn. In the one controlled study (3) of 112 trauma victims, the relative efficacies of hypnosis, desensitization, and psychodynamic psychotherapy were compared against a waiting list control group. The participants were victims of a variety of traumas who all met symptom criteria for PTSD; the majority did not directly experience the trauma but had lost a loved one. The results indicated that participants in all three treatment conditions were more improved than those in the waiting list condition, but no differences across the three treatments were observed. Inspection of the pre- and post-treatment means indicated 29% improvement on the Impact of Event Scale (IES) (4) for those in psychodynamic therapy, 34% for hypnotherapy, and 41% for desensitization, compared to about 10% improvement in the waiting list condition. The results suggest that hypnotherapy, as well as desensitization and psychodynamic therapy, may offer some help for posttrauma suffering.

Since these earlier studies, few other sufficiently powered comparative studies of hypnotherapy have been performed. The most recent large review of psychosocial therapy for PTSD from the Institute of Medicine (IOM) (1) and Cochrane Database review (5) found that hypnosis remains understudied, and that, therefore, based on this extremely limited body of evidence (little empirical support, as there are few randomized clinical trials [RCTs]), the IOM committee stated that it would be inappropriate to reach a conclusion regarding the efficacy of hypnotherapy.(1)

Psychodynamic treatments

Treatment by dynamic psychotherapy has often been advocated as a final component of crisis intervention.(6–8) However, empirical investigations of their efficacy are scarce, and those that do exist are not usually well controlled. In an attempt to account for posttrauma reactions, psychodynamic theorists, for example, (9) emphasize concepts such as denial, abreaction, catharsis, and stages of recovery from trauma. The target of Horowitz's brief psychodynamic therapy is the resolution of intrapsychic conflict arising from a traumatic experience rather than specific symptom reduction. Other psychodynamic theorists focus largely on group process.(10) Several studies have suggested that psychodynamic treatments may be useful in the treatment of PTSD, while others have not found them effective. Psychodynamic psychotherapy was not found useful in the treatment of a traumatized Vietnam veteran.(11) After 19 months of no progress with psychodynamic psychotherapy, therapy by imagery was introduced. The therapist presented a trauma-related scene and allowed the client to develop it spontaneously through associations rather than by plan. The use of the imagery technique was not planned in advance, but rather it was introduced at appropriate times in the context of a session. The client moved onto other trauma-related scenes when he was ready. Avoidance was addressed through psychodynamic techniques of dealing with transference and resistance. Ten sessions of this imagery therapy were effective in ameliorating the client's PTSD as observed by the therapist and reported by the client. Although constrained by the limitations of a single case report and unsystematic measures, this report suggests that traditional "talking" therapy was not helpful for PTSD, whereas behaviorally oriented techniques appeared to be effective.

Using psychoanalytic-oriented therapy, Bart (12) reported that trauma victims worsened following treatment. On the other hand, short-term dynamic group therapy for nine rape victims was determined to be somewhat helpful. Fear and hostility decreased significantly from pre- to post-treatment, but three of the seven victims who completed the study reported only slight change in their overall level of distress. Unfortunately, no control group was included and the content of the therapy sessions was not specified.

Twenty-eight victims of the Beverly Hills Supper Club fire were treated with individual short-term (6–12 sessions) psychodynamic psychotherapy.(13) Diagnoses included PTSD, complicated bereavement, major depressive disorder, and adjustment disorder. Patients who completed treatment showed more improvement than patients with interrupted treatment. Lindy et al. (13) subsequently observed that all treated patients "improved to a subclinical level two years after the fire" (p. 602).

As mentioned above in the section on hypnotherapy, Brom et al. (3) conducted a controlled study of Horowitz's brief psychodynamic therapy, comparing this treatment with hypnosis, desensitization, and a waiting list control group. Although the authors found no differences among the three active treatment conditions, inspection of the means on the IES suggested that psychodynamic therapy in this study yielded inferior outcome compared to desensitization (29% vs. 41% mean pre–post reduction).

The efficacy of a brief psychodynamic treatment based upon Horowitz's (9) model for bereavement was investigated in 61 women who had lost their husbands.(14) Patients were randomly assigned either to 12 weekly sessions of brief dynamic therapy or to a mutual help group led by a nonclinician. Although many of the participants in this study reported symptoms of PTSD, death of a husband does not necessarily qualify as a DSM criterion A trauma. Results indicated that patients in both conditions improved slightly on both interview and self-report ratings of PTSD symptoms, but there were no group differences. Using a quasiexperimental design, interpersonal process group therapy (IPGT) was compared with a naturally occurring waiting list control in 43 female childhood sexual abuse survivors.(15) The IPGT treatment was based on the treatment guidelines established by Courtois (16) and Yalom.(10) History of abuse was the only specified inclusion criterion. Results indicated that IPGT patients improved on several measures including PTSD diagnostic status. At pretreatment, 91% of the IPGT group and 85% of the control group met DSM criteria for PTSD; at posttreatment, only 39% of the IPGT group vs. 83% of the control group met criteria for PTSD. The IPGT group showed greater symptom reduction than did the control group on some measures (e.g., self-report measure of intrusion), whereas both groups evidenced similar symptom reduction on other measures (e.g., depression, dissociation).

In summary, most studies of psychodynamic psychotherapy were plagued by methodological flaws, including lack of controls, lack of adequate assessment of outcome, and vaguely described treatments. Similar to the data with hypnotherapy, The Institute of Medicine (1) and Cochrane Database review (5) found that psychodynamic psychotherapy approaches to PTSD remains understudied, and therefore, that based on this extremely limited body of evidence (little empirical support; there are few randomized clinical trials [RCTs]), the IOM committee stated that it would be inappropriate to reach a conclusion regarding the efficacy of psychodynamic psychotherapy.(1) Thus, the information about the efficacy of traditional interventions with PTSD from these studies is quite limited and is open to various interpretations. Clearly controlled studies need to be performed for these approaches to become more broadly validated.

COGNITIVE–BEHAVIORAL THERAPY

Cognitive–behavior therapy (CBT) includes a variety of treatment programs, including exposure procedures, cognitive restructuring procedures, anxiety management programs, and their combinations. Reviews of the extant literature on the treatment of PTSD are quite positive regarding CBT.(1, 5, 17–20) A recent meta-analysis found the largest treatment effects for cognitive–behavioral techniques and selective serotonin reuptake inhibitor (SSRI) medications.(20) One form of CBT employed with PTSD sufferers is exposure treatment, which assists patients in confronting their feared memories and situations. Another recent comprehensive review of CBT studies for PTSD found the strongest evidence for exposure therapy.(21) Both exposure in imagination and exposure in real life to trauma-related events appear to be therapeutic.

The exposure treatment that has been developed by Foa and Rothbaum (22, 23) and their colleagues typically incorporates imaginal exposure that has the patient recall the traumatic memories in the therapist's office. The patient is asked to go back in his or her mind to the time of the trauma and to relive it in his or her imagination. He or she is asked to close his or her eyes and to describe it out loud in the present tense, as if it were happening now. Very often, this narrative is tape-recorded (audiotaped) and that tape is sent home with the patient so that he or she may practice imaginal exposure daily at home between therapy sessions. Although this reliving is often painful for the patient initially, it quickly becomes less painful as exposure is repeated. The idea behind this type of treatment is that the trauma needs to be emotionally processed, or digested, so that it can become less painful.(24, 25) Also, many victims with PTSD mistakenly view the process of remembering their trauma as dangerous and, therefore, devote much effort to avoiding thinking about or processing the trauma. Imaginal reliving serves to disconfirm this mistaken belief.

Other forms of exposure involve repeatedly confronting realistically safe situations, places, or objects that are reminders of the trauma (called *in vivo*, or in real life, exposure) until they no longer elicit such strong emotions. Some therapists have patients write repeatedly about the trauma as a form of exposure.(26) In systematic desensitization (SD), the patient is taught how to relax, then presented with reminders of the trauma gradually, working up a hierarchy from the least disturbing to the most disturbing. If they become very anxious or upset, they stop the trauma imagery, relax themselves, then go back to the material for exposure, until they can encounter all memories or situations without becoming upset.

Another CBT approach, anxiety management training (AMT), involves teaching patients skills to control their anxiety and has also been helpful with PTSD. Stress inoculation training (SIT), the AMT program that has received the most attention, was developed for victims who remained highly fearful 3 months after being raped.(27) SIT typically consists of education and training of coping skills. These skills include deep muscle relaxation training, breathing control, role playing, covert modeling, thought stopping, and guided self-dialogue following SIT. The idea is that sufferers of PTSD experience a great deal of anxiety in their lives because they are frequently reminded of the trauma. Very often, when they become anxious, this is a cue for them to feel they are in danger and thus to become even more scared. SIT aims to teach skills to help decrease this anxiety in many different situations, to help "take the edge off."

Exposure therapy

The efficacy of exposure treatment for PTSD was first demonstrated with several case reports on war veterans.(28–30) Both flooding in imagination (31) and flooding *in vivo* to trauma-related events (29) appeared to be therapeutic. Most of these treatments also included additional techniques, such as anger control or relaxation training.

Prolonged exposure (PE) has been found to be highly effective in the treatment of women with PTSD following physical and sexual assault compared to waiting list or minimal attention-control conditions in five studies.(32–36) The percentage of treatment completers who no longer met criteria for PTSD ranged between 40% and 95% for PE, compared to 0% and 12% in the control conditions. The first controlled study of the treatment of PTSD in rape survivors randomly assigned PTSD rape survivors to one of four conditions: stress inoculation training (SIT), prolonged exposure (PE), supportive counseling (SC), or waiting list control (WL). Exposure treatment consisted of nine biweekly individual sessions. The first two sessions were devoted to information gathering, explaining the treatment rationale, and treatment planning including the construction of a hierarchy of feared situations for *in vivo* exposure. During the remaining sessions, survivors were instructed to relive in imagination their traumatic experiences and describe it aloud "as if it were happening now." Exposure continued for about 60 minutes and was tape-recorded so that survivors could practice imaginal exposure as homework by listening to the tape. Also for homework, survivors were instructed to approach feared situations or objects that were realistically safe. Detailed instructions for conducting exposure therapy with PTSD patients can be found in Foa and Rothbaum.(23)

SIT began with information regarding the assault and the survivor's history gathered in Session 1, followed by brief breathing retraining to alleviate anxiety aroused by the discussion of the assault. The rationale for treatment was explained in Session 2, and coping skills were taught in Sessions 3 to 9. Skills were applied first to a non-assault–related example, and then to an assault-related example. Supportive counseling focused on assisting patients in solving daily problems that may or may not be assault related. Discussion of the assault itself was largely avoided because such discussions were viewed as a form of exposure. Patients were redirected to "here and now" issues when they began discussing the assault. Patients were taught problem solving, and therapists engaged in active listening and support. Survivors in the waiting list condition were assessed at the same 5-week intervals as the treated survivors and were contacted by phone in between to maintain contact. Treatments were delivered in nine biweekly 90-minute individual sessions. All conditions produced improvement on all measures immediately posttreatment and at follow-up.

SIT produced significantly more improvement on PTSD symptoms than WL immediately following treatment. At follow-up, PE produced superior outcome on PTSD symptoms. Patients who received PE continued to improve after treatment termination, whereas patients in the SIT and SC conditions evidenced no change between posttreatment and follow-up.(37) The exposure technique studied has proven successful even in cases complicated by other diagnoses such as conversion mutism.(38)

A second study compared PE, SIT, the combination of SIT and PE, and a waiting list control group.(33) All three active treatments showed significant improvement in PTSD symptoms and depressive symptoms at posttest, and the waiting list group did not improve. These treatment effects were maintained at 6-month follow-up. On most outcome measures, PE was more effective than the other two treatments, although this difference did not always reach significance. An examination of patients who achieved good end-state functioning showed that 21% of patients in SIT, 46% of patients in PE, and 32% of patients in SIT/PE achieved this goal at posttreatment. At 6-month follow-up, 75% of patients in PE, 68% of patients in SIT, and 50% of patients in SIT/PE lost the PTSD diagnosis, whereas all waiting list patients retained the diagnosis. The hypothesis that the combined treatment would be superior was not supported. The authors suggested that these results may be due to the fact the patients in that condition actually received less prolonged imaginal exposure and SIT training than participants in the individual treatments, as treatment sessions were all equal in length. Versions of the PE program have been helpful in preventing the development of chronic PTSD following rape (39) and in treating PTSD in abused children.(40)

Additional studies also provide support for the efficacy of exposure treatment for PTSD in samples heterogeneous with regard to their traumas. Richards et al. (41) treated 14 participants with PTSD with either four sessions of imaginal exposure followed by four sessions of *in vivo* exposure, or *in vivo* followed by imaginal exposure. Patients in both treatment conditions improved considerably. The authors noted that the percentage of symptom reduction of 65% to 80% seen in this study is much higher than those of most treatment studies for other anxiety disorders. Also, at posttreatment and at 1-year follow-up, no patients met criteria for PTSD. The only notable difference between the two exposure types was in the area of phobic avoidance, on which *in vivo* exposure appeared to be more effective regardless of the order in which it was presented. In another study of outpatients with PTSD resulting from a variety of traumas, (42) exposure, cognitive therapy, and exposure plus cognitive therapy combination were all equally successful in reducing PTSD at posttreatment and 6-month follow-up. All three treatments were more effective than relaxation.

Exposure treatment was efficacious in an open trial of eight weekly sessions of imaginal and *in vivo* exposure with 23 traumatized individuals with PTSD.(43) Participants improved significantly on a variety of measures at posttreatment, with reductions of 42% on the IES, 61% on a measure of general health (General Health Questionnaire), 38% on a general symptom checklist (the Symptom Checklist-90, or SCL-90), and 35% on the Clinician-Administered PTSD Scale (CAPS).

Exposure therapy was compared to cognitive therapy in a mixed sample of trauma survivors.(44) Type of trauma included crime (52%), accident (34%), and other (15%). There was a significant improvement on all measures at posttreatment, which was maintained at follow-up for both treatments, with no significant differences between the two treatments.

Similar exposure therapy programs have been successful with different trauma populations.(45–50) In all these studies, exposure therapy programs included both imaginal and *in vivo* exposure. However, three studies have demonstrated that imaginal exposure to the traumatic memory in the absence of *in vivo* exposure produce quite good outcome. Bryant and colleagues (51) found imaginal exposure to be more effective than supportive therapy and Tarrier et. al (52) found this program to be as effective as cognitive therapy.

There are several published reports of successful treatment of PTSD in veterans with exposure therapy. In the largest and best controlled study to date of exposure therapy with veterans (53), 277 female veterans and active-duty personnel ($n = 7$) with PTSD were randomly assigned to receive 10 weekly sessions of PE or present-centered therapy (PCT). Women who received PE experienced greater reduction in PTSD symptoms and were more likely to no longer meet PTSD criteria and to achieve total remission than those who received PCT. It is also notable that PE was delivered by VA therapists, not CBT experts. In a controlled study, Keane, Fairbank, Caddell, and Zimering (54) compared the progress of 11 male veterans in an exposure therapy with 13 waiting list controls. Participants demonstrated significantly greater improvement in reexperiencing symptoms as well as trauma-related depression and anxiety than waiting list controls by the end of treatment and these gains were maintained at 6-month follow-up. In another study, Cooper and Clum (55) compared two groups of seven veterans treated for PTSD. Both groups received individual and group treatment ordinarily offered by VA psychologists at their veterans facilities. The experimental group also received nine sessions of imaginal exposure, along with several more sessions to build rapport and prepare for the exposure sessions. At 3-month follow-up, scores on measures of trait anxiety and depression were similar in both groups, but symptoms of reexperiencing, hyperarousal, and avoidance were significantly better in the exposure group. In a similar vein, Boudewyns and colleagues (56) treated 19 members of an inpatient unit with direct therapeutic exposure while 19 other patients on the same unit served as controls. At 8-month follow-up, the researchers found that there were no differences between the two groups on psychophysiological measures, but improvement in overall functioning was better in patients who had received exposure therapy. Glynn et al. (57) found that veterans who received exposure treatment, whether followed with 16 sessions of behavioral family therapy or alone, showed a significant reduction in PTSD symptoms over waiting list controls. Pitman et al. (58) found significant reductions in levels of chronic PTSD in a sample of 20 Vietnam veterans participating in 6 to 12 sessions of exposure therapy. However, no control group was available for comparison. Likewise, Frueh, Turner, Beidel, Mirabella, and Jones (59) studied the effectiveness of a 29-session treatment, held over 17 weeks, which included imaginal exposure. Overall, the study provided evidence of significant reduction in anxiety in 11 veterans who completed treatment but again the findings were limited by the absence of a control group. Finally, Bisson and Jones (60) report that 18 Gulf War veterans with PTSD showed significant reductions symptoms of PTSD, depression, and general psychiatric distress. Reductions in symptoms were maintained at 3-month follow-up, but again no comparison to a control group was made.

Exposure therapy has not been as consistently effective when delivered in a group format in a VA setting. In a large VA cooperative study of male Vietnam veterans ($n = 360$), trauma-focused group psychotherapy was not significantly more effective than a present-centered comparison group treatment that avoided trauma focus.(61) However, recent uncontrolled pilot trials at Atlanta, VA, of exposure therapy delivered in a combination of group and individual sessions have been more effective. An open trial of 102 veterans treated with Group-Based Exposure Therapy (GBET) found clinically significant and lasting reductions in the symptoms of war-related PTSD with large effect sizes on treating clinicians' assessments and moderate to large effect sizes on self-report PTSD scales.(62) Another pilot study with 37 participants using a hybrid treatment model combining individually recorded audiotapes of three traumatic memories and daily exposure practice nested in a 10-week behavioral group therapy format has been effective in treating OEF/OIF and Persian Gulf combat veterans. There were no significant differences between those with (30%) and without traumatic brain injury (TBI) on pretreatment measures nor was TBI status a predictor of significantly different treatment response.(63)

Note that the most recent large meta-analytic reviews have concluded that among all types of psychosocial therapies, the best and largest RCTs exist for exposure-based models. The recent Cochrane Database review concluded that both individual and group trauma-focused CBT/Exposure therapy were effective in the treatment of PTSD.(5) In addition, the Institute of Medicine concluded that "The committee finds that the evidence is sufficient to conclude the efficacy of exposure therapies in the treatment of PTSD."(1)

Virtual reality exposure therapy

A new medium for conducting exposure therapy has been introduced recently. Virtual reality exposure (VRE) presents the user with a computer-generated view of a virtual world that changes in a natural way with head motion. During VRE sessions patients wear the head-mounted display with stereo earphones that provide visual and audio cues consistent with being in the virtual environment that is used to reactivate their traumatic cues.

Studies have been done across a variety of anxiety disorders, with treatment for PTSD being one of the most exciting forefronts of this technology. In one investigation, Vietnam veterans with PTSD are exposed to two virtual environments, a virtual Huey helicopter flying over a "Virtual Vietnam" and a clearing surrounded by jungle. In this way, patients are repeatedly exposed to their most traumatic memories but immersed in Vietnam stimuli. The results of the first patient to complete the virtual Vietnam treatment indicate preliminary success.(64) The subject was an unemployed 50-year-old Caucasian male on 100% Veterans Administration (VA) compensation who served in Vietnam 26 years prior to the onset of this study as a helicopter pilot. He met criteria for current PTSD, current major depressive disorder, and past alcohol abuse. Treatment was delivered in fourteen 90-minute individual sessions conducted twice weekly over 7 weeks. Scores on all measures decreased from pre- to post-treatment. No statistical analyses were incorporated because this was a single subject. The following symptom measures decreased at least 30%: CAPS total (34%), CAPS reexperiencing (61%), CAPS arousal (36%), IES total (45%), IES intrusion (42%), IES avoidance (50%), and Spielberger-state anger (63%).

Following this pilot study, Rothbaum and colleagues examined 10 male patients exposed to two virtual Vietnam environments. They found that there were significant decreases in all three symptom clusters and that the patient's reported symptoms on the Impact of Events Scale were significantly decreased.(65)

Positive findings in the study of Vietnam veterans has led other groups to propose VR environments to facilitate PTSD treatment in civilians. For example, subsequent to the September 11, 2001, terrorist attacks on the World Trade Centers (WTC) in New York, Difede and Hoffman (66) constructed a scenario in which persons associated with these events could be exposed to the events again in VR. In their first report, a case study was presented using VR to provide exposure to the trauma memory with a patient who had failed to improve with traditional exposure therapy. The authors reported significant reduction of PTSD symptoms after repeatedly exposing the patient to explosions, sound effects, virtual people jumping from the burning buildings, towers collapsing, and dust clouds and attributed this success partly due to the increased realism of the VR images as compared to the mental images the patient could generate without VR. Positive treatment outcomes from a waiting list–controlled VR study with patients who were not successful in previous imaginal therapy are currently in press by this group.(67, 68) A very recent study by Difede and colleagues examined VRE for the treatment of PTSD following September 11, 2001.(69) This pilot study examined thirteen VR treatment subjects compared to eight waiting list control subjects, and determined that the VR group showed a significant decline on Clinician-Administered PTSD Scale (CAPS) scores compared to waiting list. A case study of the first Iraq veteran with PTSD treated with the Virtual Iraq indicated a 56% decrease in CAPS scores with four sessions of VRE.(70)

The results from the studies discussed above consistently support the efficacy of imaginal and *in vivo* exposure for the treatment of PTSD resulting from a variety of traumas. These results are even more impressive, given the methodological precision that was applied to many of these studies. Notably, there are now very good VR environments for the Iraq war, the Vietnam War, the World Trade Center bombings, Terrorist attacks in Israel, and a variety of other non–trauma-based environments. However, despite the fact that almost 100 papers discussing virtual reality exposure therapy for anxiety-related disorders are now in the literature, many are not optimally designed.(71) Additional randomized clinical controlled trials and trials of increased size will likely lead to exciting new uses and validation for virtual reality approaches in the future.

Anxiety management techniques (AMT)

Of the various AMT programs, stress inoculation training (SIT), (72) developed for rape survivors with chronic fear and anxiety, has received the most attention. The efficacy of SIT has been supported by several reports from Veronen, Kilpatrick, and their colleagues and others.(37, 73) In an uncontrolled investigation, a clear treatment effect emerged on rape-related fear, anxiety, phobic anxiety, tension, and depression in female rape survivors who showed elevated fear and avoidance to phobic stimuli 3 months postrape.(27) A later study was designed to compare 10 sessions each of SIT, peer counseling, and systematic desensitization (SD).(27) Survivors were permitted to select their treatment and the vast majority opted for SIT, few chose peer counseling, and none chose SD, which precluded statistical analyses. The authors reported noticeable improvement from pre- to post-treatment on most measures for the SIT completers. Case studies of rape survivors treated with SIT or its variant also indicated positive results.(74)

In a controlled study, the efficacy of six 2-hour sessions of three types of group therapy for rape-related fear and anxiety were compared to a naturally occurring waiting list control group, including SIT, assertion training, or supportive psychotherapy plus information.(73) SIT was similar to that described by Kilpatrick et al. (72) with two exceptions: (1) cognitive restructuring, assertiveness training, and role play were excluded because they were used in the comparative treatment, and (b) exposure *in vivo* was added to the application phase. Results indicated that all three treatments were highly effective in reducing rape-related fears, intrusion, and avoidance symptoms, with no group differences evident, whereas no improvements were found in the waiting list control group. Improvement was maintained at 6-month follow-up on rape-related fear measures, but not on depression, self-esteem, and social fears.

A controlled study compared three different forms of relaxation for 90 Vietnam veterans. (75) Relaxation, relaxation plus deep breathing exercises, and relaxation plus deep breathing plus biofeedback were equally, but only mildly, effective in leading to improvement. The effects of cognitive therapy and SD were studied in rape survivors, some of whom entered treatment an average of 2 weeks after their assault.(76, 77) Ratings of fear, anxiety, depression, and social adjustment, all showed significant gains for both cognitive therapy and SD.

In summary, among anxiety management approaches, SIT has received the most support for PTSD. Other AMTs such as relaxation or cognitive therapy are best viewed as treatment components of a comprehensive treatment package.

Systematic desensitization

Some of the earliest studies of behavioral treatments for PTSD adopted the SD technique pioneered by Wolpe.(78) Although participants in these studies showed improvement in posttrauma symptoms, methodological problems plagued each of these studies, rendering the results inconclusive. An exception was the Brom et al. (3) study described in detail in the section on hypnotherapy and psychodynamic therapy. In this study, patients in the desensitization condition showed a mean improvement of 41% on the IES, which was higher than the other treatments examined, although the difference did not reach statistical significance. In light of the methodological problems with the resulting lack of strong conclusions to be drawn, SD will be reviewed very briefly below.

The successful outcome of SD compared to a no-treatment control group was demonstrated in two studies with war veterans using psychophysiological measures (electromyography and heart rate), (79, 80) but the treatment required a large number of sessions over an extended period of time and PTSD was not assessed. Thirteen to eighteen sessions of SD with the last two sessions spent in *in vivo* exposure were used successfully with three automobile accident survivors.(81) Several uncontrolled studies demonstrated that SD was effective with rape survivors in reducing fear, anxiety, depression, and social maladjustment.(76, 82, 83) However, SD alone was not successful in one case study of a rape survivor.(84)

In summary, several studies examined the effects of SD with a variety of trauma survivors, most showing some beneficial results. However, the lack of adequate control conditions and/or the absence of PTSD diagnoses and measures in some of the studies limit the conclusions that can be drawn from them. With the empirical finding that relaxation during confrontation with feared material was not necessary, and with evidence for the inferiority of SD to flooding in most anxiety disorders, the use of SD for anxiety disorders, including PTSD, was largely abandoned. In its place, researchers and clinicians have used a variety of imaginal and *in vivo* exposure techniques.

Eye movement desensitization and reprocessing

Eye movement desensitization and reprocessing (EMDR) (85) is a form of exposure (desensitization) accompanied by saccadic eye movements. Briefly, the technique involves the patient's imagining a scene from the trauma, focusing on the accompanying cognition and arousal, while the therapist waves two fingers across the patient's visual field and instructs the patient to track the fingers. The sequence is repeated until anxiety decreases, at which point the patient is instructed to generate a more adaptive thought and to associate it with the scene while moving his or her eyes. After each session patients indicate their subjective units of discomfort (SUDS) level and their degree of belief in a positive cognition (validity of positive cognition; VoPC).

A number of case studies have reported positive findings with EMDR; for a comprehensive review, see.(86) In the first study of EMDR, Shapiro (87) randomly assigned trauma survivors to either one session of EMDR or an exposure control condition (EMDR without the eye movements). The results showed that patients who received EMDR reported lower SUDS ratings after the one session of EMDR than did patients in the exposure control condition, but lack of methodological rigor makes this finding difficult to interpret. Combat veterans were randomly assigned to two 90-minute EMDR sessions, an exposure control (EC; EMDR without the eye movements), both as an adjunct to standard milieu treatment for veterans with PTSD, or standard milieu treatment alone.(88) SUDS ratings to traumatic stimuli were lower in the EMDR group, and therapists rated more patients as responders in the EMDR vs. EC group. However, the three groups did not differ in their lack of response as seen on standardized self-report measures, interviews of PTSD, or on physiological responses.

Jensen (89) randomly assigned 74 veterans with PTSD to either three sessions of EMDR conducted over 10 days or to a control condition of standard VA services. Neither group improved on the PTSD severity measure. SUDS ratings decreased in the EMDR group but not in controls. Silver et al. (90) compared standard milieu treatment with milieu treatment plus EMDR, biofeedback, or group relaxation training in a sample of 100 veterans with PTSD. Results indicated that EMDR led to greater reduction of symptoms relative to the control and the biofeedback groups, but as the study was uncontrolled, the strength of the findings is limited.

In a study addressing the role of eye movement, Pitman et al. (91) compared EMDR with and without the eye movement component in a crossover design with 17 male veterans diagnosed with PTSD. Patients were randomly assigned to the two conditions. The results of this methodologically vigorous study indicated that both treatments produced modest improvement in symptoms as measured by the IES, but not on the independent assessment. In contrast to expectations, on the IES, there was slightly more improvement in the eyes-fixed condition than from EMDR. Twenty-three trauma survivors received either standard EMDR or one of two variations: an EMDR analog in which eye movements were induced by a flashing light rather than a waving finger and an analog in which a light blinked only in the center of the visual field.(92) The groups did not differ on physiological measures, SUDS, or the VoPC. No analyses on PTSD severity were reported, but following treatment, only 5 of the 23 participants met criteria for PTSD. Using a sample of 36 survivors of heterogeneous traumas, Vaughan et al. (93) compared EMDR with imagery habituation training (IHT), a procedure that involved repeated presentation of traumatic stimuli in the form of an oral scenario, and applied muscle relaxation training. The authors concluded that all three groups were equally improved on the independent assessors' rating of PTSD. Wilson et al. (94) compared EMDR to a delayed-treatment condition in a mixed sample of traumatized individuals about half of whom had PTSD. Overall, patients in the EMDR group reported decreases in presenting complaints and in anxiety, and increases in positive cognitions at posttreatment, whereas the waiting list group reported no improvement.

A well-controlled study on the efficacy of EMDR was conducted by Rothbaum (95), who randomized 21 female survivors of rape to either EMDR or a waiting list control group. Measures consisted of standardized self-report and interview instruments, with the interviews conducted by a blind evaluator. Treatment consisted of four weekly sessions conducted by a well-trained clinician, and treatment adherence was monitored and deemed acceptable by an independent evaluator designated by EMDR's originator. EMDR led to improvement on PTSD symptoms on both interview (57% reduction in symptom severity) and IES (74% reduction), and gains were maintained at a 3-month follow-up. These reductions were significantly different from the control group, who evidenced no change in symptoms. In a comparison study, participants were randomly assigned to either routine clinical care, 12 sessions of biofeedback-assisted relaxation, or 12 sessions of EMDR.(96) At posttreatment and at a 3-month follow-up, the EMDR-treated participants were more improved on self-report, psychometric, and standardized measures. However, there were no differences on psychophysiological measures. EMDR was compared to general outpatient treatment in a managed care organization (HMO).(97) On measures of PTSD, depression, and anxiety, EMDR was superior. In a well-controlled study involving EMDR, a course of nine sessions of EMDR was compared to nine sessions of a CBT treatment consisting of prolonged imaginal exposure, stress inoculation training, and cognitive therapy.(98) The results indicated that CBT was superior to EMDR at posttreatment and 1-year follow-up. Another well-controlled study evaluated the relative efficacy of Prolonged Exposure (PE) and EMDR compared to a no-treatment waiting list control (WAIT) in the treatment of PTSD in adult female rape victims (n = 74). Improvement in PTSD, as assessed by blind independent assessors, and depression, dissociation, and state anxiety was significantly greater in both PE and EMDR group than the WAIT group (20 completers per group). PE and EMDR did not differ significantly for change from baseline to either posttreatment or 6-month follow-up measurement for any quantitative scale (36), but on a measure of good end-state functioning at 6 months posttreatment, participants who had received PE were doing better than participants who had received EMDR.

In summary, several studies report beneficial effects of EMDR, although other studies report equivocal findings with EMDR not resulting in significant improvements over control conditions or comparison treatments, especially on blind, standardized PTSD measures. The recent Cochrane Database review concluded that EMDR was more effective than traditional therapies or no therapy but not different from CBT and stress management.(5) The Institute of Medicine, however, found that "the overall body of evidence for EMDR to be low quality to inform conclusion regarding treatment efficacy. Four studies, three of medium and one of small sample size, had no major limitations, but only two showed positive effect for EMDR." The committee judged that the overall evidence is inadequate to determine efficacy and that future well-designed studies are critical.(1)

COMBINED TREATMENT APPROACHES

Combined Psychosocial Treatment Programs

A modified version of Foa et al's SIT/PE combination program was adopted to treat 10 motor vehicle accident (MVA) survivors.(99) The modification consisted of the addition of pleasurable activity scheduling and discussion of existential issues. Results of this study suggest that the 9 to 12 sessions of combined treatment reduced PTSD symptoms by 68% on the CAPS.

A comprehensive treatment package was studied in an uncontrolled investigation. (100) The treatment, trauma management therapy, consisted of education, individual exposure therapy, including the "core fear," programmed practice of the exposure, and social and emotional rehabilitation (SER). SER was conducted in a group format and consisted of social skills training, anger management, and veterans' issues management. Fifteen male Vietnam combat veterans with PTSD were entered, and 11 completed 29 treatment sessions over 17 weeks. Results indicated significant improvements from pre- to post-treatment on the Clinical Global Impressions (CGI), Hamilton Rating Scale for Anxiety, heart rate reactivity to traumatic cues, total hours of sleep, number of social activities, frequency of nightmares, and trends toward significant improvement on the CAPS and flashbacks. There was no significant improvement noted on self-report measures, including the Beck Depression Inventory, Social Phobia, and Anxiety Inventory, or the Spielberger Anger Expression Inventory.

A quasiexperimental design tested a combination therapy for rape survivors with PTSD. (101) Nineteen female sexual assault survivors received cognitive processing therapy (CPT) over 12 weekly sessions in a group format. CPT includes education, exposure via writing about the assault and sharing it in a group, and cognitive restructuring components. Treated participants were not randomly assigned but rather were compared to a naturally occurring waiting list control group. Results were very encouraging for the efficacy of CPT in this population. CPT subjects improved significantly from pre- to post-treatment on PTSD and depression ratings and maintained their improvement throughout the 6-month follow-up period. The waiting list subjects evidenced no change during a comparable 12-week period.

In a later report with a larger sample, Resick (102) reported that of the 66 women who completed CPT, 97% met full criteria for PTSD at pretreatment, and of these only 12% met criteria for PTSD at posttreatment. Fifty-three women completed a 6-month follow-up and only 11% met criteria for PTSD. At pretreatment, 52% met criteria for major depression. At posttreatment, only 12.5% were still depressed. At the 6-month follow-up, 8% were depressed. In a controlled trial comparing CPT, PE, and waiting list control groups, Resick et al. (103) reported that female sexual assault survivors who received CPT or PE were significantly more improved than the waiting list control group from pre- to post-treatment on PTSD and depressive symptomatology. CPT and PE were equally effective in reducing PTSD. CPT has been found effective in a group and individual format for adult survivors of child sexual abuse compared to a waiting list control (104), in a randomized trial with military veterans (105), with incarcerated adolescents (106) and refugees, even when delivered through an interpreter.(107)

Another study testing a combination treatment approach compared self-exposure plus cognitive restructuring to progressive relaxation training in 20 female sexual assault survivors. (108) Results indicated superiority at posttreatment and follow-up for the participants treated with exposure plus cognitive restructuring.

In two randomized, controlled dismantling studies, a writing-only component for PTSD patients has fared well. In a dismantling study of CPT, the full protocol was compared to its components, cognitive therapy and written accounts, in 150 adult women with PTSD. Each treatment was delivered for 6 weeks, with 2 hours of therapy per week. Results indicated that patients in all three conditions improved substantially and equivalently on PTSD and related measures.(109) A randomized controlled trial ($n = 125$) was conducted at a Dutch outpatient clinic to evaluate the efficacy of a structured writing therapy or CBT as compared to a waiting list control condition. Treatment consisted of five 1.5-hour sessions of CBT or writing for participants with ASD or acute PTSD and ten 1.5-hour sessions for participants with chronic PTSD. Results indicated improvements with both active treatments with no differences between the two treatments.(110)

An recent meta-analytic review by Bradley and colleagues (17) examined all studies between 1980 and 2003 examining psychotherapy for PTSD. They found that across CBT, exposure therapy, EMDR, and combined treatment studies from this period, "The majority of patients treated with psychotherapy for PTSD in randomized trials recover or improve, rendering these approaches some of the most effective psychosocial treatments to date." One of the main caveats they note, however, was that polysymptomatic presentations render generalizability to the population indeterminate.

Pharmacological Augmentation of Psychotherapy

Although combining treatments with apparently different modes of action, such as SSRI antidepressant therapy, which, with psychotherapy for anxiety would seem straightforward, numerous large trials and reviews have been disappointing. These studies have suggested that standard treatment for anxiety or depression with combined chronic pharmacotherapy and psychotherapy provide little benefit over either treatment alone.(111–114)

In one of the only studies to combine antidepressant medication with CBT for PTSD, outpatient men and women with chronic PTSD completed 10 weeks of open-label sertraline and then were randomly assigned to five additional weeks of sertraline alone ($n = 31$) or sertraline plus 10 sessions of twice-weekly PE ($n = 34$). Results indicated that sertraline led to a significant reduction in PTSD severity after 10 weeks but was associated with no further reductions after 5 more weeks. Participants who received PE showed further reduction in PTSD severity. This augmentation effect was observed only for participants who showed a partial response to medication. Thus, the addition of PE to sertraline for PTSD improves outcome for individuals experiencing a less than full response to the medication.(115)

An alternative approach to both standard chronic pharmacological treatments that tend to target symptom clusters but not necessarily the root cause of the disorder, is the possibility of enhancing the specific new learning that occurs with psychotherapy. The pathways mediating this learning are on the one hand very complex, but on the other hand, specific learning processes that utilize brain regions such as the amygdala and PFC that are involved with extinction of fear are well understood. The sections below will discuss evidence that those with disorders of aversive emotion respond to behavioral therapy and utilize new emotional learning to compete with or inhibit the aversive memories, a process known as extinction that may be enhanced with specific pharmacotherapy. Together these approaches offer tantalizing future ways in which fear, aversive, and traumatic memories may be modulated to alleviate suffering due to negative memories.

The inhibition of fear acquired by associative learning has been studied in both animals and humans. Following the pairing of an aversive unconditioned stimulus (UCS) to a neutral conditioned stimulus (CS), a conditioned fear response is established. If the neutral CS is then repeatedly presented in the absence of the UCS, a procedure known as extinction training, the result is an inhibition of the conditioned fear response to the neutral CS. From an operational perspective, extinction may thus be defined as "a reduction in the strength or probability of a conditioned fear response as a consequence of repeated presentation of the CS in the absence of the UCS."(116)

A variety of behavioral observations support the hypothesis that extinction is a form of learning and not "unlearning" or the forgetting of a conditioned association reviewed in.(117) Thus, Davis and colleagues tested the hypothesis that enhancing neurotransmission at NMDA receptors would facilitate extinction.(118) D-cycloserine (DCS) is a partial NMDA agonist, acting at the strychnine-insensitive glycine recognition site of the NMDA receptor complex to enhance NMDA receptor activity.(119, 120) The central findings of this study were that both systemic and amygdala-specific administration of DCS dose-dependently enhanced extinction of previously conditioned fear but did not influence fear in rats that had not received extinction training. The general findings of this study have been replicated by numerous groups with extinction of fear with startle and freezing and with extinction of appetitive cues, such as cocaine-conditioned place preference.(121–128) Collectively, data from rodent studies suggest that DCS, a drug already shown to be safe for use in humans for treating tuberculosis, may have potential use in the facilitation of extinction-based therapies for human anxiety disorders.

From a therapeutic standpoint, the behavior therapies for different anxiety disorders generally involve some form of extinction training.(116) This involves graded exposure to the feared object or event in the absence of actual harm. This exposure may be *imaginal* or *in vivo* where the feared stimulus is directly encountered by the patient, or in virtual reality. Considering the similarity between extinction training in rodents and exposure therapy for anxiety disorders in humans, novel ways to integrate pharmacotherapy with psychotherapy seemed plausible. Historically, there has been hope to combine these two approaches into a treatment more effective than either alone, but unfortunately this has not generally been achieved.(112, 129) In fact, sometimes, combining pharmacotherapy with psychotherapy can make a bad situation worse. (111, 130) However, extinction-based therapies for anxiety may be an exception to this trend.

To determine whether DCS would also improve extinction of fear in human patients with fear-related disorders, a double-blind, placebo-controlled trial in a controlled exposure paradigm was performed.(131) Twenty-eight subjects with fear of heights (acrophobia) were treated with two sessions of behavioral exposure therapy using virtual reality exposure to heights within a virtual glass elevator. Single doses of placebo or DCS were taken prior to each of the two sessions of virtual reality exposure therapy. Exposure therapy combined with DCS resulted in significantly larger reductions of acrophobia symptoms on all main outcome measures, including fear within the virtual environment, acrophobia symptoms outside of the environment, and acrophobia-related anxiety. In addition, subjects receiving DCS showed significantly greater decreases in a physiological measure of anxiety during the Behavioral Avoidance Test (BAT). These preliminary data provided initial support for the use of acute dosing of DCS as an adjunct to exposure-based psychotherapy to accelerate the associative learning processes that contribute to correcting psychopathology.

Since that experiment, DCS has also been used in a double-blind, placebo-controlled trial for the treatment of social anxiety disorder, utilizing exposure therapy as well. In this study, 27 subjects received 4 exposure therapy sessions combined with DCS or placebo. Those receiving DCS in addition to exposure therapy reported significantly less social anxiety compared with patients receiving exposure therapy plus placebo. Controlled effect sizes were in the medium to large range.(132, 133) An additional recent study has also examined using DCS to accelerate obsession-related distress reduction in patients with obsessive–compulsive disorder (OCD) undergoing extinction-based exposure therapy. DCS given prior to the therapy was found to decrease both the number of exposure sessions required to achieve clinical milestones and the rate of therapy dropout. After four exposure sessions, patients in the DCS group reported significantly greater decreases in obsession-related distress compared to the placebo group.(134)

There are currently two negative findings of DCS use in the augmentation of extinction in humans. However, in both studies, one utilizing exposure therapy for the treatment of spider phobia (135) and the second utilizing extinction for a conditioned cue in healthy human subjects (136), the placebo-controlled groups had good recovery as well. This suggests, as has been found in the animal studies, that if a "floor effect" of complete extinction is accomplished, then DCS may not augment extinction any further. Rather it appears that DCS may be most useful in disorders in which either a large number of therapy sessions is normally needed for a response or in which the nature of the disorder is quite refractory to normal exposure-based therapy approaches.

At least four randomized clinical trials of DCS augmentation of treatment for PTSD are currently ongoing but none yet published. There is a great deal of excitement as to whether these new approaches will lead to advances in psychosocial treatment methodologies. It is hoped that, with progress in the neurobiology and neuropharmacology of extinction of fear, previously undiscovered approaches to pharmacotherapy will significantly enhance treatment for refractory mood and anxiety disorders, including PTSD.

SUMMARY AND CONCLUSIONS

Overall, the most controlled studies of psychosocial treatments for PTSD have been conducted on cognitive–behavioral treatments. These studies demonstrate that techniques such as prolonged exposure procedures, stress inoculation training, and cognitive processing therapy are effective in reducing symptoms of PTSD. Systematic desensitization has largely been abandoned in favor of pure exposure techniques. Relaxation and cognitive therapy are best viewed as treatment components rather than standalone treatments. Contrary to clinical intuition, there is no evidence indicating the superiority of programs that combine different cognitive–behavioral techniques.

Many of the studies examining EMDR have methodological flaws and the results are mixed. Reports on the efficacy of psychodynamic interventions on posttrauma problems are equivocal: some report negative results, and others are more optimistic, but the majority of the reports are not well controlled. Because these interventions are widely employed with trauma survivors, it is imperative that their efficacy be examined in well-controlled studies.

New approaches combining the neuroscience of exposure/extinction therapy with pharmacotherapy aimed at specifically enhancing the emotional learning process that occurs with psychotherapy are also quite promising and very exciting.

In summary, results suggest that psychotherapy for PTSD leads to large improvements from baseline and that these are among the most powerful types of approaches for treating psychiatric disorders. Notably, the Institute of Medicine (1) report states that "evidence is sufficient to conclude the efficacy of exposure therapy in the treatment of PTSD" in contrast to current medication approaches for PTSD where "the committee found the evidence for all classes of drugs reviewed inadequate to determine efficacy for patients with PTSD." (1) Thus, psychosocial treatment approaches, particularly exposure therapy, is the most validated form of treatment for PTSD. The importance of future randomized clinical trials for different types of treatment and combinations of pharmacotherapy and psychotherapy are of utmost importance going forward.

REFERENCES

1. Institutes of Medicine. Treatment of Posttraumatic Stress Disorder: An Assessment of the Evidence. Washington, DC: National Academies Press; 2008.
2. Spiegel D. Hypnosis in the treatment of victims of sexual abuse. Psychiatr Clin North Am 1989; 12(2): 295–305.
3. Brom D, Kleber RJ, Defares PB. Brief psychotherapy for posttraumatic stress disorders. J Consult Clin Psychol 1989; 57(5): 607–12.
4. Horowitz M, Wilner N, Alvarez W. Impact of Event Scale: a measure of subjective stress. Psychosom Med 1979; 41(3): 209–18.
5. Bisson J, Andrew M. Psychological treatment of post-traumatic stress disorder (PTSD). Cochrane Database Syst Rev 2007(3): CD003388.
6. Burgess AW, Holmstrom LL. Rape trauma syndrome. Am J Psychiatry. 1974; 131(9): 981–6.
7. Evans HI. Psychotherapy for the rape victim: some treatment models. Hosp Community Psychiatry 1978; 29(5): 309–12.
8. Fox S, Scherl D. Crisis intervention with victims of rape. Social Work 1972; 17: 37–42.
9. Horowitz MJ. Stress-Response Syndromes. Northvale, NJ: Jason Aronson; 1976.
10. Yalom I. The Theory and Practice of Group Psychotherapy. 4th ed. New York: Basic; 1995.
11. Grigsby JP. The use of imagery in the treatment of posttraumatic stress disorder. J Nerv Ment Dis 1987; 175(1): 55–59.
12. Bart P. Unalienating Abortion, Demystifying Depression, and Restoring Rape Victims. Paper Presented at: 128th Annual Meeting of the American Psychiatric Association. Anaheim, CA; 1975.
13. Lindy JD, Green BL, Grace M, Titchener J. Psychotherapy with survivors of the Beverly Hills Supper Club fire. Am J Psychother 1983; 37(4): 593–610.
14. Marmar CR, Horowitz MJ, Weiss DS, Wilner NR, Kaltreider NB. A controlled trial of brief psychotherapy and mutual-help group treatment of conjugal bereavement. Am J Psychiatry 1988; 145(2): 203–9.
15. Scarvalone P, Cloitre M, Difede J. Interpersonal Process Therapy for Incest Survivors: Preliminary Outcome Data. Paper Presented at: Society for Psychotherapy Research. Vancouver, British Columbia; 1995.
16. Courtois C. Healing the incest wound: adult survivors in therapy. New York: W.W. Norton; 1988.
17. Bradley R, Greene J, Russ E, Dutra L, Westen D. A multidimensional meta-analysis of psychotherapy for PTSD. Am J Psychiatry 2005; 162(2): 214–27.
18. Rothbaum BO, Meadows EA, Resick P, Foy DW. Cognitive-behavioral Treatment Position Paper for the ISTSS Treatment Guidelines Committee.
19. Solomon SD, Gerrity ET, Muff AM. Efficacy of treatments for posttraumatic stress disorder. An empirical review. JAMA 1992; 268(5): 633–8.
20. Van Etten ML, Taylor S. Comparative efficacy of treatments for posttraumatic stress disorder: a meta-analysis. Clin Psychol Psychotherapy 1998; 5: 126–45.
21. Rothbaum BO, Meadows EA, Resick PA, Foy DW. Cognitive-behavioral therapy. In: Foa EB, Keane TM, Friedman MJ, eds. Effective Treatments for PTSD: Practice Guidelines from the International Society for Traumatic Stress Studies. New York: Guilford, 2000: 60–83.
22. Foa EB, Rothbaum BO. Treating the Trauma of Rape: Cognitive-Behavioral Therapy for PTSD. New York: The Guilford Press; 1998.
23. Foa EB, Hembree E, Rothbaum BO. Prolonged Exposure Therapy for PTSD: Emotional Processing of Traumatic Experiences, Therapist Guide. New York: Oxford University Press; 2007.
24. Foa E, Sketetee G, Rothbaum BO. Behavioral/cognitive conceptualizations of post-traumatic stress disorder. Behav Ther 1989; 20: 155–76.
25. Foa EB, Kozak MJ. Emotional processing of fear: exposure to corrective information. Psychol Bull 1986; 99(1): 20–35.
26. Resick P, Schnicke MK. Cognitive Processing Therapy for Rape Victims: A Treatment Manual. Newbury Park: Sage; 1993.
27. Veronen LJ, Kilpatrick DG. Stress management for rape victims. In: Meichenbaum D, Jaremko ME, eds. Stress Reduction and Prevention. New York: Plenum; 1983.
28. Fairbank JA, Gross RT, Keane TM. Treatment of posttraumatic stress disorder. Evaluating outcome with a behavioral code. Behav Modif 1983; 7(4): 557–68.
29. Johnson CH, Gilmore JD, Shenoy RS. Use of a feeding procedure in the treatment of a stress-related anxiety disorder. J Behav Ther Exp Psychiatry 1982; 13(3): 235–7.

30. Keane TM, Kaloupek DG. Imaginal flooding in the treatment of a posttraumatic stress disorder. J Consult Clin Psychol 1982; 50(1): 138–40.

31. Keane TM, Fairbank JA, Caddell JM, Zimering RT. Implosive (flooding) therapy reduces symptoms of PTSD in Vietnam combat veterans. Behav Ther 1989; 20: 245–60.

32. Foa EB, Rothbaum BO, Riggs D, Murdock T. Treatment of posttraumatic stress disorder in rape victims: a comparison between cognitive-behavioral procedures and counseling. J Consult Clin Psychol 1991; 59: 715–23.

33. Foa EB, Dancu CV, Hembree EA. A comparison of exposure therapy, stress inoculation training, and their combination for reducing posttraumatic stress disorder in female assault victims. J Consult Clin Psychol 1999; 67(2): 194–200.

34. Foa EB, Hembree EA, Cahill SP et al. Randomized trial of prolonged exposure for posttraumatic stress disorder with and without cognitive restructuring: outcome at academic and community clinics. J Consult Clin Psychol 2005; 73(5): 953–64.

35. Resick PA, Nishith P, Weaver TL, Astin MC, Feurer CA. A comparison of cognitive-processing therapy with prolonged exposure and a waiting condition for the treatment of chronic posttraumatic stress disorder in female rape victims. J Consult Clin Psychol 2002; 70: 867–79.

36. Rothbaum BO, Astin MC, Marsteller F. Prolonged exposure vs. eye movement desensitization and reprocessing (EMDR) for PTSD rape victims. J Trauma Stress 2005; 18: 607–16.

37. Foa EB, Rothbaum BO, Riggs DS, Murdock TB. Treatment of posttraumatic stress disorder in rape victims: a comparison between cognitive-behavioral procedures and counseling. J Consult Clin Psychol 1991; 59(5): 715–23.

38. Rothbaum BO, Foa E. Exposure treatment of PTSD concomitant with conversion mutism: a case study. Behav Ther 1991; 22: 449–56.

39. Foa EB, Hearst-Ikeda D, Perry KJ. Evaluation of a brief cognitive-behavioral program for the prevention of chronic PTSD in recent assault victims. J Consult Clin Psychol 1995; 63(6): 948–55.

40. Deblinger E, McLeer SV, Henry D. Cognitive behavioral treatment for sexually abused children suffering post-traumatic stress: preliminary findings. J Am Acad Child Adolesc Psychiatry 1990; 29(5): 747–52.

41. Richards DA, Lovell K, Marks IM. Post-traumatic stress disorder: evaluation of a behavioral treatment program. J Trauma Stress 1994; 7(4): 669–80.

42. Marks I, Lovell K, Noshirvani H, Livanou M, Thrasher S. Treatment of posttraumatic stress disorder by exposure and/or cognitive restructuring: a controlled study. Arch Gen Psychiatry 1998; 55(4): 317–25.

43. Thompson JA, Charlton PF, Kerry R, Lee D, Turner SW. An open trial of exposure therapy based on deconditioning for post-traumatic stress disorder. Br J Clin Psychol 1995; 34: 407–16.

44. Tarrier N, Pilgrim H, Sommerfield C et al. A randomized trial of cognitive therapy and imaginal exposure in the treatment of chronic posttraumatic stress disorder. J Consult Clin Psychol 1999; 67(1): 13–8.

45. Gillespie K, Duffy M, Hackman A, Clark DM. Community based cognitive therapy in the treatment of posttraumatic stress disorder following the Omagh bomb. Behavior Research and Therapy 2002; 40(4): 345–57.

46. Difede J, Eskra D. Adaptation of Cognitive Processing Therapy for the treatment of PTSD following terrorism: A case study of a World Trade Center (1993) survivor. J Trauma Practice 2002; 1(3/4): 155–65.

47. Marks I, Lovell K, Noshirvani H, Livanou M, Thrasher S. Treatment of posttraumatic stress disorder by exposure and/or cognitive restructuring. Arch Gen Psychiatry 1998; 55: 317–25.

48. Taylor S, Thordarson DS, Maxfield L et al. Efficacy, speed, and adverse effects of three PTSD treatments: exposure therapy, relaxation training, and EMDR. J Consult Clin Psychol 2003; 71: 330–8.

49. Thompson JA, Charlton PF, Kerry R, Lee D, Turner SW. An open trial of exposure therapy based on deconditioning for post-traumatic stress disorder. Br J Clin Psychol 1995; 34: 407–16.

50. Paunovic N, Ost LG. Cognitive-behavior therapy vs exposure in the treatment of PTSD in refugees. Behav Res and Ther 2001; 39: 1183–97.

51. McNally RJ, Bryant RA, Ehlers A. Does early psychological intervention promote recovery from posttraumatic stress? Psychological Science in the Public Interest 2003; 4: 45–79.

52. Tarrier N, Pilgrim H, Sommerfield C et al. A randomized trial of cognitive therapy and imaginal exposure in the treatment of chronic posttraumatic stress disorder. J Consult Clin Psychol 1999; 67: 13–8.

53. Schnurr PP, Friedman MJ, Engel CC et al. Cognitive behavioral therapy for posttraumatic stress disorder in women. J Am Med Assoc 2007; 297: 820–30.

54. Keane TM, Fairbank JA, Caddell JM, Zimering RT. Implosive (flooding) therapy reduces symptoms of PTSD in Vietnam combat veterans. Behav Ther 1989; 20: 245–60.

55. Cooper NA, Clum GA. Imaginal flooding as a supplementary treatment for PTSD in combat veterans: A controlled study. Behav Ther 1989; 3: 381–91.

56. Boudewyns PA, Hyer LA, Woods MG, Harrison W, McCannie EW. PTSD among Vietnam veterans: An early look at treatment outcome using direct therapeutic exposure. J Trauma Stress 1990; 3: 359–68.

57. Glynn SM, Eth S, Randolph ET et al. A test of behavioral family therapy to augment exposure for combat-related posttraumatic stress disorder. J Consult Clin Psychol 1999; 67(2): 243–51.

58. Pitman RK, Orr SP, Altman B et al. Emotional processing and outcome of imaginal flooding therapy in Vietnam veterans with chronic posttraumatic stress disorder. Compr Psychiatry 1996; 37: 409–18.

59. Frueh BC, Turner SM, Beidel DCC, Mirabella RF, Jones WJ. Trauma management therapy: A preliminary evaluation of a multi-component behavioral treatment for chronic combat-related PTSD. Behav Res and Ther 1996; 34: 533–43.

60. Bisson JI, Jones N. Taped imaginal exposure as a treatment for post-traumatic stress reactions. J R Army Med Corps 1995; 141(1): 20–4.

61. Schnurr PP, Friedman MJ, Foy DW et al. Randomized trial of trauma-focused group therapy for posttraumatic stress disorder: Results from a department of veterans affairs cooperative study. Arch Gen Psychiatry 2003; 60: 481–9.

62. Ready DJ, Brown-Thomas KB, Worley V et al. A Field Test of Group Based Exposure Therapy with 102 Veterans with War-Related Posttraumatic Stress Disorder. J Traumatic Stress; in press.

63. Crowe CM, Price M, Bradley R. Preliminary findings from an uncontrolled pilot of a novel delivery model for exposure therapy in OEF/OIF and Persian Gulf combat veterans. Unpublished manuscript; 2007.

64. Rothbaum BO, Hodges L, Alarcon R et al. Virtual Vietnam: a Virtual Environment for the Treatment of Vietnam War Veterans with Posttraumatic Stress Disorder. Paper Presented at: Lake George Research Conference on Posttraumatic Stress Disorder, Lake George, NY; 1998.

65. Rothbaum BO, Hodges LF, Ready D, Graap K, Alarcon RD. Virtual reality exposure therapy for Vietnam veterans with posttraumatic stress disorder. J Clin Psychiatry 2001; 62(8): 617–22.

66. Difede J, Hoffman HG. Virtual reality exposure therapy for World Trade Center posttraumatic stress disorder: a case report. Cyberpsychol Behav 2002; 5: 529–35.

67. Difede J, Cukor J, Jayasinghe N et al. Virtual reality exposure therapy for the treatment of posttraumatic stress disorder following September 11, 2001. J Clin Psychiatry 2007; in press.

68. Difede J, Hoffman H, Jaysinghe N. Innovative use of virtual reality technology in the treatment of PTSD in the aftermath of September 11. Psychiatr Serv 2002; 53(9): 1083–5.

69. Difede J, Cukor J, Jayasinghe N et al. Virtual reality exposure therapy for the treatment of posttraumatic stress disorder following September 11, 2001. J Clin Psychiatry 2007; 68(11): 1639–47.

70. Gerardi M, Rothbaum BO, Ressler K, Heekin M, Rizzo A. Virtual reality exposure therapy Using a virtual Iraq: Case report. J Traumatic Stress; in press.

71. Parsons TD, Rizzo AA. Affective outcomes of virtual reality exposure therapy for anxiety and specific phobias: a meta-analysis. J Behav Ther Exp Psychiatry; 2007.

72. Kilpatrick DG, Veronen LJ, Resick PA. Psychological sequelae to rape: assessment and treatment strategies. In: Dolays DM, Meredith RL, eds. Behavioral Medicine: Assessment and Treatment Strategies. New York: Plenum; 1982: 473–97.

73. Resick PA, Jordan CG, Girelli SA et al. A comparative victim study of behavioral group therapy for sexual assault victims. Behav Ther 1988; 19: 385–401.

74. Pearson MA, Poquette BM, Wasden RE. Stress inoculation and the treatment of post-rape trauma: a case report. Behav Ther 1983; 6: 58–9.

75. Watson CG, Tuorila JR, Vickers KS, Gearhart LP, Mendez CM. The efficacies of three relaxation regimens in the treatment of PTSD in Vietnam War veterans. J Clin Psychol 1997; 53(8): 917–23.

76. Frank E, Anderson B, Stewart BD et al. Efficacy of cognitive behavior therapy and systematic desensitization in the treatment of rape trauma. Behav Ther 1988; 19: 403–20.

77. Frank E, Stewart BD. Depressive symptoms in rape victims. A revisit. J Affect Disord 1984; 7(1): 77–85.

78. Wolpe J. Psychotherapy by reciprocal inhibition. Stanford, CA: Stanford University Press; 1988.

79. Bowen GR, Lambert JA. Systematic desensitization therapy with post-traumatic stress disorder cases. In: Figley CR, ed. Trauma and its Wake. New York: Brunner/Mazel; 1986; 2: 280–91.

80. Peniston EG. EMG biofeedback-assisted desensitization treatment for Vietnam combat veteran's post-traumatic stress disorder. Clinical Biofeedback Health 1986; 9: 35–41.

81. Muse M. Stress-related, posttraumatic chronic pain syndrome: behavioral treatment approach. Pain 1986; 25: 389–94.

82. Frank E, Stewart BD. Treating depression in victims of rape. Clin Psychol 1983; 8: 65–74.

83. Turner SM. Systematic Desensitization of Fears and Anxiety in Rape Victims. Paper Presented at: Advancement of Behavior Therapy. San Francisco, CA; 1979.

84. Becker JV, Abel GG. Behavioral treatment of victims of sexual assault. In: Turner SM, Calhoun KS, Adams HE, eds. Handbook of Clinical Behavior Therapy. New York: Wiley; 1981: 347–79.

85. Shapiro F. Eye Movement Desensitization and Reprocessing: Basic Protocols, Principles, and Procedures. New York: Guilford; 1996.

86. Lohr JM, Tolin DF, Lilienfeld SO. Efficacy of eye movement desensitization and reprocessing: implications for behavior therapy. Behav Ther 1998; 29: 123–56.

87. Shapiro F. Efficacy of the eye movement desensitization procedure in the treatment of traumatic memories. J Trauma Stress 1989; 2: 199–223.

88. Boudewyns PA, Stwertka SA, Hyer LA. Eye movement desensitization for PTSD of combat: a treatment outcome pilot study. Behav Ther 1993; 16: 29–33.

89. Jensen JA. An investigation of eye movement desensitization and reprocessing (EMDR) as a treatment for posttraumatic stress disorder (PTSD) symptoms of Vietnam combat veterans. Behav Ther 1994; 25: 311–25.

90. Silver SM, Brooks A, Obenchain J. Treatment of Vietnam war veterans with PTSD: a comparison of eye movement desensitization and reprocessing, biofeedback, and relaxation training. J Trauma Stress 1995; 8(337–42).

91. Pitman RK, Orr SP, Altman B et al. Emotional processing during eye movement desensitization and reprocessing therapy of Vietnam veterans with chronic posttraumatic stress disorder. Compr Psychiatry 1996; 37(6): 419–29,

92. Renfrey G, Spates CR. Eye movement desensitization: a partial dismantling study. J Behav Ther Exp Psychiatry 1994; 25(3): 231–9.

93. Vaughan K, Armstrong MS, Gold R et al. A trial of eye movement desensitization compared to image habituation training and applied muscle relaxation in post-traumatic stress disorder. J Behav Ther Exp Psychiatry 1994; 25(4): 283–91.

94. Wilson SA, Becker LA, Tinker RH. Eye movement desensitization and reprocessing (EMDR) treatment for psychologically traumatized individuals. J Consult Clin Psychol 1995; 63(6): 928–37.

95. Rothbaum BO. A controlled study of eye movement desensitization and reprocessing in the treatment of posttraumatic stress disordered sexual assault victims. Bull Menninger Clin 1997; 61(3): 317–34.

96. Carlson JG, Chemtob CM, Rusnak K, Hedlund NL, Muraoka MY. Eye movement desensitization and reprocessing (EDMR) treatment for combat-related posttraumatic stress disorder. J Trauma Stress 1998; 11(1): 3–24.

97. Marcus SV, Marquis P, Sakai C. Controlled study of treatment of PTSD using EMDR in an HMO setting. Psychotherapy 1997; 34: 307–15.

98. Devilly GJ, Spence SH. The relative efficacy and treatment distress of EMDR and a cognitive-behavior trauma treatment protocol in the amelioration of posttraumatic stress disorder. J Anxiety Disord 1999; 13(1–2): 131–57.

99. Hickling EJ, Blanchard EB. The private practice psychologist and manual-based treatments: post-traumatic stress disorder secondary to motor vehicle accidents. Behav Res Ther 1997; 35(3): 191–203.

100. Frueh BC, Turner SM, Beidel DC, Mirabella RF, Jones WJ. Trauma management therapy: a preliminary evaluation of a multicomponent behavioral treatment for chronic combat-related PTSD. Behav Res Ther 1996; 34(7): 533–43.

101. Resick PA, Schnicke MK. Cognitive processing therapy for sexual assault victims. J Consult Clin Psychol 1992; 60(5): 748–56.

102. Resick P. Does Prior History of Victimization Affect Rape Therapy Outcome? Paper Presented at: Research Workshop on Violence in the Lives of Women: Impact and Treatment. NIMH, Washington, DC; 1994.

103. Resick PA, Nishith P, Astin M. A Controlled Trial Comparing Cognitive Processing Therapy and Prolonged Exposure: Preliminary Findings. Paper Presented at: Lake George Research Conference On Posttraumatic Stress Disorder. Lake George, NY; 1998.

104. Chard KM. An evaluation of cognitive processing therapy for the treatment of posttraumatic stress disorder related to childhood sexual abuse. J Consult Clin Psychol 2005; 73: 965–71.

105. Monson CM, Schnurr PP, Resick PA et al. Cognitive processing therapy for veterans with military-related posttraumatic stress disorder. J Consult Clin Psychol 2006; 74(5): 898–907.

106. Ahrens J, Rexford L. Cognitive processing therapy for incarcerated adolescents with PTSD. J aggression, maltreatment and trauma 2002; 6(1): 201–16.

107. Schulza PM, Hubera CL, Resick PA. Practical adaptations of cognitive processing therapy with Bosnian refugees: Implications for adapting practice to a multicultural clientele. Cogn Behav Pract 2006; 13(4): 310–21.

108. Echeburua E, de Corral P, Zubizarreta I, Sarasua B. Psychological treatment of chronic posttraumatic stress disorder in victims of sexual aggression. Behav Modif 1997; 21(4): 433–56.

109. Resick PA, Galovski TE, Uhlmansiek MO et al. A randomized clinical trial to dismantle components of cognitive processing therapy for posttraumatic stress disorder in female victims of interpersonal violence. J Consult Clin Psychol, in press.

110. van Emmerik AAP, Kamphuis JK, Emmelkamp PMG. Treating acute stress disorder and posttraumatic stress disorder with cognitive behavioral therapy or structured writing therapy: a randomized controlled trial. Psychother Psychosom 2008; 77: 93–100.

111. Barlow DH, Gorman JM, Shear MK, Woods SW. Cognitive-behavioral therapy, imipramine, or their combination for panic disorder: A randomized controlled trial. JAMA 2000; 283(19): 2529–36.

112. Foa E, Franklin ME, Moser J. Context in the clinic: How well do cognitive-behavioral therapies and medications work in combination? Biol Psych 2002; 52: 987–97.

113. Foa EB, Liebowitz MR, Kozak MJ et al. Randomized, placebo-controlled trial of exposure and ritual prevention, clomipramine, and their combination in the treatment of obsessive-compulsive disorder. Am J Psychiatry 2005; 162(1): 151–61.

114. Otto MW, Basden SL, Leyro TM, McHugh RK, Hofmann SG. Clinical perspectives on the combination of D-cycloserine and cognitive-behavioral therapy for the treatment of anxiety disorders. CNS Spectr 2007; 12(1): 51–6, 59–61.

115. Rothbaum BO, Cahill S, Foa EB et al. Augmentation of sertraline with prolonged exposure in the treatment of PTSD. J Traumatic Stress 2006; 19: 625–38.

116. Rothbaum BO, Davis M. Applying learning principles to the treatment of post-trauma reactions. Ann N Y Acad Sci 2003; 1008: 112–21.

117. Myers KM, Davis M. Behavioral and neural analysis of extinction. Neuron 2002; 36(4): 567–84.

118. Walker DL, Ressler KJ, Lu KT, Davis M. Facilitation of conditioned fear extinction by systemic administration or intra-amygdala infusions of D-cycloserine as assessed with fear-potentiated startle in rats. J Neurosci 2002; 22(6): 2343–51.

119. Monahan JB, Handelmann GE, Hood WF, Cordi AA. D-cycloserine, a positive modulator of the N-methyl-D-aspartate receptor, enhances performance of learning tasks in rats. Pharmacol Biochem Behav 1989; 34(3): 649–53.

120. Hood W, Compton R, Monahan J. D-cycloserine: a ligand for the N-methyl-D-aspartate coupled glycine receptor has partial agonist characteristics. Neurosci Lett 1989; 98(1): 91–5.

121. Lee JL, Milton AL, Everitt BJ. Reconsolidation and extinction of conditioned fear: inhibition and potentiation. J Neurosci 2006; 26(39): 10051–6.

122. Botreau F, Paolone G, Stewart J. d-Cycloserine facilitates extinction of a cocaine-induced conditioned place preference. Behav Brain Res 2006; 172(1): 173–8.

123. Ledgerwood L, Richardson R, Cranney J. D-cycloserine facilitates extinction of learned fear: effects on reacquisition and generalized extinction. Biol Psychiatry 2005; 57(8): 841–7.

124. Richardson R, Ledgerwood L, Cranney J. Facilitation of fear extinction by D-cycloserine: theoretical and clinical implications. Learn Mem 2004; 11(5): 510–6.

125. Ledgerwood L, Richardson R, Cranney J. D-cycloserine and the facilitation of extinction of conditioned fear: consequences for reinstatement. Behav Neurosci 2004; 118(3): 505–13.

126. Ledgerwood L, Richardson R, Cranney J. Effects of D-cycloserine on extinction of conditioned freezing. Behav Neurosci 2003; 117(2): 341–9.

127. Yang YL, Chao PK, Ro LS, Wo YY, Lu KT. Glutamate NMDA receptors within the amygdala participate in the modulatory effect of glucocorticoids on extinction of conditioned fear in rats. Neuropsychopharmacology 2007; 32(5): 1042–51.

128. Yang YL, Lu KT. Facilitation of conditioned fear extinction by d-cycloserine is mediated by mitogen-activated protein kinase and phosphatidylinositol 3-kinase cascades and requires de novo protein synthesis in basolateral nucleus of amygdala. Neuroscience. 2005; 134(1): 247–60.

129. Otto M. Learning and "Unlearning" Fears: Preparedness, Neural Pathways, and Patients. Biol Psych 2002; 52: 917–20.

130. Marks I, Swinson R, Basoglu M et al. Alprazolam and exposure alone and combined in panic disorder with agoraphobia. A controlled study in London and Toronto. Br J Psychiatry 1993; 162: 776–87.

131. Ressler KJ, Rothbaum BO, Tannenbaum L et al. Cognitive enhancers as adjuncts to psychotherapy: use of D-cycloserine in phobic individuals to facilitate extinction of fear. Arch Gen Psychiatry 2004; 61(11): 1136–44.

132. Hofmann SG, Pollack MH, Otto MW. Augmentation treatment of psychotherapy for anxiety disorders with D-cycloserine. CNS Drug Rev. Fall-Winter 2006; 12(3–4): 208–17.

133. Hofmann SG, Meuret AE, Smits JA et al. Augmentation of exposure therapy with D-cycloserine for social anxiety disorder. Arch Gen Psychiatry 2006; 63(3): 298–304.

134. Kushner MG, Kim SW, Donahue C et al. D-Cycloserine augmented exposure therapy for obsessive compulsive disorder. Biol Psychiatry 2007; in press.

135. Guastella AJ, Dadds MR, Lovibond PF, Mitchell P, Richardson R. A randomized controlled trial of the effect of d-cycloserine on exposure therapy for spider fear. J Psychiatr Res 2007; 41(6): 466–71.

136. Guastella AJ, Lovibond PF, Dadds MR, Mitchell P, Richardson R. A randomized controlled trial of the effect of d-cycloserine on extinction and fear conditioning in humans. Behav Res Ther 2007; 45(4): 663–72.

9 | Pharmacotherapy of posttraumatic stress disorder

Lakshmi N Ravindran and Murray B Stein

INTRODUCTION

With vivid descriptions dating back to ancient Greece, the battlefield phenomenon, known In its various incarnations as "soldier's heart," "shell shock," and "combat fatigue," is not just limited to military populations. Studies on the more recent construct of "posttraumatic stress disorder" (PTSD), initially accepted by the psychiatric community in 1980, (1) now suggest a lifetime prevalence of 6.8% in the general U.S. population.(2) With recent world events and media coverage bringing increased awareness to this disabling disorder, the drive to find effective treatments for this condition is even greater.

This goal of this chapter is to review the evidence base of pharmacological interventions for PTSD. Wherever possible, the review is reliant on randomized, double-blind, placebo-controlled trials to provide the most meaningful information. However, in cases where this is not feasible, other evidence (e.g., open-label or active-control trials) may be mentioned. The use of pharmacotherapy to prevent development of PTSD following trauma is discussed in a subsequent chapter (see the chapter by Bisson and Zohar, this volume). Effective psychotherapeutic interventions for PTSD also exist and are commonly used either as monotherapy or in conjunction with pharmacological agents. Details substantiating these management strategies are also discussed in another chapter (see chapter by Ressler and Rothbaum, this volume)

ANTIDEPRESSANTS

Selective Serotonin Reuptake Inhibitors

The class of medications known as the selective serotonin reuptake inhibitors (SSRIs) has largely replaced all other classes of antidepressants as first-line agents for the acute treatment of PTSD. At this time, only paroxetine and sertraline have official FDA approval for treatment of this disorder; however, clinically all SSRIs are generally used for this purpose. Although each SSRI is structurally distinct with varying effects on the different neurotransmitters, as a class they serve to enhance serotonin function in the brain. The exact mechanism by which they accomplish this remains uncertain, but it is thought to involve effects on 2nd messenger systems and/or neuropeptides, such as brain-derived neurotrophic factor (BDNF).(3)

One of the earliest reports of SSRI efficacy in chronic PTSD came from van der Kolk and colleagues (4) who reported results of a 5-week placebo-controlled trial of fluoxetine in both civilian and combat populations. They found fluoxetine resulted in significant decreases in overall PTSD symptomatology following the treatment period, particularly in the symptom clusters of hyperarousal and numbing. The other notable finding from this trial was the marked difference in symptom severity change between civilians (40%) and combat veterans (15%), although it should be noted that the severity of PTSD symptoms at baseline was significantly worse in the veteran population. Nevertheless, this discrepancy may have been responsible in part for the contention that combat-related PTSD is less responsive to pharmacological intervention. Since then, two other placebo-controlled studies have confirmed the utility of fluoxetine in PTSD, with one study finding it effective even for combat-related symptoms.(5, 6) In contrast, two placebo-controlled trials failed to find positive effects for treatment with fluoxetine. The authors of the first study (7) suggested that the lack of effect may have been due to the severe, chronic nature of the combat-related trauma in their subjects, while the authors of the second study (8) wondered whether the use of lower doses and a predominantly female population may have played a role in the decreased response rates found in their results.

Following the early reports of successful use of SSRIs for this disorder, several other large placebo-controlled trials have since been conducted with a number serving as the basis for regulatory approval of two particular SSRIs, sertraline and paroxetine. Two large multicenter trials comparing placebo and sertraline treatment over 12 weeks found moderate effects for active drug (effect sizes ≈0.5) (9, 10), with the former study also noting particular effects for sertraline on the hyperarousal and numbing/avoidance clusters of symptoms. Similarly, two large trials found that paroxetine significantly decreased PTSD symptoms in all three symptoms clusters, following 12 weeks of treatment compared to placebo.(11, 12) More recently, Marshall et al. (13) provided additional support for the efficacy of paroxetine when they studied an urban population with a high minority quotient. They noted that paroxetine appeared to be helpful for treatment of core PTSD symptoms along with associated features of PTSD, which included significant dissociative symptoms and interpersonal issues.

Currently, there is only one double-blind study involving the use of citalopram that compares it to sertraline and placebo; (14) however, although citalopram was able to demonstrate an overall improvement in the PTSD symptoms by the end of this study, the results failed to demonstrate significant differences in efficacy between the three treatment arms. Nevertheless, open-label trials have suggested a role for citalopram in the treatment of PTSD, in adults as well as children and adolescents.(15–18) Similarly, open-label trials have also demonstrated moderate success using escitalopram (19) and fluvoxamine.(20–23).

While the findings from the above trials support specific PTSD symptom reduction with SSRIs, evidence in the literature also suggests that SSRIs may be useful in improving and sustaining amelioration in quality of life for this population, with the majority of the recovery occurring during the acute treatment phase.(24)

At this time, SSRIs represent the most extensively investigated class of medications in PTSD research. A recent report from the Institute of Medicine (IOM) concluded that evidence for SSRI efficacy in PTSD was inconclusive, citing the less-than-robust effect overall effect sizes. (25) Nonetheless, many studies, as cited above, suggest a beneficial role for SSRIs in the treatment of PTSD—though the magnitude of benefits varies widely among individuals and, generally, is less than would be desired of a first-line treatment. Among the SSRIs, there is every reason to believe that efficacy is shared by the entire class. As such, the use of a particular SSRI for PTSD should take into consideration factors such as side effects, prior response, and perhaps family history of response. Dosages of SSRIs for the treatment of PTSD are in the same range as those recommended for major depressive disorder. Because many patients with PTSD suffer from comorbid MDD, (26) the use of SSRIs is expected to benefit both conditions.

Duration of treatment with SSRIs

There is evidence from several studies that extended treatment with SSRIs may provide additional benefit in PTSD. Londberg and colleagues (27) studied a cohort of patients who had previously completed one of two double-blind, placebo-controlled trials using sertraline as an acute-phase treatment for PTSD. Of these, 252 subjects were enrolled into a 24-week, open-label, continuation-phase study, again using sertraline. The investigators observed that not only did 54% of nonresponders during the original 12-week acute-phase trials convert to responders, but 92% of the original acute-phase responders maintained their recovery. Subsequent analyses of investigational measures also showed that 20% to 25% of the overall improvement in PTSD symptoms occurred during this extended continuation phase and similarly that 41% of the improvement in depressive symptoms and 31% of the improvement in quality of life also occurred during this period. Finally, when a subsample ($N = 96$) of the responders from this continuation-phase study were rerandomized to double-blind maintenance treatment with either sertraline or placebo for an additional 28 weeks, both relapse (sertraline 5.3% vs. placebo 26.1%) and discontinuation (sertraline 15.8% vs. placebo 45.7%) rates were significantly higher in the placebo group.(28) A similar study was conducted by Martenyi and colleagues (29) using fluoxetine. Following an initial 12 week, acute-phase, placebo-controlled trial, fluoxetine responders were subsequently rerandomized for continuation treatment of a further 24 weeks. At endpoint, SSRI treatment was found to be superior to placebo with respect to time to relapse ($p = 0.027$), and once again patients receiving active treatment had significantly greater improvement in their PTSD symptoms compared to those on placebo ($p = 0.011$). Overall, there were also fewer dropouts from the fluoxetine group (5.8%) compared to those receiving placebo (16.1%)

This collection of studies highlights the importance of providing extended treatment for PTSD in order to elicit maximal improvement of symptoms, maintain recovery, and prevent relapse. The noteworthy finding from Londberg et al. (27) regarding conversion of nonresponders to responders only *after* the acute-phase treatment also serves to underline the necessity for patience when treating this population (although this may be clinically feasible only when there is at least some initial response to SSRI treatment). At present, guidelines for duration of pharmacotherapy treatment recommend continuing medications for 6 to 12 months in cases of acute PTSD or 12 to 24 months for chronic PTSD; under certain circumstances, such as persistent residual symptoms or poor psychosocial functioning, an even longer treatment period may be of benefit.(30, 31)

Dual Reuptake Inhibitors

There are two serotonin/norepinephrine reuptake inhibitors currently available on the market. There are currently only two placebo-controlled trials assessing the use of Venlafaxine extended-release (XR) in PTSD. In the first, Davidson and colleagues (32) conducted an acute-phase, three-arm treatment study comparing venlafaxine XR to sertraline and placebo. At endpoint, venlafaxine XR was found to be significantly more efficacious than placebo on the primary outcome measure of PTSD symptom reduction, specifically on the subscales measuring symptoms of avoidance-numbing and hyperarousal; these differences in improvement were seen as early as Week 2. Furthermore, the results of an analysis to control for depression severity and severity by treatment suggested that the improvement in PTSD symptoms was not mediated by improvement in depressive symptoms, which was an important finding as the two conditions are so often comorbid. There were no significant differences in efficacy on primary or secondary outcome measures between venlafaxine XR and sertraline.

In one of the few longer-term pharmacotherapy studies investigating medications other than SSRIs, Davidson et al. (33) carried out a 6-month placebo-controlled trial using venlafaxine. Once again, venlafaxine was found to be superior to placebo with respect to improvement in overall PTSD symptoms ($p = 0.006$), in particular for symptom clusters of reexperiencing ($p = 0.008$) and avoidance-numbing ($p = 0.006$), with a trend toward significance for symptoms of hyperarousal ($p = 0.06$). The authors also noted that the superior efficacy of the drug was sustained from Week 12 (the typical end of an acute-phase trial) to endpoint. Finally, Venlafaxine XR-treated patients also showed greater improvement on measures of resilience, stress-vulnerability, and quality of life relative to their placebo-treated counterparts. Although there are relatively few randomized clinical trials to support its use in PTSD, it probably represents a very reasonable 1st or 2nd line pharmacotherapy option.

The other dual reuptake inhibitor, duloxetine, has only recently been approved for use in the United States, Canada, and parts of Europe. At present, there are no published, randomized clinical trials investigating its efficacy in the treatment of PTSD. However, based on its putative mechanism of action and some preliminary evidence from trials investigating its use in depression and other anxiety disorders (34–37), there is reason to believe duloxetine may be useful and that it merits investigating for treatment of PTSD.

Tricyclic Antidepressants

The tricyclic antidepressants (TCAs) represent one of the earliest classes of antidepressant to be used in a widespread fashion. They are still commonly used and quite effective (for depression), although they have largely been relegated to second- or third-line agents as a result of their adverse-effect profile, which includes a number of anticholinergic effects.

In one of the earliest controlled trials investigating antidepressant efficacy in PTSD, 18 hospitalized male veterans completed a double-blind, crossover trial consisting of two 4-week treatment periods with an intervening 4-day switchover period.(38) The trial, which employed desipramine (up to 200 mg daily) did not find significant differences in PTSD symptom change between the two treatments, although there did seem to be an improvement in observer-rated depression symptoms with desipramine. Of note is that the period of active treatment was quite short (only 4 weeks) and the investigators did not utilize observer-rated scales for PTSD but rather employed substitute items chosen post hoc from more general depression and anxiety scales. A larger trial, comparing amitriptyline and placebo in 46 veterans with chronic PTSD, was conducted by Davidson and colleagues in 1990.(39) In this case, amitriptyline showed some benefit over placebo on certain measures but not on the structured interview for PTSD. One notable result from this trial was the overall relative lack of response in both treatment groups, even after 12 weeks of treatment, with 64% of the amitriptyline-treated group and 72% of the placebo group still meeting criteria for PTSD. This finding highlights the common situation of persistent residual symptoms, with significant clinical impact, even in patients who may have had a degree of response to treatment. Two other placebo-controlled trials using TCAs have also been conducted. These are discussed below in the section of the chapter entitled "Monoamine Oxidase Inhibitors."

Monoamine Oxidase Inhibitors

The monoamine oxidase inhibitors (MAOIs) represent an older class of antidepressants that works to increase monoamine availability by irreversibly inhibiting the enzyme, monoamine oxidase, responsible for their breakdown. Although MAOIs are effective antidepressants, their use is mainly limited by the need to maintain a strict low-tyramine diet to decrease the risk of hypertensive crises. Consequently, MAOIs are rarely first-line agents for treatment of psychiatric disorders. Nevertheless, there have been placebo-controlled trials using these medications. Frank et al. (40) compared phenelzine, imipramine, and placebo in 34 Vietnam veterans with PTSD. Both active treatment groups displayed significantly improved PTSD symptoms compared to placebo, with the phenelzine-treated group showing particular improvement in intrusive or reexperiencing symptoms. A subsequent study by Kosten et al. (41) examining the same medications, but in a slightly larger sample of 60 veterans, found similar results in terms of active treatment vs. placebo. This time, however, there seemed to be a more pronounced advantage for the subjects receiving phenelzine. In contrast to these two trials, findings from a smaller, double-blind, crossover study ($N = 13$) in which patients were randomized to treatment with either phenelzine or placebo did not reveal differences between treatment groups.(42) There are no other placebo-controlled trials of irreversible MAOIs in PTSD. We are unaware of more recent trials with MAOIs or of trials that compare MAOIs to SSRIs. It is, therefore, difficult to specify where in the PTSD therapeutic armamentarium MAOIs should be used. Would MAOIs be useful for SSRI- or SNRI-refractory patients? There are no data to support such a contention at this time.

A subtype of MAOIs, called reversible inhibitors of monoamine oxidase A (RIMAs) have also been available. The selectivity and reversibility of the RIMAs are thought to render them safer to use. An initial trial of the RIMA, brofaromine, found it to be effective over placebo in individuals suffering from PTSD for $\geq$ 1 year.(43) However, outcomes from a subsequent, large, placebo-controlled trial failed to differentiate active treatment from placebo, although both groups did demonstrate significant symptom reduction. Moclobemide, another RIMA, was compared to fluoxetine and tianeptine (a drug thought to work by selectively accelerating serotonin reuptake) in a study comparing different classes of antidepressants in PTSD.(44) All three treatment groups showed significant improvement in severity of PTSD symptoms with no between-group differences. However, this was a head-to-head trial with no placebo-control group.

At this time, neither brofaromine nor moclobemide is commercially available in the United States, although the latter is available in Canada, Europe, and other parts of the world.

Bupropion

The proposed mechanism of action for the antidepressant bupropion involves dual reuptake inhibition of both norepinephrine and dopamine, although with negligible serotonergic activity. (45) Due to its nicotinic antagonist activity, it is also commonly used as a smoking cessation aid. In the only placebo-controlled trial investigating change in PTSD symptoms as a primary outcome measure, subjects treated with bupropion sustained release (SR) could not be distinguished from the placebo group.(46) An earlier study that compared bupropion SR to placebo for smoking cessation in veterans with chronic PTSD found the active drug helpful for this purpose, but no differences were found between groups on the secondary measures of PTSD outcome.(47)

Mirtazapine

In 1994, mirtazapine was introduced to the psychiatric pharmacopoeia. It is thought to enhance both serotonin and norepinephrine release via blockade of presynaptic α_2-adrenergic receptors. At the same time, mirtazapine also exerts a significant blocking effect at the both the 5-HT$_2$ and

5-HT$_3$ serotonergic receptors and notably at the H$_1$ histaminic receptor.(48) At this time, only a single 8-week, placebo-controlled pilot trial exists to study the use of mirtazapine in PTSD.(49) In the sample of 29 patients, the authors claimed mirtazapine (up to 45 mg daily) produced a significant treatment effect on the global improvement item of their primary outcome measure, as well as amelioration on a number of secondary measures. For patients on mirtazapine, statistical analyses showed moderate (0.42) to strong (1.06) effect sizes with respect to change in PTSD symptoms. However, the conclusions of the study were limited by the small sample size, and unfortunately, there have been no subsequent larger trials to substantiate the findings.

Nefazodone

Nefazodone is an antidepressant that works via antagonist activity at the postsynaptic 5-HT2A receptor and inhibition of presynaptic serotonin and norepinephrine reuptake, as well as displaying relatively potent antagonism of the alpha-1-adrenergic receptor.(50)

Although a number of open trials have suggested a utility for nefazodone in PTSD, there is a dearth of randomized clinical trials to support this. In the only published placebo-controlled trial (51), there was a significant decline in PTSD symptom scores in nefazodone-treated subjects compared to those receiving placebo, but the population studied was relatively small. Another double-blind, head-to-head comparison of nefazodone to sertraline demonstrated efficacious reduction of PTSD symptoms over time in both treatment arms, with no differences between groups.(52) The lack of larger published trials is most likely due to the recent withdrawal of nefazodone from the market in Europe, Canada, Australia, and New Zealand, following reports of its association with hepatotoxicity in a number of patients. Given these concerns, the use of nefazodone is effectively a more academic consideration rather than a practical one.

ANTICONVULSANTS

Numerous anticonvulsant medications are known to have mood-stabilizing properties and have thus found a role in the treatment of various psychiatric disorders. While their value has been most pronounced in treating bipolar disorder, there is also evidence to support some utility in the depressive disorders and certain anxiety disorders.(53) The hypothesis then that a kindling and sensitization mechanism may figure in the development of PTSD (54) has naturally led researchers to question their possible effectiveness for treatment of this particular anxiety disorder. Within this class, the medications that have been of most interest include carbamazepine, valproic acid, lamotrigine, gabapentin, topiramate, tiagabine, and levetiracetam. Although literature from case reports and open trials suggest they may be helpful, controlled studies investigating the usefulness of these medications has only been conducted in a limited way for PTSD, and with mixed results.

A preliminary 12-week placebo-controlled trial of 15 subjects suggested that lamotrigine may be helpful for the reexperiencing and avoidance/numbing symptoms clusters of PTSD. (55) However, the limited sample size precluded more definitive conclusions. In 2006, Connor and colleagues conducted a 12-week, open-label trial of tiagabine, thought to function as a selective GABA reuptake inhibitor.(56) Responders following the open-label treatment period ($N = 18$) were then randomized to continuation treatment or placebo for a further 12 weeks. Although there was no difference in relapse rates between treatment groups, there did appear a trend of increased remission in the tiagabine group (p=0.08). However, in a subsequent double-blind, placebo-controlled trial with much more substantial numbers ($N = 232$), no differences were found between groups in any of the primary or secondary outcome measures. (57) Likewise, Davis et al. (58) were unable to find any differences in PTSD outcomes between 85 veterans randomized to 8 weeks of placebo or divalproex monotherapy. However, it is possible that the relatively briefer duration of the trial and the chronicity of illness in these subjects ($M = 24.4$ years) may have played a role in the lack of response seen. Finally, a randomized, placebo-controlled trial of topiramate augmentation therapy of 40 male veterans failed to find any treatment effect for active medication after 7 weeks (59), although it should be acknowledged that the dropout rate, mainly due to adverse events (topiramate $N = 8$, placebo $N = 2$), for this trial was quite high. In contrast, the only double-blind, placebo-controlled topiramate monotherapy trial found that topiramate was actually helpful in reducing reexperiencing symptoms of PTSD ($p = 0.038$), although there was no statistically significant difference between treatment groups in overall PTSD scores.(60) Nevertheless, the authors suggested that the results warranted further investigation in larger trials.

At best the results of these limited numbers of trials are mixed and no definitive conclusions on the utility of anticonvulsants for PTSD can be drawn. As such, the role of anticonvulsants for the treatment of PTSD remains uncertain, and only future controlled trials with larger and more diverse study populations will help in illuminating their function for this disorder.

BENZODIAZEPINES AND OTHER HYPNOTICS

Benzodiazepines and sedative–hypnotic medications are among the commonest adjunctive therapies for antidepressants in the treatment of PTSD.(61) Their use is mainly directed toward symptomatic treatment of the chronic sleep difficulties and other hyperarousal symptoms, such as irritability, so common in PTSD. Surprisingly, despite their widespread clinical use for this disorder, there are few controlled trials in the literature to support these practices.

A randomized, single-blind, crossover study of clonazepam (up to 2 mg daily) failed to find significant differences in outcome compared to placebo, although the study population was limited to only six subjects.(62) Braun et al. (63) chose to study a relatively larger sample of 16 subjects with chronic PTSD, who were randomized to either alprazolam or placebo for 5 weeks with subsequent crossover following an intervening 2-week washout period. In this case, the investigators found that alprazolam conferred benefit in terms of improvement in PTSD symptoms.

The paucity of clinical trials investigating benzodiazepines is of concern given the prevalent use of these medications in the PTSD population. Further, the "mixed" results even from this limited sample, serve to underline the need for more definitive investigations to support and reinforce effective clinical decision making.

ANTIPSYCHOTICS

The use of adjunctive antipsychotic use, particularly atypical antipsychotics, for PTSD is becoming increasingly common in clinical practice. Multiple rationales for this practice can be found in the literature. Among individuals suffering from PTSD, it has been estimated that up to 40% may experience psychotic symptoms, typically positive symptoms such as hallucinations and delusions (64), and the presence of these symptoms is not entirely explained by the presence of comorbid psychotic disorders or medical problems. (65) In addition, it has been hypothesized that dopamine dysfunction may not only trigger the production of these psychotic symptoms but may also play a role in mediation of hyperarousal symptoms, such as hypervigilance, exaggerated startle, and irritability.(66, 67) Together these lines of thought suggest an initial rational neurochemical basis for the use of atypical antipsychotics in PTSD. These medications have also been shown to have anxiolytic properties themselves, thought to be based in part in the enhanced noradrenergic transmission that results from antagonism of the 5-HT2A receptors. Additional anxiolytic activity has been attributed to antagonism of the α_2-adrenergic receptor and partial agonism at the 5-HT$_{1A}$ receptor.(68) Finally, the sedating effects of the atypical antipsychotics, mainly ascribed to histaminic H$_1$ receptor blockade, are often used to target the sleep difficulties so characteristic of PTSD. Given the multitude of effects, it is not surprising that atypical use is so widespread for this disorder. Although not reviewed here, there certainly appears to be both theoretical and substantial evidentiary bases to support the use of atypicals as adjunctive therapy in certain subpopulations suffering from PTSD (69–71); however, the question remains as to whether there is evidence to substantiate their use as a monotherapy treatment in this disorder.

Despite the availability of 6 different atypical antipsychotics (olanzapine, risperidone, quetiapine, ziprasidone, clozapine, and aripiprazole) currently available on the market, there are only two published double-blind, placebo-controlled trials of atypical antipsychotic monotherapy for PTSD. In the first, Butterfield et al. (72) conducted a 10-week, placebo-controlled trial of olanzapine (up to 20 mg daily) and found that although both treatment groups improved over time, there were no notable differences in outcome between groups. Potential shortcomings suggested to explain this included the small sample size ($N = 15$) with unusually elevated placebo response rate, shorter than customary treatment duration that may have missed delayed responders, a primarily female population (gender may affect treatment response), diverse trauma types included, and the presence of comorbidity in all but one subject. A more recent 12-week pilot study (73) compared flexibly dosed risperidone monotherapy (mean daily dose = 2.62 mg) to placebo. In this case, low-dose risperidone appeared to confer a significant therapeutic benefit in treatment of PTSD symptoms relative to placebo, as well as being reasonably well tolerated. Once again, however, limited conclusions can be drawn because of the small sample size ($N = 20$).

These trials notwithstanding, there does seem to be a role for atypical antipsychotics in the treatment of PTSD and their use in clinical practice is likely to continue. However, that does not mitigate the need for larger research trials exploring the use of olanzapine, risperidone, and the other atypicals to validate these practices. The main limitations to their current use include the presence of significant metabolic effects, such as glucose and lipid dysregulation. As such, these side effects should be carefully and routinely monitored, even when these drugs are administered in low doses.

ADRENERGIC AGENTS

A number of brief reports in the literature have suggested a utility for adrenergic agents in the treatment of PTSD (74–77), particularly for the symptoms of hyperarousal. One of these, clonidine, works as an agonist at the postsynaptic α_2-adrenergic receptor, most commonly used as an antihypertensive, but it has also been reported, when used in conjunction with impramine, to have a role in decreasing nightmares.(78) However, at this time there are no placebo-controlled trials to substantiate this. Guanfacine is another centrally acting alpha adrenergic agent that works in much the same way as clonidine. In the case of guanfacine, there is a single placebo-controlled trial for its use in veterans with chronic PTSD, but the results of the trial did not support a positive effect on posttraumatic symptoms, sleep disturbance, or general mood disturbance.(79) In contrast, the antihypertensive agent, prazosin, a centrally acting selective $_1$-antagonist, has shown more promise. Raskind et al. (80) carried out a 20-week, placebo-controlled, crossover trial with prazosin in 10 veterans with chronic PTSD and severe nightmares. The superiority of prazosin was seen on all primary outcome measures that included change in levels of distressing dreams and overall PTSD severity. These findings were subsequently replicated using a larger sample of veterans ($N = 40$) and a parallel group design over 8 weeks.(81) Most recently, Taylor et al. (82) noted similar results in a smaller outpatient sample ($N = 13$) of civilians with chronic PTSD, nightmares, and sleep disturbance who underwent a 7-week crossover trial (each treatment period was 3 weeks). Noteworthy findings during prazosin treatment included a substantial increase in total sleep time (94 minutes), shorter REM latency with increased REM sleep time, and a change toward normal dream content. Hopefully, additional studies of longer duration will continue to substantiate these results.

NOVEL AGENTS

The quest to discover and develop novel pharmacological agents to treat PTSD is an ongoing pursuit. Although several agents are under investigation, two agents that may be promising include d-cycloserine and hydrocortisone.

D-cycloserine, a partial agonist of the n-methyl-d-aspartate (NMDA) receptor, has been of interest in certain anxiety disorders, including social anxiety disorder (83, 84) and obsessive–compulsive disorder (85). A single pilot study (86) of 11 outpatients with chronic PTSD compared d-cycloserine to placebo in a 12-week, double-blind, crossover design (each treatment period was 4 weeks). The active treatment did appear to cause improvement of numbing/avoidance symptoms of PTSD, although placebo patients also registered improvement of these symptoms. D-cycloserine also appeared to improve certain neurocognitive measures compared to placebo. Larger, parallel group design studies may help to further elucidate the utility of this medication for PTSD.

Interest in glucocorticoid dysregulation mechanisms in PTSD has prompted the investigation of hydrocortisone as a possible early intervention to prevent PTSD and more recently as a potential treatment for PTSD. A preliminary, placebo-controlled, crossover trial (3-month duration) of low-dose hydrocortisone (10 mg daily) appeared to show some benefit in reducing PTSD symptoms, particularly of the reexperiencing and avoidance type.(87) However, the results of this study should be interpreted with extreme caution as the sample consisted of only three subjects, with two subjects on concurrent sleep medication and one also receiving concurrent psychotherapy. Nevertheless, if a larger trial were able to replicate these findings, the results would certainly be intriguing.

CONCLUSIONS

Pharmacological agents represent an important and effective tool in the clinician's armamentarium for treatment of PTSD. Although the evidence base to support the success of different medication classes to treat this illness continues to expand and develop, there are always additional areas of research that remain to be explored. In particular, there is a need to develop better predictors of response to specific drug classes or psychotherapy, as well as a better understanding of situations in which combination treatment with medication and psychotherapy might be most appropriate. Also helpful would be improved strategies to enhance compliance and tolerability of pharmacological interventions, as well as developing more definitive guidelines around the necessity for continuation and maintenance treatment over more extended periods. Although there is certainly a preliminary evidence base to support the use of many medications for PTSD, it is equally evident that there is a relative dearth of well-powered, definitive, randomized controlled trials and consequent need to conduct such trials, of both acute and long-term outcomes and in a variety of populations (e.g., recent combat veterans and persons exposed to childhood trauma) to substantiate and validate many of the findings, including their generalizability. And finally there is a pressing need to develop well-tolerated pharmacological treatments that work better, that is, those that have a more profound impact on symptom reduction and restoration of functioning.

Establishing successful treatment strategies for PTSD remains a crucial and active area of research with psychotherapy and pharmacotherapy representing the twin cornerstones of intervention for this disorder. Deciding on which technique is the most appropriate for a given patient depends on many factors, including but not limited to illness severity, comorbidity, previous response to treatment, and preference of both patient and clinician. Regardless of what type of treatment is eventually chosen, the ultimate goals of intervention should be symptom reduction, and ideally, resolution, as well as a full return of optimal psychosocial functioning.

ACKNOWLEDGMENTS

Several authoritative reviews (88, 89) provided invaluable assistance during the compilation and synthesis of the literature for this chapter. We are grateful to the authors of those reviews for making their work available as extremely useful sources of reference.

REFERENCES

1. American Psychiatric Association. Diagnostic and statistical manual of mental disorders (DSM-III). 3rd ed. Washington DC: American Psychiatric Association; 2008.
2. Kessler RC, Berglund P, Demler O et al. Lifetime prevalence and age-of-onset distributions of DSM-IV disorders in the National Comorbidity Survey Replication. Arch Gen Psychiatry 2005; 62(6): 593–602.
3. Duman RS. Novel therapeutic approaches beyond the serotonin receptor. Biol Psychiatry 1998; 44(5): 324–35.
4. van der Kolk BA, Dreyfuss D, Michaels M et al. Fluoxetine in posttraumatic stress disorder. J Clin Psychiatry 1994; 55(12): 517–22.
5. Connor KM, Sutherland SM, Tupler LA, Malik ML, Davidson JR. Fluoxetine in post-traumatic stress disorder. Randomised, double-blind study. Br J Psychiatry 1999; 175: 17–22.

6. Martenyi F, Brown EB, Zhang H, Prakash A, Koke SC. Fluoxetine vs. placebo in posttraumatic stress disorder. J Clin Psychiatry 2002; 63(3): 199–206.

7. Hertzberg MA, Feldman ME, Beckham JC, Kudler HS, Davidson JR. Lack of efficacy for fluoxetine in PTSD: a placebo controlled trial in combat veterans. Ann Clin Psychiatry 2000; 12(2): 101–5.

8. Martenyi F, Brown EB, Caldwell CD. Failed efficacy of fluoxetine in the treatment of posttraumatic stress disorder: results of a fixed-dose, placebo-controlled study. J Clin Psychopharmacol 2007; 27(2): 166–70.

9. Brady K, Pearlstein T, Asnis GM et al. Efficacy and safety of sertraline treatment of posttraumatic stress disorder: a randomized controlled trial. JAMA 2000; 283(14): 1837–44.

10. Davidson JR, Rothbaum BO, van der Kolk BA, Sikes CR, Farfel GM. Multicenter, double-blind comparison of sertraline and placebo in the treatment of posttraumatic stress disorder. Arch Gen Psychiatry 2001; 58(5): 485–92.

11. Marshall RD, Beebe KL, Oldham M, Zaninelli R. Efficacy and safety of paroxetine treatment for chronic PTSD: a fixed-dose, placebo-controlled study. Am J Psychiatry 2001; 158(12): 1982–8.

12. Tucker P, Zaninelli R, Yehuda R et al. Paroxetine in the treatment of chronic posttraumatic stress disorder: results of a placebo-controlled, flexible-dosage trial. J Clin Psychiatry 2001; 62(11): 860–8.

13. Marshall RD, Lewis-Fernandez R, Blanco C et al. A controlled trial of paroxetine for chronic PTSD, dissociation, and interpersonal problems in mostly minority adults. Depress Anxiety 2007; 24(2): 77–84.

14. Tucker P, Potter-Kimball R, Wyatt DB et al. Can physiologic assessment and side effects tease out differences in PTSD trials? A double-blind comparison of citalopram, sertraline, and placebo. Psychopharmacol Bull 2003; 37(3): 135–49.

15. Seedat S, Stein DJ, Emsley RA. Open trial of citalopram in adults with post-traumatic stress disorder. Int J Neuropsychopharmacol 2000; 3(2):135–40.

16. Seedat S, Lockhat R, Kaminer D, Zungu-Dirwayi N, Stein DJ. An open trial of citalopram in adolescents with post-traumatic stress disorder. Int Clin Psychopharmacol 2001; 16(1): 21–5.

17. Seedat S, Stein DJ, Ziervogel C et al. Comparison of response to a selective serotonin reuptake inhibitor in children, adolescents, and adults with posttraumatic stress disorder. J Child Adolesc Psychopharmacol 2002; 12(1): 37–46.

18. English BA, Jewell M, Jewell G, Ambrose S, Davis LL. Treatment of chronic posttraumatic stress disorder in combat veterans with citalopram: an open trial. J Clin Psychopharmacol 2006; 26(1): 84–8.

19. Robert S, Hamner MB, Ulmer HG, Lorberbaum JP, Durkalski VL. Open-label trial of escitalopram in the treatment of posttraumatic stress disorder. J Clin Psychiatry 2006; 67(10): 1522–6.

20. De Boer M, Op den Velde W, Falger PJ et al. Fluvoxamine treatment for chronic PTSD: a pilot study. Psychother Psychosom 1992; 57(4): 158–163.

21. Marmar CR, Schoenfeld F, Weiss DS et al. Open trial of fluvoxamine treatment for combat-related posttraumatic stress disorder. J Clin Psychiatry 1996; 57(8): 66–70.

22. Davidson JR, Weisler RH, Malik M, Tupler LA. Fluvoxamine in civilians with posttraumatic stress disorder. J Clin Psychopharmacol 1998; 18(1): 93–5.

23. Escalona R, Canive JM, Calais LA, Davidson JR. Fluvoxamine treatment in veterans with combat-related post-traumatic stress disorder. Depress Anxiety 2002; 15(1): 29–33.

24. Rapaport MH, Endicott J, Clary CM. Posttraumatic stress disorder and quality of life: results across 64 weeks of sertraline treatment. J Clin Psychiatry 2002; 63(1): 59–65.

25. Committee on Treatment of Posttraumatic Stress Disorder (Institute of Medicine). Treatment of Posttraumatic Stress Disorder: An Assessment of the Evidence. Washington, DC: The National Academies Press; 2007.

26. Shalev AY, Freedman S, Peri T et al. Prospective study of posttraumatic stress disorder and depression following trauma. Am J Psychiatry 1998; 155(5): 630–7.

27. Londborg PD, Hegel MT, Goldstein S et al. Sertraline treatment of posttraumatic stress disorder: results of 24 weeks of open-label continuation treatment. J Clin Psychiatry 2001; 62(5): 325–31.

28. Davidson J, Pearlstein T, Londborg P et al. Efficacy of sertraline in preventing relapse of posttraumatic stress disorder: results of a 28-week double-blind, placebo-controlled study. Am J Psychiatry 2001; 158(12): 1974–81.

29. Martenyi F, Brown EB, Zhang H, Koke SC, Prakash A. Fluoxetine v. placebo in prevention of relapse in post-traumatic stress disorder. Br J Psychiatry 2002; 181: 315–20.

30. Foa EB, Davidson JR, Frances A. The expert consensus guidelines series: treatment of posttraumatic stress disorder. J Clin Psychiatry 1999; 60 (Suppl 16): 3–76.

31. Stein DJ, Bandelow B, Hollander E et al. WCA Recommendations for the long-term treatment of posttraumatic stress disorder. CNS Spectr 2003; 8(8 Suppl 1): 31–9.

32. Davidson J, Rothbaum BO, Tucker P et al. Venlafaxine extended release in posttraumatic stress disorder: a sertraline- and placebo-controlled study. J Clin Psychopharmacol 2006; 26(3): 259–67.

33. Davidson J, Baldwin D, Stein DJ et al. Treatment of posttraumatic stress disorder with venlafaxine extended release: a 6-month randomized controlled trial. Arch Gen Psychiatry 2006; 63(10): 1158–65.

34. Goldstein DJ, Mallinckrodt C, Lu Y, Demitrack MA. Duloxetine in the treatment of major depressive disorder: a double-blind clinical trial. J Clin Psychiatry 2002; 63(3): 225–31.

35. Raskin J, Goldstein DJ, Mallinckrodt CH, Ferguson MB. Duloxetine in the long-term treatment of major depressive disorder. J Clin Psychiatry 2003; 64(10): 1237–44.

36. Hartford J, Kornstein S, Liebowitz M et al. Duloxetine as an SNRI treatment for generalized anxiety disorder: results from a placebo and active-controlled trial. Int Clin Psychopharmacol 2007; 22(3): 167–74.

37. Endicott J, Russell JM, Raskin J et al. Duloxetine treatment for role functioning improvement in generalized anxiety disorder: three independent studies. J Clin Psychiatry 2007; 68(4): 518–24.

38. Reist C, Kauffmann CD, Haier RJ et al. A controlled trial of desipramine in 18 men with posttraumatic stress disorder. Am J Psychiatry 1989; 146(4): 513–6.

39. Davidson J, Kudler H, Smith R et al. Treatment of posttraumatic stress disorder with amitriptyline and placebo. Arch Gen Psychiatry 1990; 47(3): 259–66.

40. Frank JB, Kosten TR, Giller EL Jr, Dan E. A randomized clinical trial of phenelzine and imipramine for posttraumatic stress disorder. Am J Psychiatry 1988; 145(10): 1289–91.

41. Kosten TR, Frank JB, Dan E, McDougle CJ, Giller EL Jr. Pharmacotherapy for posttraumatic stress disorder using phenelzine or imipramine. J Nerv Ment Dis 1991; 179(6): 366–70.

42. Shestatzky M, Greenberg D, Lerer B. A controlled trial of phenelzine in posttraumatic stress disorder. Psychiatry Res 1988; 24(2): 149–55.

43. Katz RJ, Lott MH, Arbus P et al. Pharmacotherapy of post-traumatic stress disorder with a novel psychotropic. Anxiety 1994; 1(4): 169–74.

44. Onder E, Tural U, Aker T. A comparative study of fluoxetine, moclobemide, and tianeptine in the treatment of posttraumatic stress disorder following an earthquake. Eur Psychiatry 2006; 21(3): 174–9.

45. Davidson JR, Connor KM. Bupropion sustained release: a therapeutic overview. J Clin Psychiatry 1998; 59(4): 25–31.

46. Becker ME, Hertzberg MA, Moore SD et al. A placebo-controlled trial of bupropion SR in the treatment of chronic posttraumatic stress disorder. J Clin Psychopharmacol 2007; 27(2): 193–7.

47. Hertzberg MA, Moore SD, Feldman ME, Beckham JC. A preliminary study of bupropion sustained-release for smoking cessation in patients with chronic posttraumatic stress disorder. J Clin Psychopharmacol 2001; 21(1): 94–8.

48. Stimmel GL, Dopheide JA, Stahl SM. Mirtazapine: an antidepressant with noradrenergic and specific serotonergic effects. Pharmacotherapy 1997; 17(1): 10–21.

49. Davidson JR, Weisler RH, Butterfield MI et al. Mirtazapine vs. placebo in posttraumatic stress disorder: a pilot trial. Biol Psychiatry 2003; 53(2): 188–91.

50. Davis R, Whittington R, Bryson HM. Nefazodone. A review of its pharmacology and clinical efficacy in the management of major depression. Drugs 1997; 53(4): 608–36.

51. Davis LL, Jewell ME, Ambrose S et al. A placebo-controlled study of nefazodone for the treatment of chronic posttraumatic stress disorder: a preliminary study. J Clin Psychopharmacol 2004; 24(3): 291–7.

52. McRae AL, Brady KT, Mellman TA et al. Comparison of nefazodone and sertraline for the treatment of posttraumatic stress disorder. Depress Anxiety 2004; 19(3): 190–6.

53. Mula M, Pini S, Cassano GB. The role of anticonvulsant drugs in anxiety disorders: a critical review of the evidence. J Clin Psychopharmacol 2007; 27(3): 263–72.

54. Post RM, Weiss SR, Smith M, Li H, McCann U. Kindling vs. quenching. Implications for the evolution and treatment of posttraumatic stress disorder. Ann N Y Acad Sci 1997; 821: 285–95.

55. Hertzberg MA, Butterfield MI, Feldman ME et al. A preliminary study of lamotrigine for the treatment of posttraumatic stress disorder. Biol Psychiatry 1999; 45(9): 1226–9.

56. Connor KM, Davidson JR, Weisler RH, Zhang W, Abraham K. Tiagabine for posttraumatic stress disorder: effects of open-label and double-blind discontinuation treatment. Psychopharmacology (Berl) 2006; 184(1): 21–5.

57. Davidson JR, Brady K, Mellman TA, Stein MB, Pollack MH. The efficacy and tolerability of tiagabine in adult patients with post-traumatic stress disorder. J Clin Psychopharmacol 2007; 27(1): 85–8.

58. Davis LL, Davidson JR, Ward LC et al. Divalproex in the treatment of posttraumatic stress disorder: a randomized, double-blind, placebo-controlled trial in a veteran population. J Clin Psychopharmacol 2008; 28(1): 84–8.

59. Lindley SE, Carlson EB, Hill K. A randomized, double-blind, placebo-controlled trial of augmentation topiramate for chronic combat-related posttraumatic stress disorder. J Clin Psychopharmacol 2007; 27(6): 677–81.

60. Tucker P, Trautman RP, Wyatt DB et al. Efficacy and safety of topiramate monotherapy in civilian posttraumatic stress disorder: a randomized, double-blind, placebo-controlled study. J Clin Psychiatry 2007; 68(2): 201–6.

61. Mellman TA, Clark RE, Peacock WJ. Prescribing patterns for patients with posttraumatic stress disorder. Psychiatr Serv 2003; 54(12): 1618–21.

62. Cates ME, Bishop MH, Davis LL, Lowe JS, Woolley TW. Clonazepam for treatment of sleep disturbances associated with combat-related posttraumatic stress disorder. Ann Pharmacother 2004; 38(9): 1395–9.

63. Braun P, Greenberg D, Dasberg H, Lerer B. Core symptoms of posttraumatic stress disorder unimproved by alprazolam treatment. J Clin Psychiatry 1990; 51(6): 236–8.

64. Hamner MB, Frueh BC, Ulmer HG, Arana GW. Psychotic features and illness severity in combat veterans with chronic posttraumatic stress disorder. Biol Psychiatry 1999; 45(7): 846–52.

65. Sareen J, Cox BJ, Goodwin RD, Asmundson JG. Co-occurrence of posttraumatic stress disorder with positive psychotic symptoms in a nationally representative sample. J Trauma Stress 2005; 18(4): 313–22.

66. Charney DS, Deutch AY, Krystal JH, Southwick SM, Davis M. Psychobiologic mechanisms of posttraumatic stress disorder. Arch Gen Psychiatry 1993; 50(4): 295–305.

67. Seedat S, Stein MB, Oosthuizen PP, Emsley RA, Stein DJ. Linking posttraumatic stress disorder and psychosis: a look at epidemiology, phenomenology, and treatment. J Nerv Ment Dis 2003; 191(10): 675–81.

68. Philip NS, Carpenter LL, Tyrka AR, Price LH. Augmentation of antidepressants with atypical antipsychotics: a review of the current literature. J Psychiatr Pract 2008; 14(1): 34–44.

69. Hamner MB, Robert S. Emerging roles for atypical antipsychotics in chronic post-traumatic stress disorder. Expert Rev Neurother 2005; 5(2): 267–75.

70. Gao K, Muzina D, Gajwani P, Calabrese JR. Efficacy of typical and atypical antipsychotics for primary and comorbid anxiety symptoms or disorders: a review. J Clin Psychiatry 2006; 67(9): 1327–40.

71. Pae CU, Lim HK, Peindl K et al. The atypical antipsychotics olanzapine and risperidone in the treatment of posttraumatic stress disorder: a meta-analysis of randomized, double-blind, placebo-controlled clinical trials. Int Clin Psychopharmacol 2008; 23(1): 1–8.

72. Butterfield MI, Becker ME, Connor KM et al. Olanzapine in the treatment of post-traumatic stress disorder: a pilot study. Int Clin Psychopharmacol 2001; 16(4): 197–203.

73. Padala PR, Madison J, Monnahan M et al. Risperidone monotherapy for post-traumatic stress disorder related to sexual assault and domestic abuse in women. Int Clin Psychopharmacol 2006; 21(5): 275–80.

74. Horrigan JP. Guanfacine for PTSD nightmares. J Am Acad Child Adolesc Psychiatry 1996; 35(8): 975–6.

75. Horrigan JP, Barnhill LJ. The suppression of nightmares with guanfacine. J Clin Psychiatry 1996; 57(8): 371.

76. Porter DM, Bell CC. The use of clonidine in post-traumatic stress disorder. J Natl Med Assoc 1999; 91(8): 475–7.

77. Raskind MA, Dobie DJ, Kanter ED et al. The alpha1-adrenergic antagonist prazosin ameliorates combat trauma nightmares in veterans with posttraumatic stress disorder: a report of 4 cases. J Clin Psychiatry 2000; 61(2): 129–33.

78. Kinzie JD, Leung P. Clonidine in cambodian patients with posttraumatic stress disorder. J Nerv Ment Dis 1989; 177(9): 546–50.

79. Neylan TC, Lenoci M, Samuelson KW et al. No improvement of posttraumatic stress disorder symptoms with guanfacine treatment. Am J Psychiatry 2006; 163(12): 2186–8.

80. Raskind MA, Peskind ER, Kanter ED et al. Reduction of nightmares and other PTSD symptoms in combat veterans by prazosin: a placebo-controlled study. Am J Psychiatry 2003; 160(2): 371–3.

81. Raskind MA, Peskind ER, Hoff DJ et al. A parallel group placebo controlled study of prazosin for trauma nightmares and sleep disturbance in combat veterans with post-traumatic stress disorder. Biol Psychiatry 2007; 61(8): 928–34.

82. Taylor FB, Martin P, Thompson C et al. Prazosin effects on objective sleep measures and clinical symptoms in civilian trauma posttraumatic stress disorder: a placebo-controlled study. Biol Psychiatry 2008; 63(6): 629–32.

83. Hofmann SG, Meuret AE, Smits JA et al. Augmentation of exposure therapy with D-cycloserine for social anxiety disorder. Arch Gen Psychiatry 2006; 63(3): 298–304.

84. Guastella AJ, Richardson R, Lovibond PF et al. A randomized controlled trial of D-cycloserine enhancement of exposure therapy for social anxiety disorder. Biol Psychiatry 2008; 63(6): 544–9.

85. Kushner MG, Kim SW, Donahue C et al. D-cycloserine augmented exposure therapy for obsessive-compulsive disorder. Biol Psychiatry 2007; 62(8): 835–8.

86. Heresco-Levy U, Kremer I, Javitt DC et al. Pilot-controlled trial of D-cycloserine for the treatment of post-traumatic stress disorder. Int J Neuropsychopharmacol 2002; 5(4): 301–7.

87. Aerni A, Traber R, Hock C et al. Low-dose cortisol for symptoms of posttraumatic stress disorder. Am J Psychiatry 2004; 161(8): 1488–90.

88. Zhang W, Davidson JR. Post-traumatic stress disorder: an evaluation of existing pharmacotherapies and new strategies. Expert Opin Pharmacother 2007; 8(12): 1861–70.

89. Ipser J, Seedat S, Stein DJ. Pharmacotherapy for post-traumatic stress disorder - a systematic review and meta-analysis. S Afr Med J 2006; 96(10): 1088–109.

10 | Early interventions following traumatic events

Jonathan I Bisson, Arieh Y Shalev, and Joseph Zohar

It is well recognized that traumatic events can cause significant psychological reactions. However, research published in recent years has suggested that individual responses vary greatly and range from a very limited or absent psychological reaction through to marked distress.(1, 2) Such work has convincingly challenged the notion that most individuals involved in traumatic events experience significant distress initially that gradually reduces over time. This trajectory appears to be one of several that can occur. Four distinct types of response have been described (2, 3): a *resilient response* in which no psychological symptoms are present shortly after the event or subsequently, a *delayed response* in which psychological symptoms gradually develop over time, a *prolonged response* in which psychological symptoms manifest immediately and do not reduce over time, and a *recovery response* in which individuals experience psychological symptoms initially that then gradually reduce over time.

Creamer et al. (2) found that around a third of individuals admitted to hospital in Australia as a result of traumatic injury described a *resilient response*, a third a *prolonged response*, with a sixth reporting a *delayed response*, and a sixth a *recovery response*. Creamer et al's. results are not entirely consistent with other studies that have found a trend for reduction of psychological symptoms over time if mean symptom levels are tracked.(4, 5) However, the Galea et al. study concerned an entire cohort of survivors and would still accommodate Creamer's four subgroups, and Foa and Rothbaum (5) mainly reported on survivors with a significant initial response, essentially limiting the possible responses to *prolonged* or *recovery* types.

There appears to be no indication to intervene with individuals who have a *resilient response* but a strong indication to intervene effectively with those with *prolonged responses*. The decision as to whether and when to intervene with those with a *delayed* or *recovery response* is more challenging. If effective preventative interventions exist, these would be ideal for those with delayed responses, if effective interventions are available that speed up recovery in the recovery group these would be indicated. Sadly these decisions are further complicated by our current inability to accurately predict who will follow which trajectory (6, 7, 8) and everyone would have to be monitored longitudinally to determine this.

The development of an intervention effective at preventing the development of post-traumatic stress disorder (PTSD) and other psychological difficulties following traumatic events has become something of a holy grail for researchers and clinicians. Sadly the task is proving to be difficult. Multiple attempts to develop effective interventions have now proved unsuccessful, despite many having had excellent face validity and several being grounded in a sound theoretical base.(9) One of the problems in many early intervention studies has been lack of initial diagnosis and measurement of severity of symptoms, resulting in the treatment of a mixed bag of subjects with both high and low risk of developing PTSD. Thankfully there remains considerable energy to develop effective early interventions and more recent attempts appear to have been helpfully informed by previous work.

Early interventions following traumatic events now represent a heterogeneous group of approaches, delivered at a variety of different time points to various populations. They include pharmacological interventions commenced within a few hours of the traumatic event (10), single session psychological interventions for everybody involved within one month of a traumatic events (11, 12), responses directed at whole communities (13), brief psychological interventions for those with marked symptoms within one month of the traumatic event (14), and longer psychological interventions for individuals suffering from acute PTSD between 1 and 3 months after a traumatic event.(15)

There is no single widely accepted definition of early intervention, a limited number of identifiable candidate interventions, and an absence of information regarding the optimal timing of early intervention. We have, therefore, considered the term early intervention to include *any intervention delivered within three months of a traumatic event* and limited our focus to *early interventions that primarily aim to prevent or treat symptoms of acute stress disorder or post-traumatic stress disorder.*

THEORETICAL MODELS

Social, psychological, and biological models have been developed to explain the responses of individuals following traumatic events. Early interventions address factors considered important in all three models although, to date, the best researched interventions have primarily focused on the psychological and biological models. The three models described below are helpful, although when considered in isolation they may inhibit the development of more holistic approaches to early intervention. It seems likely to us that an optimal response would encompass social, psychological, and biological factors. Social factors such as lack of social support and subsequent stressors may have a role as markers of those with little early response who require follow-up or targeted social interventions.(7)

SOCIAL MODELS

The social model of emotional response to a traumatic event considers mental distress to represent the best coping strategy available to an individual at that time. It does not view responses as pathological but rather as a reflection of an individual's own coping in the context of their situation. Social models regard the wider influence of social forces as more important than other influences as causes or precipitants of mental illness (16) and assert that the abilities of individuals with distress are constrained by barriers set up by others, for example, responses to disability. The social model would consider important factors to include self-management, advocacy, human rights, self-defined needs, community development, nonmedicalization, education, employment, and employment support.

Treating emerging mental disorders, including PTSD, is not an inherent goal of social models of responses to traumatic events. However, social models do address putative mediators of PTSD symptom trajectories following traumatic exposure. Their main thrust is to provide individuals who were exposed to a potentially traumatic event with the kind of interpersonal and social responses that might increase the likelihood of better adaptation, better use of social resources, and thereby sustain the recovery in those with initial symptoms and reduce the likelihood of delayed responses.

PSYCHOLOGICAL MODELS

Unfortunately most of the current psychological models are concerned within individual factors (as opposed to between individual factors) and among those mainly ones that explain the occurrence of PTSD, but not the occurrence of recovery. Consequently, most of the interventions that have been derived from these models address individuals (rather than groups, families, confidants, or attachment networks), who already have symptoms, and follow the general therapeutic model of an encounter between a professional (usually highly skilled) and a "patient" or a "client." Within that kind of "psychology" the following knowledge has been gained.

The earliest psychological models were based on PTSD being a fear-based condition, characterized by excessive response elements such as avoidance, physiological reactivity, and a resistance to modification, for example (17). Foa and Kozak (18) built on this work to develop a respected theory that argued for a breakdown in emotional processing following traumatic events. Cognitive-based theories consider the importance of preexisting beliefs and models of the world and the difficulty assimilating the information provided by a traumatic experience into them. For example, Janoff Bullman (19) described PTSD sufferers as having their assumptions shattered about the world being a meaningful and benevolent place.

Brewin et al. (20) developed the dual representation theory of PTSD, proposing that various factors affect the outcome of emotional processing, including severity and length of trauma, its meaning to the person, accompanying emotions such as shame and guilt, and the availability of appropriate emotional support. The theory distinguishes between memories that are easily verbally recalled and give rise to emotions related to the trauma and memories that cannot be deliberately accessed and give rise to symptoms such as dreams and flashbacks. It has received some support from recent replicated findings of reduced verbal declarative memory in PTSD sufferers.(21) Ehlers and Clark (22) subsequently proposed a cognitive model of PTSD in which the trauma memory has not been integrated into the context of preceding and subsequent experience. Problematic appraisals of the trauma and/or its aftermath have occurred with the development of dysfunctional behavior and cognitive strategies, preventing memory elaboration, exacerbating symptoms, and hindering reassessment of problematic appraisals. They argue that PTSD develops when the traumatic memory induces a sense of current threat promoted by excessive negative reappraisals of what happened.

Psychological models addressing interaction between individuals are badly missing, as are those that combine the effect of traumatic fear responses with those of the often experienced traumatic loss or grief.

BIOLOGICAL MODELS

Our understanding of the neurobiology of PTSD has undoubtedly advanced in recent years, although many findings require further replication to confirm them. The amygdala is believed to play a key role in the development and maintenance of PTSD. It receives information about external stimuli and determines their emotional relevance.(23) The amygdala triggers emotional responses, including the fight, flight, or freezing response, and alterations in stress hormones and catacholemines. The hippocampus and medial prefrontal cortex are believed to influence the response of the amygdala by exerting an inhibitory control over the initial alarm responses (e.g., (24)). Hippocampal lesions have been associated with a stronger fear response, and smaller hippocampal volumes have been associated with PTSD (25), possibly as a vulnerability factor for developing the disorder.(26) Decreased activity in medial prefrontal and anterior cingulate areas has been found to be correlated with increased activity in the amygdala, leading to the suggestion that PTSD represents a failure of these areas to regulate the activity of the amygdala, which results in hyperreactivity to threat.(27) Several studies have found alteration of the cortisol responses in people with posttraumatic stress disorder and an enhanced response to the dexamethasone suppression test.(28) Increased adrenergic response to the traumatic event has arguably been associated with PTSD, for example (29, 30), with the suggestion that an initial adrenergic surge may be associated with the consolidation of traumatic memories.(31) Altered cortisol levels may promote the development and symptomatology of PTSD by disinhibiting traumatic memory retrieval and also failing to contain a sympathetic stress response.(32) Pitman (33) suggested that a positive feedback cycle is formed with overconsolidation of memories as a result of this (see Figure 10.1).

Another biological model focuses on memory and speculates about what would have happened had we interfered with either the consolidation of traumatic emotional memory or with the maintenance of those memories. An elegant work by Cohen, Zohar et al. (34) looking at Lewis rats and comparing them to Fischer rats, looked at this more closely, providing support for this notion (see chapter 7). They used an animal model looking at anisomycin, the protein inhibiting consolidation, and found that, if given right after the exposure, it is associated with a reduction in the rates of PTSD-like symptoms.(34) Moreover, other interventions that also interfere with memory consolidation were found to be effective, including galanin administration and exploring the effect of increased cortisol secretion (intact HPA axis plasticity) as an effective way to decrease the impact of memory consolidation. The potential role of PKMzeta is being explored in a preliminary study as well.

All of the data converge to probably support the potential role in regard to early intervention or manipulation of memory consolidation process (i.e., trying to prevent the consolidation) as a potential tool for future early intervention in the first few hours or weeks after trauma, assuming that it might have a potential preventive effect.

Positive Feedback Cycle
(after Pitman, 1989)

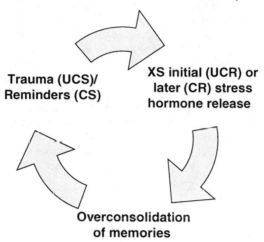

Trauma (UCS)/ **XS initial (UCR) or**
Reminders (CS) **later (CR) stress**
hormone release

Overconsolidation
of memories

Too much significance leads to too much remembrance

Figure 10.1 Positive Feedback Cycle (after Pitman,
1989).

TYPES OF EARLY INTERVENTION

Various early interventions have been developed as described above. The exact nature of the intervention depends on several factors, not least the nature of the traumatic event. If the event is a disaster then interventions at an organizational and community level are required, with a focus on immediate practical and pragmatic support, the reinstatement of normal roles within communities, and the move toward restoration of a normal social structure. Hobfoll et al. (13) have recently published an authoritative paper in this area reviewing the limited evidence for specific approaches but concluding that there are five empirically supported intervention principles. These are promoting sense of safety, sense of self- and community-efficacy, connectedness, calming, and hope. Other important work in this area has been produced by the Inter-Agency Standing Committee.(35)

Early interventions that have focused on individuals or small groups of people affected by traumatic events have been subjected to better designed trials to determine their efficacy. During the 1980s there was a growth in attempts to offer everybody involved in traumatic events a group or individual intervention to reduce the risk of later psychological sequelae. The most widely quoted intervention has been that of psychological debriefing, although this term has been used to cover such a wide range of different interventions that, without description of the actual nature of the intervention being described, it is impossible to determine from the term *psychological debriefing* alone what is actually meant. Since the early 1980s such interventions have been used with groups and individuals, the majority being based either loosely or more strictly on a process originally described for use in groups of ambulance personnel called Critical Incident Stress Debriefing (CISD).(36) This involved a seven-stage approach in which individuals were guided through a vivid description of what actually happened; their emotional reactions at the time; and then educated about the possible consequences, how to deal with them, and where to seek further support if necessary. It was later argued that CISD should be given as one component of a more complex package of interventions, known as critical incident stress management (CISM).(37)

In the last decade the focus has moved from single-session interventions to more complex approaches designed for all individuals involved, including CISM, trauma risk management (38), and psychological first aid.(39) These interventions have potential but have not yet been subjected to randomized controlled trials to determine their true efficacy. More efficacy research has been done with multiple-session psychological treatments ranging from supportive counseling and education approaches to more formal cognitive behavioral therapy (CBT) interventions increasingly targeting symptomatic individuals. (14, 15) The CBT approaches have been trauma focused and contain various well recognized techniques from effective trauma-focused cognitive behavioural therapy (TFCBT) interventions for chronic PTSD. Most of them contain some form of prolonged imaginal exposure to the traumatic event, *in vivo* exposure to feared situations, and a variable amount of cognitive therapy techniques. The pharmacological agents tested have largely adhered to the biological theories of the development of PTSD. For example propranolol has been used in an attempt to reduce the adrenergic surge (10), and hydrocortisone has been used to address the lowered cortisol hypothesis.(40)

THE EFFICACY OF EARLY INTERVENTIONS

Given the limited space available in a single chapter, we have restricted our assessment of the efficacy of early interventions to randomized controlled trial research. That is not to say that some interventions not described may be shown to be effective in the future or to claim that the evidence available from randomized controlled trials is beyond criticism. Indeed much of it can be criticized when scrutinized closely, and it is important to be cautious when scrutinizing the results, particularly with regard to the generalizability of them across different populations than those considered.

Given the differences between the interventions and populations included in randomized controlled trials, we have separated them into seven groups based on the categories adopted by the United Kingdom's National Institute of Health and Clinical Excellence Guidelines on PTSD (9):

1. Single session interventions provided to any individual exposed to a traumatic event with the aim of preventing PTSD

Systematic reviews and meta-analyses of this data have been conducted by various groups (41, 12) and have consistently shown that there is no convincing evidence to suggest that providing a single-session individual psychological intervention, following traumatic events, is useful for most people. Indeed some studies have found that individual psychological debriefing may exacerbate traumatic stress symptoms in some people (42), particularly those who are most distressed.(43) Randomized controlled trials (RCTs) of group psychological debriefing have not produced convincing evidence of its effectiveness (44, 45) but have not suggested the possibility of a harmful effect. Indeed, a post hoc analysis found that soldiers exposed to a large number of traumatic events may experience some benefit from group debriefing.(45) Table 10.1 summarizes the trials included in a recent systematic review.(46) A subsequent RCT that considered the distribution of an educational pamphlet shortly after attendance at an emergency unit (47) failed to demonstrate superiority over no intervention.

2. Multiple session interventions provided to any individual exposed to a traumatic event with the aim of preventing PTSD

Tables 10.2 and 10.3 summarize the RCTs included in the recent Cochrane Systematic Review.(48) The only statistically significant differences found were in favor of the wait list control group over adapted critical incident stress debriefing for self-reported PTSD symptoms immediately postintervention, and for preventive counseling over monitoring/usual care for self-reported PTSD symptoms immediately postintervention.

3. Multiple-session interventions begun in the first month with the aim of preventing PTSD or ongoing distress in individuals with acute stress disorder

Tables 10.2 and 10.3 summarize the RCTs included in a recent Systematic Review. (49) Statistically significant differences were found in favor of TFCBT over wait list and supportive counseling, TFCBT plus anxiety management over supportive counseling, TFCBT plus hypnosis over supportive counseling, and TFCBT over cognitive restructuring.

4. Multiple-session interventions begun in the first month with the aim of preventing PTSD or ongoing distress based on other risk factors

Tables 10.2 and 10.3 summarize the RCTS included in a recent Systematic Review. (49) No statistically significant differences were found between the interventions and controls.

Table 10.1 Summary of randomized controlled trials of one-off early psychological interventions (need permission to reproduce from Guildford).

Authors (Year)	Treatment Tested	Target Population	Comparison Group	Sample (n)	Time post-trauma	Duration (mins)	Main Outcome Measure	Outcome	Effect Size (Hedges's unbiased g)	Follow-up Period
Bordow & Porritt (1979) (53)	Immediate Review 3 month Social Worker input	MVA victims	Standard Care	70	< 1 week	60	Traumatic neurosis symptoms	Social Worker input fared best followed by immediate review	Unable to calculate	3–4 months
Bunn & Clarke (1979) (54)	Individual Counselling	Relatives of seriously ill/injured	Standard Care	30	<12 hours	20	Composite of anxiety scores	Intervention group fared better	Unable to calculate	5 minutes
Hobbs et al (1996) (55) / Mayou et al (2000) (56)	Debriefing	MVA victims	Standard Care	106	24–48 hours	60	IES	Intervention group fared worse	0.21	4 months
Lee et al (1996) (57)	Debriefing	Miscarriage	Standard Care	39	14 days	60	IES	No significant difference	-0.12	4 months
Stevens & Adshead (1996) (58)	Individual Counselling	MVA, Assault or Dog Bite	Standard Care	42	<24 hours	60	IES	No significant difference	Unable to calculate	3 months
Bisson et al (1997) (42)	Debriefing	Acute Burn Trauma Victims		103	2–19 days	30–120	IES	Intervention group fared worse	0.22	3 months
Conlon et al (unpublished) (59)	Debriefing	MVA victims	Advice and Leaflet	40	< 14 days	30	IES	No significant difference	-0.02	3 months
Dolan et al (unpublished) (60)	Debriefing	Accident and Emergency Attenders	Standard Care	69	< 14 days	45–120	IES	No significant difference	0.04	1 month
Rose et al (1999) (61)	Debriefing Education	Victims of violence	Standard Care	105	< 1 month	60	PSS	No significant difference	Psychological debriefing vs. standard care - 0.06. Psychological debriefing vs. education - 0.24	6 months

(Continued)

Table 10.1 (Continued)

Authors (Year)	Treatment Tested	Target Population	Comparison Group	Sample (n)	Time post-trauma	Duration (mins)	Main Outcome Measure	Outcome	Effect Size (Hedges's unbiased g)	Follow-up Period
Campfield & Hills (2001) (62)	Individual or small group debriefing	Victims of robbery	Delayed debriefing	77	< 10 hours or > 48 hours	60–120	PDS	< 10 hours group fared better	-2.56	2 weeks
Litz et al (unpublished) (44)	Group CISD Stress Education class	Soldiers deployed on a peacekeeping mission	No Intervention	1,050	In Kosovo pre redeployment	48–148 mins Mean = 88.1 (sd 25.2) mins	PCL	No significant difference	Unable to calculate	9 months
Sijbrandij et al (in press) (63)	Emotional debriefing Psychoeducational debriefing	Civilian survivors of various traumatic events	No intervention	236	11–19 days (median = 15)	45–60	SI-PTSD	No significant differences. Some evidence worse outcome in emotional debriefing	Emotional Debriefing – 0.18 Educational debriefing - 0.03	6 weeks
Marchand et al (2006) (64)	Ind'l debriefing over two sessions a week apart	Victims of an armed robbery	No intervention	75	First session 2 – 22 days (mean 11.21, sd = 6.75)	? duration	IES	No significant difference	Completers - 0.5 Intention to Treat (ITT) - 0.48	Post Rx 3 months

Table 10.2 Summary of randomized controlled trials of multiple session early psychological interventions (need permission to reproduce from Journal).

Source	Intervention and control conditions	Population	Time since trauma at start of intervention	Severity Criterion	T Stress outcomes	Randomized (n) : completers (n)	Follow-up period	Significant differences
Andre (1997) (65)	Up to 6 sessions of CBT vs. usual care	Assaulted bus drivers	At least 14 days	None	IES	132 :	6 months	Insufficient data
Bisson (2003) (66)	Four 60 min. sessions of exposure based CBT vs. standard care	Physical injury from civilian trauma	5–10 weeks	Acute psychol'l distress	CAPS, IES	152 : 124 completed to 3 months	3 and 13 months	TFCBT better than standard care at 13 months only
Brom (1993) (67)	Up to six sessions of individual preventative counselling vs. monitoring group	Outpatient victims of MVA	Not reported	None	IES, TSI	738 randomized, 151 agreed to enter study : 21 completed	3 months	Neutral
Bryant (1998) (14)	Five 90 min. weekly sessions of exposure based CBT vs. supportive counselling	Outpatients following MVA or industrial accident	Mean 9.9 days (CBT); 10.3 days SC	Acute Stress Disorder	IES, CIDI PTSD module	24: 24 completed	6 months and 4 years	TFCBT better than SC
Bryant (1999) (68)	Five 90 min. weekly sessions of prolonged exposure or prolonged exposure plus anxiety management vs. supportive counselling	Outpatients following MVA or non- sexual assault	Mean 10.3 days (exposure plus anx mgmt), 10.0 days (PE), 10.6 days (SC)	Acute Stress Disorder	CAPS, IES	56: 45 completed	6 months and 4 years	TFCBT and TFCBT plus AM better than SC
Bryant (2003) (69)	Five 90 min. weekly sessions of exposure based CBT vs. supportive counselling	Outpatients with mild trauamatic brain injury om MVA or non-sexual assault	2 weeks	Acute Stress Disorder	CAPS, IES	24: 24 completed	6 months	TFCBT better than SC
Bryant (2005) (70)	Six 90 min. sessions of exposure based CBT or CBT plus hypnosis vs. supportive counselling	Outpatients following MVA or non-sexual assault	Mean 15.8 days (CBT); 13.5 days (CBT-hypnosis); 14.0 days (SC)	Acute Stress Disorder	CAPS, IES	87: 69 completed	6 months and 3 years	TFCBT and TFCBT plus hypnosis better than SC.
Bryant (2008) (71)	Five 90 min sessions of exposure therapy or cognitive restructuring vs. waiting list	Outpatient victims of civilian trauma	Mean 22.8 days	Acute Stress Disorder	CAPS, IES	69 completed	6 months	Exposure therapy and Cognitive restructuring better than WL. ET better than CR

(Continued)

Table 10.2 (Continued)

Source	Intervention and control conditions	Population	Time since trauma at start of intervention	Severity Criterion	T Stress outcomes	Randomized (n) : completers (n)	Follow-up period	Significant differences
Bugg (submitted)(72)	One face to face and two telephone sessions with a writing task and information intervention vs information only	Outpatient victims of MVA, occupational injury or assault	5–6 weeks	Acute Stress Disorder	PDS	148 randomized: 67 available to initial follow-up	3 and 6 months post trauma	Neutral
Echeburua (1996) (73)	Five 60 min. session of exposure based CBT vs. relaxation	Female victims of rape or sexual assault	1.4 months	Acute PTSD	Scale of Severity of PTSD Symptoms	20: 20 completed	3, 6 and 12 months	TFCBT better than relaxation at 12 month f'up only
Ehlers (2003) (74)	Twelve plus three 90 min. sessions of trauma focused CBT or self help booklet vs. wating list	Outpatient victims of MVA	4 months	Acute and chronic PTSD	CAPS, PDS	85: 80 completed 12 participants met criteria for acute PTSD and were included in this review. All 12 completed	3 and 9 months	TFCBT better than self help booklet and WL
Foa (2006) (75)	Four 2 hour sessions of exposure based CBT or supportive counselling vs. continuous assessment.	Female victims of sexual and non-sexual assault	20.5 days to assessment	PTSD symptom criteria	SCID-PTSD, PSSI	90: 66 completed	3 and 9 months	Neutral
Gamble (2005) (76)	1 session of face to face counselling and 1 session of telephone counselling lasting up to 60 mins vs treatment as usual.	Mothers following traumatic birth.	Within 72 hours	None	MINI-PTSD	103: 102 completed initial follow-up, 103 completed 3 month follow-up	3 months	Intervention better than treatment as usual at 3 months only
Gidron (2001) (77)	Two sessions of Memory structuring intervention vs. supportive listening	Outpatient victims of an MVA.	24 hours	Heart rate greater than 95 beats per minute in emergency room.	PDS	Number randomized unclear: 17 completed	3–4 months	Neutral

(Continued)

Table 10.2 (Continued)

Source	Intervention and control conditions	Population	Time since trauma at start of intervention	Severity Criterion	T Stress outcomes	Randomized (*n*) : completers (*n*)	Follow-up period	Significant differences
Gidron (2007) (78)	Two sessions of Memory structuring intervention vs. supportive listening	Outpatient victims of an MVA.	Within 48 hours	Heart rate greater than 95 beats per minute in emergency room.	PDS	Number randomized unclear: 34 completed	3 months	Neutral
Kazak (2005) (79)	Three 45min sessions of adapted CBT and family therapy intervention vs treatment as usual	38 caregivers and parents of children newly diagnosed with cancer.	Median 6 days, range 0–10 days	None	IES-R	38: 31 completed available to follow-up	2 months	Neutral
Marchand (2006) (80)	Two 1 hour sessions of adapted critical incident stress debriefing vs a no intervention control group	Outpatient victims of armed robbery.	11.21 days	Meet criterion A1 and A2 for PTSD	SCID, IES	75: 61 available at 1 month follow-up	3 months	No intervention better than adapted CISD initially only
Öst unpublished (81)	Sixteen 60 min. sessions of exposure based CBT vs. waiting list	Outpatient victims of violent crime.	6.8 weeks	Acute PTSD	CAPS, IES-R	43: 41 completed	Follow-up data not yet available	TFCBT better than wait list
Ryding (1998) (82)	Two group sessions of counselling and education vs treatment as usual.	Women following emergency caesarean section.	Not clearly stated, a few days after giving birth	None	IES	106: 100 completed	6 months post partum	Neutral
Ryding (2004) (83)	Two group sessions of counselling and education vs treatment as usual.	Women following emergency caesarean section.	2 months	None	IES	162: 147 available at initial follow-up	6 months post partum	Neutral

(Continued)

Table 10.2 (Continued)

Source	Intervention and control conditions	Population	Time since trauma at start of intervention	Severity Criterion	T Stress outcomes	Randomized (n) : completers (n)	Follow-up period	Significant differences
Sijbrandij (2007) (43)	Four 2 hour weekly sessions of exposure based CBT vs. waiting list	Outpatient victims of civilian traumatic events.	40 days	Acute PTSD, (some participants did not meet the onset criterion)	SI-PTSD	143: 117 completed	4 months	Neutral
Shalev et al. (in press) (49)	Twelve weekly 1.5 hour sessions of prolonged exposure, cognitive therapy, SSRI, Placebo, and waitlist	Adult survivors of traumatic events admitted to a general hospital ER (83% motor vehicle accidents; 11% terrorist attacks; 6% work accidents and other events)	29.5±5.5 days	Full or partial ASD (partial = ASD without dissociation or ASD without avoidance criterion)	CAPS, PSS-SR	Randomized PE: 72 CT: 52 WL: 120 SSRI/PBO: 52 Completers: PE: 53 CT: 46 WL: 103 SSRI/PBO: 44	Five (early interventions) Eight (Early and delayed interventions) and fourteen months.	PE and CT better than other groups
Van Emmerick (2008) (84)	Five 90 minute sessions of exposure based CBT, or a writing intervention vs. waiting list condition.	Outpatients following civilian trauma	Mean of 119.40 days	ASD, acute PTSD Or chronic PTSD	IES	125: 85 completed 66 eligible for this review: 47 completed	No consistent point of long term follow-up	TFCBT and writing intervention better than wait list
Wagner (2007) (85)	Up to six 90 min. sessions of behavioural activation and treatment as usual vs. treatment as usual.	Inpatients following civilian trauma	> 4 weeks	Acute PTSD	PCL	8: 8 completed	3 months post-trauma	Neutral
Zatzick (2001) (86)	Collaborative care intervention, including assignment to trauma support specialist vs usual care	Physically injured hospitalized MVA & assault victims.	Within 1 month	All hospitalized individuals	PCL	34: 26 completed	3 months	Neutral
Zatzick (2004) (87)	Multifaceted collaborative care for PTSD and alcohol abuse	Physically injured hospitalized MVA & assault victims.	Not clearly stated but soon after admission	Significant symptoms of PTSD and/or depression	PCL	121: 106 retained at 1 month, 99 retained at 12 months	1, 3, 6 and 12 months	Neutral

Table 10.3 Summary of outcomes for randomized controlled trials of multiple session early psychological interventions (need permission to reproduce from Journal).

Comparison	Follow-up	Trials (*n*)	Sample (*n*)	RR, SMD or WMD (95% CI)
Interventions within one month for all exposed to the trauma				
Adapted Critical Incident Stress Debriefing vs Usual Care (PTSD symptoms self-report)	Post Rx	1	75	7.34 (0.04, 14.64)*
	3 months post trauma	1	75	5.77 (-1.03, 12.57)
Adapted Critical Incident Stress Debriefing vs Usual Care (PTSD diagnosis)	Post Rx	1	75	3.82 (0.42, 35.04)
	3 months post trauma	1	75	2.55 (0.24, 26.87)
Preventive Counselling vs Monitoring/ usual care (PTSD symptoms Clinician administered)	Post Rx	1	103	-0.64 (-1.94, 0.66)
	3 months post trauma	1	103	-1.29 (-2.47, -0.11)*
Preventive Counselling vs Monitoring/ usual care (PTSD diagnosis)	Post Rx	2	202	1.24 (0.72, 2.13)
	3 months post trauma	1	103	0.35 (0.10, 1.23)
Group counselling vs control group (PTSD diagnosis)	6 months post trauma	1	147	0.53 (0.25, 1.10)
Group counselling vs control group (PTSD symptoms self-report)	6 months post trauma	1	147	-1.30 (-6.11, 3.51).
Brief family intervention vs treatment as usual (PTSD symptoms self-report for primary caregivers)	? follow-up	1	16	-3.63 (-18.22, 10.96)
Brief family intervention vs treatment as usual (PTSD symptoms self-report for secondary caregivers)	? follow-up	1	13	-11.20 (-33.75, 11.35)
Collaborative Care vs Usual Care for an inpatient service (PTSD diagnosis)	1 month post trauma	1	29	0.36 (0.09, 1.48)
	4 months post trauma	1	26	0.39 (0.10, 1.48)
Collaborative Care vs Usual Care for an inpatient service (PTSD symptoms self-report)	1 month post trauma	1	29	-6.60 (-15.93, 2.73) 6.40
	4 months post trauma	1	26	(-5.58, 18.38)
Interventions within one month for individuals with specific risk factors other than acute stress disorder				
Memory structuring intervention vs supportive listening (PTSD diagnosis)	3 months post trauma	1	17	0.28 (0.04, 2.02)
Interventions for individuals with acute stress disorder				
Therapist Guided Self Help plus Psycho-education vs Psycho-education only (PTSD symptoms self-report)	Post treatment	1	104	1.83 (-2.57, 6.23)
	3 months post trauma	1	104	1.10 (-3.80, 6.00)
Trauma focused CBT vs waitlist (PTSD symptoms clinician rated)	Post treatment	1	60	-24.40 (-37.20, -11.60)*
Trauma focused CBT vs waitlist (PTSD diagnosis)	Post treatment	1	60	0.43 (0.25, 0.75)
Trauma Focused CBT vs Supportive Counselling (PTSD symptoms clinician rated) - completers	Post treatment	3	100	-21.51 (-30.24, -12.77)*
	3 months post trauma	3	98	-21.42 (-31.42, -11.42)*
	2–4 year post trauma	3	76	-13.66 (-20.56, -6.77)*
Trauma Focused CBT vs Supportive Counselling (PTSD diagnosis) - ITT	Post treatment	4	142	0.41 (0.28, 0.90)
	6 months post trauma	4	142	0.40 (0.19, 0.82)
	2–4 years	3	137	0.72 (0.48, 1.07)

(Continued)

Table 10.3 (Continued)

Comparison	Follow-up	Trials (n)	Sample (n)	RR, SMD or WMD (95% CI)
Trauma Focused CBT vs Trauma Focused CBT plus Anxiety Management (PTSD symptoms clinician rated) – completers	Post treatment	1	29	-4.46 (-19.28, 10.36)
	6 months post trauma	1	26	-4.77 (-24.40, 14.86)
Trauma Focused CBT vs Trauma Focused CBT plus Anxiety Management ((PTSD diagnosis) – ITT	Post treatment	1	29	1.40 (0.27, 4.18)
	6 months post trauma	1	26	0.67 (0.13, 3.35).
Trauma Focused CBT plus Anxiety Management vs Supportive Counselling (PTSD symptoms clinician rated) – completers	Post treatment	1	31	-17.44 (-13.12, -1.76)*
	6 months post trauma	1	28	-25.85 (-42.61, -9.09)*
Trauma Focused CBT plus Anxiety Management vs Supportive Counselling (PTSD diagnosis) – ITT	Post treatment	1	31	0.36 (0.12, 1.07)
	6 months post trauma	1	28	0.35 (0.12, 0.99)*
Trauma Focused CBT vs Trauma Focused CBT plus Hypnosis (PTSD symptoms clinician rated) – completers	Post treatment	1	47	-0.22 (-11.84, 11.40)
	6 months post trauma	1	47	-0.42 (-15.65, 14.81)
	Longer ? post trauma	1	37	-0.68 (-16.40, 15.04)
Trauma Focused CBT vs Trauma Focused CBT plus Hypnosis (PTSD diagnosis) – ITT	Post treatment	1	63	1.21 (0.60, 2.46)
	6 months post trauma	1	63	0.91 (0.52, 1.58)
	Longer ? post trauma	1	63	0.84 (0.48, 1.49)
Trauma Focused CBT plus Hypnosis vs Supportive Counselling (PTSD symptoms clinician rated) – completers	Post treatment	1	45	-21.77 (-35.71, -7.83)*
	6 months post trauma	1	45	-15.49 (-31.62, 0.64)
	Longer ? post trauma	1	34	-18.05 (-35.58, -0.52)*
Trauma Focused CBT plus Hypnosis vs Supportive Counselling (PTSD diagnosis) – ITT	Post treatment	1	54	0.60 (0.30, 1.18)
	6 months post trauma	1	54	0.69 (0.39, 1.19)
	Longer ? post trauma	1	54	0.70 (0.43, 1.13)
Trauma focused CBT vs cognitive restructuring (without exposure) (PTSD symptoms clinician rated) – ITT	Post treatment	1	60	-11.50 (-25.39, 2.39)
	6 months post trauma	1	60	-17.70 (-32.50, -2.90)*
Trauma focused CBT vs cognitive restructuring (without exposure) (PTSD diagnosis) – ITT	Post treatment	1	60	0.53 (0.30, 0.94)*
	6 months post trauma	1	60	0.58 (0.34, 1.00)
Cognitive restructuring (without exposure) vs waitlist (PTSD symptoms clinician rated) – ITT	Post treatment	1	60	-12.90 (-25.78, -0.02)
Cognitive restructuring (without exposure) vs waitlist (PTSD diagnosis) – ITT	Post treatment	1	60	0.83 (0.59, 1.16)

Interventions beginning within three months for individuals with traumatic stress symptoms other than acute stress disorder

Comparison	Follow-up	Trials (n)	Sample (n)	RR, SMD or WMD (95% CI)
Trauma Focused CBT vs Waitlist (PTSD symptoms clinician rated) – ITT	Post treatment	4	268	-0.54 (-1.12, 0.03)
	3–5 months post trauma	1	61	-1.22 (-8.05, 5.61)
	9–11 months post trauma	2	73	-0.85 (-2.49, 0.79)
	13 months post trauma	1	152	-6.01 (-12.44, 0.42)

(Continued)

Table 10.3 (Continued)

Comparison	Follow-up	Trials (n)	Sample (n)	RR, SMD or WMD (95% CI)
Trauma Focused CBT vs Waitlist (PTSD diagnosis) – ITT	Post treatment	6	455	0.81 (0.56, 1.18)
	3-5 months post trauma	2	141	0.64 (0.42, 0.99)*
	9–11 months post trauma	2	54	0.42 (0.03, 5.23)
	13 months post trauma	1	115	0.74 (0.36, 1.51)
Trauma Focused CBT vs Supportive Counselling (PTSD symptoms clinician rated) – ITT	Post treatment	1	60	-1.65 (-8.36, 5.06)
	3–5 months post trauma	1	60	-2.01 (-9.17, 5.15)
	9–11 months post trauma	1	60	2.51 (-4.79, 9.81)
Trauma Focused CBT vs Supportive Counselling (PTSD diagnosis) – ITT	Post treatment	1	60	1.16 (0.78, 1.71)
Supportive Counselling vs Waitlist (PTSD symptoms clinician rated) – ITT	Post treatment	1	59	1.17 (-5.70, 8.04)
	3–5 months post trauma	1	59	0.79 (-6.27, 7.85)
	9–11 months post trauma	1	59	-4.67 (-11.93, 2.59)
Supportive Counselling vs Waitlist (PTSD diagnosis) – ITT	Post treatment	1	59	0.93 (0.61, 1.39)
Stepped collaborative care vs usual care for an inpatient service (PTSD diagnosis)	1 month post trauma	1	101	0.85 (0.42, 1.69)
	3 months post trauma	1	101	0.90 (0.44, 1.85)
	6 months post trauma	1	102	0.64 (0.33, 1.23)
	12 months post trauma	1	95	0.73 (0.34, 1.60)
Interventions for individuals with acute post traumatic stress disorder				
Behavioural activation vs treatment as usual (PTSD symptoms self-report) – ITT	Post treatment	1	8	-18.70 (-43.41, 6.01)
Trauma Focused CBT vs Waitlist (PTSD symptoms clinician rated) – ITT	Post treatment	3	150	-0.86 (-1.60, -0.12)*
	3–5 months post trauma	1	95	-0.88 (-6.52, 4.76)
	9–11 months post trauma	1	12	-33.67 (-52.77, -14.57)*
Trauma Focused CBT vs Waitlist (PTSD diagnosis) – ITT	Post treatment	4	193	0.56 (0.27, 1.18)
	3–5 months post trauma	1	95	0.85 (0.50, 1.44)
	9–11 months post trauma	1	12	0.09 (0.01, 1.35)
Structured writing therapy vs waitlist (PTSD symptoms self-report) – ITT	Post treatment	1	42	-14.22 (-25.48, -2.96)*
Structured writing therapy vs waitlist (PTSD diagnosis) – ITT	Post treatment	1	42	0.61 (0.25, 1.47)
Trauma Focused CBT vs Relaxation (PTSD symptoms clinician administered) – ITT	Post treatment	1	20	-6.70 (-13.84, 0.44)
	6 months post trauma	1	20	-4.30 (-9.02, 0.42)
	12 months post trauma	1	20	-5.50 (-10.20, -0.80)*
Trauma Focused CBT vs Relaxation (PTSD diagnosis) – ITT	Post treatment	1	20	0.40 (0.10, 1.60)
	6 months post trauma	1	20	0.33 (0.02, 7.32)
	12 months post trauma	1	20	0.20 (0.01, 3.70)

5. Studies beginning within 3 months, offering intervention to individuals with traumatic stress symptoms (other than acute stress disorder (ASD))

Tables 10.2 and 10.3 summarize the RCTs included in a recent Systematic Review. (49) The only statistically significant difference found was in favor of TFCBT over the wait list control group for PTSD diagnosis 3 to 5 months postintervention.

6. Studies offering intervention to individuals with a diagnosis of acute PTSD

Tables 10.2 and 10.3 summarize the RCTs included in the recent Systematic Review. (49) Statistically significant differences were found in favor of TFCBT over a wait list control group and TFCBT over relaxation but only at 12 months posttrauma. A recent RCT (49) randomized 289 individuals with acute PTSD to 12 sessions of trauma-focused prolonged exposure (PE), trauma-focused cognitive therapy (CT), escitalopram (a selective serotonin reuptake inhibitor), a placebo medication, or a wait list control group. Participants of the wait list started 12 sessions of "delayed" PE, 5 months from the traumatic event. At 5 months, the PE and CT groups fared statistically significantly better than the other three groups. The early and delayed PE groups did not differ, 8 months after the traumatic event. The results were maintained 14 months after the traumatic event.

7. Pharmacological interventions provided within 3 months of a traumatic event with the aim of preventing or treating PTSD

Table 10.4 summarizes the pharmacological trials. There is no good evidence that a pharmacological intervention can prevent the development of PTSD even in those perceived to be at higher risk, that is, individuals with raised heart rate (10) or significant symptoms shortly after a traumatic event.(50, 51) The limited evidence of greater reduction in symptoms and physiological response to a trigger in the Pitman study is compromised by the higher rate of dropouts in the propranolol group and the absence of an intention to treat analysis. A promising result was of hydrocortisone in the Schelling et al. (40) study, but again the sample size was very small and the extreme nature of the study group severely limits generalizability. The one RCT of medication for acute PTSD (49) described above found no positive effect over placebo or wait list and a statistically significant inferior performance than the two trauma-focused psychological treatments used. However, it was not sufficiently powered to examine the efficacy of escitalopram per se.

Currently, Zohar, Shalev et al. are finalizing a large study that will include 200 patients, randomized to receive escitalopram (120mg/day for 24 weeks) or placebo, beginning within 1 month of trauma. This study is carried out in hospital emergency rooms and related to civilians (mostly car accidents). This type of study will be able to give us a better indication of what might or might not be effective.

Despite the disappointing results to date, efforts to discover pharmacological interventions for PTSD should be energetically pursued, as pharmacotherapy can be dispensed to large numbers of survivors at risk without the inherent limitations of delivering psychological therapies in mass casualty disasters.(52)

SUGGESTED MODEL OF CARE

With the information available at present, there is no good evidence to suggest that any formal intervention should be recommended or made available on a routine basis to everybody involved in a traumatic event. This has led to the majority of guidelines to be cautious in their recommendations. They largely advise against individual psychological debriefing (9, 13), but caution against doing nothing, and argue for the delivery of supportive practical and pragmatic input. This will often involve basic needs such as housing, finances, food, and nutrition in the first instance and follow a hierarchy of needs. The only good evidence for the effectiveness for early interventions at present concerns multiple-session cognitive–behavioral therapy interventions for acute stress disorder and acute PTSD. However, methodological issues, such as comparing to waiting list vs. placebo and being single-blind, hamper the interpretation and generalizability of those studies.

A pragmatic approach to early intervention grounded in the research evidence available would develop social care systems that provide basic pragmatic, practical support in a

Table 10.4 Summary of randomized controlled trials of early pharmacological interventions.

Authors (Year)	Treatment Tested	Population	Sample (n)	Time post-trauma	Duration	Main Outcome Measure	Outcome
Schelling et al (2001) (40)	Intravenous hydrocortisone vs. placebo	Septic shock victims on ITU	20	< 24 hours	12 days	PTSS-10	HC group better than placebo at 31 months
Pitman et al (2002) (10)	Propranolol 40mg qds vs. placebo	Emergency Unit trauma victims	31	<6 hours	19 days	CAPS	No significant difference at 1 and 3 months
Mellman et al (2002) (88)	Temazepam 30 mg 5 days, 15mg 2 days vs. placebo	MVA, Assault, Industrial accident	22	14 days	7 days	PTSD	No significant difference at 6 weeks, trend in favour of placebo
Shalev et al., in press (49)	Twelve weeks of escitalopram (SSRI; up to 20mg) placebo (PBO) and waitlist (WL) control	Adult survivors of traumatic events admitted to a general hospital ER with full or partial ASD	SSRI: 26 PBO: 26 WL: 120	29.5+/-5.5 days	12 weeks	CAPS	No significant differences between any group at 5 months
Stein et al (2007) (89)	Propranolol 40mg tds vs. Gabapentin 400mg tds vs. placebo	Physically injured	48	< 48 hours	14 days	PCL-C	No significant differences at 8 months

sympathetic and empathic manner and allows follow-up and identification of trauma survivors who need further care. Despite the absence of conclusive research, easily accessible, accurate information that identifies normal reactions seems likely to be reassuring, encourages self-support and social support, and attempts to identify individuals who are developing difficulties. Individuals who are developing difficulties should be monitored and, if their symptoms do not resolve within 1 month of the traumatic event, should be offered trauma-focused cognitive-behavioral therapy. This would usually comprise up to 12 sessions, with some sessions at 90 minutes. If individuals do not respond to this, they should be reassessed and alternative interventions planned. By this time an individual will probably be suffering from chronic PTSD. There is no evidence for the use of medication as an early intervention to prevent or treat traumatic stress symptoms. However, in cases of marked depressive responses, antidepressants can be justified.(9)

SERVICE/ORGANIZATION IMPLICATIONS

There is a clear need to develop services with a focus on ensuring all first responders have an understanding of normal reactions to traumatic events; how to deal with distressed people in a sympathetic, empathic manner; and to acknowledge the importance of practical, pragmatic support and the lack of need for formal interventions for everybody. This means that mental health professionals' key role in the immediate aftermath of disaster is to prepare and provide ongoing support and supervision to those individuals providing the immediate support. As time goes on services need staff who are able to fully assess traumatized individuals to determine their needs and then deliver evidence-based interventions (trauma-focused cognitive-behavioral therapy interventions with the current evidence).

FUTURE RESEARCH DIRECTIONS

There is an urgent need for further research into this area. Of particular importance is research into early biological changes and the development of pharmacological approaches based on these. Likewise, other trauma-focused interventions that have been shown to be effective in chronic PTSD, in particular eye movement desensitization and reprocessing, should be subjected to formal evaluation as an early intervention, particularly for symptomatic individuals. There is also a need to develop better systems and community responses, as it appears that a comprehensive community response and public health approach offers the best hope of reducing the overall impact of traumatic events on society.

REFERENCES

1. Bonano G, Galea S, Bucciarelli A et al. Psychological resilience after disaster: New York City in the aftermath of the September 11th terrorist attacks. Psychol Sci 2006; 17: 181–6.
2. Creamer M, O'Donnell ML, Parslow R. Predicting healthy adjustment resistance and resilience following traumatic injury. Presented at ISTSS annual conference, Baltimore; 2007.
3. Bonanno GA. Loss, trauma and human resilience: Have we underestimated the human capacity to thrive after extremely aversive events? Am Psychol 2004; 59(1): 20–8.
4. Galea S, Vlahov D, Resnick H et al. Trends of probable post-traumatic stress disorder in New York City after the September 11 terrorist attacks. Am J Epidemiol 2003; 158: 514–24.
5. Foa E, Rothbaum B. Treating the trauma of rape: Cognitive-behavioral therapy for PTSD. New York: Guilford Press; 1998.
6. Bryant R. Early predictors of posttraumatic stress disorder. Biol Psychiatry 2003; 53(9): 789–95.
7. Brewin CR, Andrew B, Valentine JD. Meta-analysis of risk factors for posttraumatic stress disorder in trauma-exposed adults. J Consult Clin Psychol 2000; 68: 748–66.
8. Shalev A, Freedman S, Peri T et al. Predicting PTSD in trauma survivors: prospective evaluation of self-report and clinician-administered instruments. Br J Psych 1997; 170: 558–64.
9. [NCCMH] National Collaborating Centre for Mental Health. Post-traumatic stress disorder: The management of PTSD in adults and children in primary and secondary care. London and Leicester: Gaskell and BPS; 2005.
10. Pitman RK, Sanders KM, Zusman RM et al. Pilot study of secondary prevention of posttraumatic stress disorder with propranolol. Biol Psychiatry 2002; 51: 189–92.

11. Rose S, Bisson J, Churchill R et al. Psychological debriefing for preventing post traumatic stress disorder (PTSD). Cochrane Database Syst Rev 2005; 2: CD002946.

12. Van Emmerik A, Kamphuis J, Hulsbosch A et al. Single session debriefing after psychological trauma: a meta analysis. Lancet 2002; 360(9335): 766–71.

13. Hobfoll SE, Watson P, Bell CC et al Five Essential Elements of Immediate and Mid–Term Mass Trauma Intervention: Empirical Evidence. Psychiatry 2007; 70: 283–315.

14. Bryant R, Harvey A, Basten C et al. Treatment of acute stress disorder: a comparison of cognitive-behavioural therapy and supportive counselling. J Consult Clin Psychol 1998; 66(5): 862–6.

15. Ehlers A, Clark D, Hackmann A et al. A randomized controlled trial of cognitive therapy, a self-help booklet, and repeated assessments as early interventions for posttraumatic stress disorder. Arch Gen Psychiatry 2003; 60: 1024–31.

16. Tyrer P, Steinberg, D. Models for Mental Disorders: Conceptual models in Psychiatry. Chichester: John Wiley and Sons; 2003.

17. Keane T, Zimering R, Caddell J. A behavioural formulation of post-traumatic stress disorder in Vietnam veterans. Behav Ther 1985; 8: 9–12.

18. Foa E, Kozak M. Emotional processing of fear: exposure to corrective information. Psychol Bull 1986; 99: 20–35.

19. Bullman J. Shattered Assumptions: Towards a New Psychology of Trauma. New York: Free Press; 1992.

20. Brewin C, Dalgleish T, Joseph S. A dual representation theory of posttraumatic stress disorder. Psychol Rev 1996; 103: 670–86.

21. Brewin CR, Kleiner JS, Vasterling JJ et al. Memory for emotionally neutral information in posttraumatic stress disorder: A meta-analytic investigation. J Abnorm Psychol 2007; 116(3): 448–63.

22. Ehlers A, Clark DM. A cognitive model of posttraumatic stress disorder. Behav Res Ther 2000; 38: 319–45.

23. Davis M. Neural systems involved in fear and anxiety measured with fear-potentiated startle. Am Psychol 2006; 61(8): 741–56.

24. Armony JL, LeDoux JE. How the brain processes emotional information. Ann N Y Acad Sci 1997; 821: 259–70.

25. Bremner JD, Staib LH, Kaloupek D et al. Neural correlates of exposure to traumatic pictures and sound in Vietnam combat veterans with and without posttraumatic stress disorder: a positron emission tomography study. Biol Psychiatry 1999; 45: 806–16.

26. Gilbertson MW, Shenton ME, Ciszewski A, Kasai et al. Smaller hippocampal volume predicts pathologic vulnerability to psychological trauma. Nat Neurosci 2002; 5(11): 1242–7.

27. Shin L, Rauch S, Pitman R. Amygdala, medial prefrontal cortex and hippocampal function in PTSD. Ann N Y Acad Sci 2006; 1071: 67–79.

29. Yehuda R, Golier JA, Halligan SL et al. The ACTH response to dexamethasone in PTSD. Am J Psychiatry 2004; 161(8): 1397–403.

29. Delahanty DL, Nugent NR, Christopher NC et al. Initial urinary epinephrine and cortisol levels predict acute PTSD symptoms in child trauma victims. Psychoneuroendocrinology 2005; 30(2): 121–8.

30. Videlock EJ, Peleg T, Segman R et al. Stress hormones and post-traumatic stress disorder in civilian trauma victims: a longitudinal study. Part II: The adrenergic response. Int J Neuropsychopharmacol 2007; 11(3): 373–80.

31. Pitman RK, Delahanty DL. Conceptually driven pharmacologic approaches to acute trauma. CNS Spectr 2005; 10(2): 99–106.

32. Pitman RK, Altman B, Greenwald E et al. Psychiatric complications during flooding therapy for post-traumatic stress disorder. J Clin Psychiatry 1991; 52: 17–20.

33. Pitman RK. Post-traumatic stress disorder, hormones, and memory. Biol Psychiatry 1989; 26: 221–3.

34. Cohen H, Zohar J, Gidron Y et al. Blunted HPA axis response to stress influences susceptibility to posttraumatic stress response in rats. Biol Psychiatry 2006; 59(12): 1208–18.

35. Inter-agency standing committee (IASC). IASC guidelines on mental health and psychosocial input support in emergency situations. Geneva: IASC; 2007.

36. Mitchell J. When disaster strikes…the critical incident stress debriefing process. J Emerg Med Serv 1983; 8: 36–39.

37. Mitchell J, Everly G. The scientific evidence for critical incident stress management. J Emerg Med Serv 1997; 22: 86–93.

38. Jones N, Roberts P, Greenberg N. Peer-group risk assessment: a post-traumatic management strategy for hierarchical organizations. Occup Med 2003; 53: 469–475.

39. National child traumatic stress network and national center for PTSD. 2nd ed. Psychological First Aid: Field operations guide; 2006.

40. Schelling G, Briegel J, Roozendaal B et al. The effect of stress doses of hydrocortisone during septic shock on posttraumatic stress disorder in survivors. Biol Psychiatry 2001; 50(12): 978–85.

41. Rose S, Bisson J, Wessely S et al. A systematic review of brief psychological interventions ("debriefing") for the treatment of immediate trauma related symptoms and the prevention of post traumatic stress disorder. Cochrane Library. (major revision), 2005.

42. Bisson J, Jenkins P, Alexander J et al. Randomised controlled trial of psychological debriefing for victims of acute burn trauma. Br J Psychiatry 2005; 171(1): 78–81.

43. Sijbrandij M, Olff M, Reitsma J et al. Treatment of acute posttraumatic stress disorder with brief cognitive behavioural therapy: a randomized controlled trial. Am J Psychiatry 2007; 164: 82–90.

44. Litz B, Gray M, Bryant R et al. Early intervention for trauma: current status and future directions. Clinical Psychology – Science & Practice 2002; 9: 112–34.

45. Adler A, Litz B, Castro C et al. A group randomized trial of critical incident stress debriefing provided to U.S. peacekeepers. J Trauma Stress 2008; 21: 253–63.

46. Bisson JI, McFarlane AC, Rose S et al. Psychological debriefing for adults. Effective Treatments for PTSD. In Foa E, Keane T, Friedman M et al, eds. Effective Treatments for PTSD. New York: Guilford; 2009, pages 83-105.

47. Turpin G, Downs M, Mason S. Effectiveness of providing self-help information following acute traumatic injury: randomised controlled trial. Br J Psychiatry 2005; 187: 76–82.

48. Roberts NP, Kitchiner N, Kenardy J, Bisson JI. Systematic review and meta-analysis of multiple session early interventions following traumatic events. Cochrane Library; 2009, Issue 3.

49. Roberts NP, Kitchiner N, Kenardy J, Bisson JI. Systematic review and meta-analysis of multiple session early interventions following traumatic events. Am J Psych 2009; 166: 293-301.

50. Mellman T, Clark R, Peacock W. Prescribing patterns for patients with posttraumatic stress disorder. Psychiatr Serv 2003; 54: 1618–21.

51. Gelpin E, Bonne O, Peri T et al. Treatment of recent trauma survivors with benzodiazepines: a prospective study. J Clin Psychiatry 1996; 57(9): 390–4.

52. Norris FH, Friedman MJ, Watson PJ et al. 60,000 disaster victims speak: part 1. An empirical review of the empirical literature, 1981–2001. Psychiatry 2002; 65(3): 207–39.

53. Bordow S, Porritt D. An experimental evaluation of crisis intervention. Soc Sci Med [A] 1979; 13: 251–6.

54. Bunn B, Clarke A. Crisis intervention: an experimental study of the effects of a brief period of counselling on the anxiety of relatives of seriously injured or ill hospital patients. Br J Med Psychol 1979; 52(2): 191–5.

55. Hobbs M, Mayou R, Harrison B et al. A randomised controlled trial of psychological debriefing for victims of road traffic accidents. Br Med J 1996; 313(7070): 1438–9.

56. Mayou R, Ehlers A, Hobbs M. Psychological debriefing for road traffic accident victims: three year follow-up of a randomised controlled trial. Br J Psychiatry 2000; 176(6): 589–93.

57. Lee C, Slade P, Lygo V. The influence of psychological debriefing on emotional adaptation in women following early miscarriage: a preliminary study. Br J Med Psychol 1996; 69(1): 47–58.

58. Stevens and Adshead 1996 in Hobbs M, & Adshead G. Preventive psychological intervention for road crash survivors. In: Mitchell M, ed. The Aftermath of Road Accidents: Psychological, Social and Legal Perspectives. London: Routledge, 1996: 159–71.

59. Conlon L, Fahy T, Conroy R. PTSD in ambulant RTA victims: prevalence, predictors and a randomised controlled trial of psychological debriefing in prophylaxis; unpublished.

60. Dolan L, Bowyer D, Freeman C et al. Critical incident stress debriefing after trauma: is it effective?; unpublished.

61. Rose S, Brewin C, Andrews B et al. A randomized controlled trial of individual psychological debriefing for victims of violent crime. Psychol Med 1999; 29: 793–9.

62. Campfield K, Hills A. Effect of timing of critical incident stress debriefing (CISD) on post-traumatic symptoms. J Trauma Stress 2001; 14(2): 327–40.

63. Sijbrandij M, Olff M, Reitsma J et al. Emotional or educational debriefing after psychological trauma. Randomised controlled trial. Br J Psychiatry 2006; 189: 150–5.

64. Marchand A, Guay S, Boyer R et al. A Randomized controlled trial of an adapted form of individual critical incident stress debriefing for victims of an armed robbery. Brief Treat Crisis Interven 2006; 6(2): 122–9.

65. Andre C, Lelord F, Legeron P et al. Etude controlee sur l'efficacite a 6 mois d'une prise en charge precoce de 132 conducteurs d'autobus victims d'agression [Effectiveness of early intervention on 132 bus drivers victims of aggressions: a controlled trial]. L'Encephale 1997; 23: 65–71.

66. Bisson JI, Shepherd JP, Joy D et al. Early cognitive-behavioural therapy for post-traumatic stress symptoms after physical injury. Br J Psychiatry 2004; 184: 63–9.

67. Brom D, Kleber RJ, Hofman MC. Victims of traffic accidents incidence and prevention of post-traumatic stress disorder. J Clin Psychol 1993; 49: 131–9.

68. Bryant RA, Sackville T, Dang ST, Moulds M, Guthrie R. Treating acute stress disorder: an evaluation of cognitive behavior therapy and supportive counseling techniques. Am J Psychiatry 1999; 156(11): 1780–6.

69. Bryant R, Moulds M, Guthrie R et al. Imaginal exposure alone and imaginal exposure with cognitive restructuring in treatment of posttraumatic stress disorder. J Consult Clin Psychol 2003; 71(4): 706–12.

70. Bryant R, Moulds M, Guthrie R et al. The additive benefit of hypnosis and cognitive-behavioural therapy in treating acute stress disorder. J Consult Clin Psychol 2005; 73(2): 334–40.

71. Bryant RA, Mastrodomenico J, Felmingham KL et al. Treatment of acute stress disorder: a random-ized controlled trial. Arch Gen Psychiatry 2008; 65: 659–67.

72. Bugg A, Turpin G, Mason S et al. A randomised controlled trial of the effectiveness of writing as a self-help intervention for traumatic injury patients at risk of developing post-traumatic stress disorder; unpublished.

73. Echeburua E, de Corral P, Sarasua B et al. Treatment of acute posttraumatic stress disorder in rape victims: an experimental study. J Anxiety Disord 1996; 10(3): 185–99.

74. Ehlers A, Clark D, Hackmann A et al. A randomized controlled trial of cognitive therapy, a self-help booklet and repeated assessments as early interventions for posttraumatic stress disorder. Arch Gen Psychiatry 2003; 60(10): 1024–32.

75. Foa EB, Zoellner LA, Feeny NC. An evaluation of three brief programs for facilitating recovery after assault. J Trauma Stress 2006; 19(1): 29–43.

76. Gamble J, Creedy D, Moyle W et al. Effectiveness of a counselling intervention after a traumatic child-birth: a randomized controlled trial. Birth 2005; 32(1): 11–9.

77. Gidron Y, Gal R, Freedman S et al. Translating research findings to PTSD prevention: results of a randomized-controlled pilot study. J Trauma Stress 2001; 14(4): 773–80.

78. Gidron Y, Gal R, Givati G et al. Interactive effects of memory structuring and gender in preventing posttraumatic stress symptoms. J Nerv Ment Dis 2007; 195(2): 1–4.

79. Kazak AE, Simms S, Alderfer MA et al. Feasibility and preliminary outcomes from a pilot study of a brief psychological intervention for families of children newly diagnosed with cancer. J Pediatr Psychol 2005; 30(8): 644–55.

80. Marchand A, Guay S, Boyer R et al. A randomized controlled trial of an adapted form of individual critical incident stress debriefing for victims of an armed robbery. Brief Treat Crisis Interv 2006; 6(2): 122–9.

81. Ost L, Paunovic N, Gillow A. Cognitive-behavior therapy in the prevention of chronic PTSD in crime victims; unpublished.

82. Ryding E, Wijma K, Wijma B. Postpartum counselling after an emergency caesarean. Clin Psychol Psychother 1998; 5: 231–7.

83. Ryding El, Wiren E, Johansson G et al. Group counselling for mothers after emergency cesarean sec-tion: a randomized controlled trial of intervention. Birth 2004; 31(4): 247–53.

84. van Emmerik AAP, Kamphuis JH, Emmelkamp PMG. Treating acute stress disorder and posttrau-matic stress disorder with cognitive behavioural therapy or structured writing therapy: a random-ized controlled trial. Psychother Psychosom 2008; 77(2): 93–100.

85. Wagner AW, Zatzick DF, Ghesquiere A et al. Behavioural activation as an early intervention for post-traumatic stress disorder and depression. Cogn Behav Pract 2007; 4: 341–9.

86. Zatzick D, Roy-Byrne P, Russo JE et al. Collaborative interventions for physically injured trauma survivors: a pilot randomized effectiveness trial. Gen Hosp Psychiatry 2001; 23(3): 114–23.

87. Zatzick D, Roy-Byrne P, Russo J et al. A randomized effectiveness trial of stepped collaborative care for acutely injured trauma survivors. Arch Gen Psychiatry 2004; 61(5): 498–506.

88. Mellman TA, Bustamante V, David D et al. Hypnotic medication in the aftermath of trauma. J Clin Psychiatry 2002; 63: 1183–4.

89. Stein MB, Kerridge C, Dimsdale JE et al. Pharmacotherapy to prevent PTSD: results from a ran-domized controlled proof-of-concept trial in physically injured patients. J Trauma Stress 2007; 20(6): 923–32.

11 | Traumatic stress disorders in children

Soraya Seedat

INTRODUCTION

Pediatric posttraumatic stress disorder (PTSD) is unique among disorders of childhood and adolescence in its requirement of an etiopathogenic agent with enduring sequelae.(1) As in adults it is characterized by a cluster of symptoms that develop in the aftermath of traumatic events that involve actual or threatened death or injury or threat to the physical integrity of one's self or others. Traumatic events include physical or sexual abuse or maltreatment, road traffic injuries, violence, war-related trauma, severe burns, and natural disasters, among others.(1) These events are considered trauma-tic because they overwhelm a child or adolescent's perceived ability to cope. During the traumatic event, there is recruitment of adaptive, stress-mediating neural systems (e.g., hypothalamic–pituitary–adrenal axis and sympathetic nervous system) that, in turn, produces adaptive physiological, behavioral, emotional, and cognitive responses necessary for survival.(2) By definition and according to the *DSM-IV-TR*, traumatic events should evoke acute subjective reactions of intense fear, horror, or helplessness.(1, 3)

However, the *DSM-IV-TR* includes a qualifier for children and adolescents who may instead show responses of disorganized or agitated behavior.(3) The *DSM-IV-TR* requirement of a subjective response acknowledges that individual traumatic reactions play a crucial role in determining the development of PTSD.

At the time that the diagnosis was first formulated more than 25 years ago(4), the question of whether PTSD could manifest in children and adolescents was hotly debated. Since then the multitude of studies that have emerged in parallel with subsequent iterations of the DSM have consistently have found that the disorder can be reliably detected in preschool and school-going children and adolescents, and that youth with chronic PTSD may have a more unremitting course than adults with the disorder.(5–10) While the *DSM-IV-TR* has made progress in recognizing that children and adolescents with PTSD may have different symptom patterns compared with adults,(3) more recent studies using alternative PTSD criteria have suggested the need for optimal diagnostic algorithms that are more developmentally sensitive, valid, and stable for making the diagnosis in preschool children.(10, 11) This chapter provides a conceptual overview of PTSD in childhood—its diagnosis, epidemiology, phenomenology, psychobiology, as well as current psychotherapeutic and psychopharmacologic treatment approaches.

EPIDEMIOLOGY

In community surveys of PTSD, prevalence rates using *DSM-III-R* criteria range from 0.1% among preschool children (age range: 2–5 years)(12) to 3%–6% in older adolescents (age range: 16–22 years).(6, 13) Estimates of PTSD prevalence in children and adolescents who have experienced trauma are considerably higher with most reported rates in the order of 30% to 40%. (1, 14–16) Consistent with this, a meta-analysis by Fletcher (16) (2003) of 34 studies of 2,697 children and adolescents found that, overall, across a wide range of trauma, 36% of children met criteria for PTSD. Of note, the rate of PTSD did not differ markedly across age and developmental level (<7 years: 39%, 6–12 years: 33%, >12 years: 27%).

The majority of studies of PTSD have been conducted following motor accidents, sexual abuse, natural disasters, criminal violence, burns, and war. Rates of PTSD in children and young people (based on studies that have used *DSM-III* and *DSM-III-R* criteria) show a similar pattern to those in adults. They are high following sexual abuse (48%–90%), (17, 18) violent crime (27%–33%),(19, 20) and war (27%–33%).(21, 22) In contrast, natural disasters give rise to considerably lower rates of PTSD (0%–5%).(23–26) In addition to the type of trauma, prevalence rates by a variety of other factors are to be considered, including the severity and chronicity of the trauma; the child's proximity to the trauma; the personal impact on the child; time lapsed since the event; and the presence of parental psychopathology, especially parental PTSD.(1, 16)

An important and challenging issue in the trauma field involves early identification of individuals who will later develop PTSD. Although it was initially thought that a diagnosis of acute stress disorder (ASD) would address this challenge, studies in adults have found that approximately three quarters of trauma survivors who meet diagnostic criteria for ASD go on to develop PTSD; it is also true that only a minority of individuals who develop PTSD after trauma meet criteria initially for ASD (for review).(27) Several studies have now investigated the relationship between acute stress disorder (ASD) and longer-term PTSD in children and adolescents. Similarly, a number of prospective studies of the predictive validity of ASD in children and adolescents suggest that current ASD diagnostic criteria are not optimal for identifying younger children at high risk for the development of PTSD. (10, 28–30) Bryant et al. (31) indexed the relationship between ASD and subsequent PTSD in injured children aged 7–13 years. At 6 months posttrauma, PTSD was diagnosed in 25% of children who were diagnosed with ASD. In terms of those children with full ASD, 33% met criteria for PTSD and 50% met criteria for subsyndromal PTSD, while 11% of those without ASD developed PTSD. Acute stress reactions that did not include dissociation provided better prediction of PTSD than full ASD criteria.

Similarly, a study in preschool children in the age group of 2 to 6 years and 7 to 10 years ($N = 60$) exposed to motor vehicle accidents where assessments for ASD and PTSD, respectively, were conducted at 2 to 4 weeks and again at 6 months using both *DSM-IV* criteria and alternative criteria (i.e., reduction in the requisite number of endorsed avoidance symptoms from 3 to 1 and removal of the *DSM-IV* criterion A2 concerning emotional responsiveness to the event), found that the rate of PTSD was 10% using the alternative criteria compared with 1.7% using standard *DSM-IV* criteria.(10) The alternative criteria also showed better predictive validity and stability over time with 69% of children diagnosed with ASD after trauma retaining a diagnosis of PTSD at 6 months. Dalgeish et al.,(30) in a large sample of child and adolescent road-accident survivors who were homogeneous for trauma type, found that the acute stress disorder dissociation criterion did not have a unique role in predicting later PTSD, indicating that the significant association between acute stress disorder and later PTSD "may therefore simply reflect persistence or chronicity in the symptom clusters that acute stress disorder and PTSD have in common." Of note, subacute stress disorder (acute stress disorder minus dissociation) was approximately three times more sensitive in predicting PTSD than the full acute stress disorder syndrome in the study, while the full syndrome did not incrementally increase the ability to predict PTSD in children and adolescents.

PHENOMENOLOGY OF PEDIATRIC PTSD AND ACUTE STRESS DISORDER

The core symptoms of PTSD span three clusters: intrusion/reexperiencing, avoidance and numbing, and hyperarousal (3). For each of these clusters, the *DSM-IV-TR* includes qualifiers for children and adolescents although the overall number of qualifiers are few. It is noteworthy that 8 of the 17 criteria require verbal descriptions of symptoms and feeling states.(8) Moreover, evidence suggests that children with subthreshold symptoms who do not meet full criteria for PTSD may experience significant levels of disability.(7) Debate, therefore, continues about whether more distinct criteria should be applied considering that youth's understanding and recall of their traumatic experiences may differ substantially from adults and be colored by developmental aspects. For example, reexperiencing symptoms (recurrent, intrusive recollections, memories, nightmares, or other senses of reliving the traumatic experience) in young children, for which at least one symptom must be present, may comprise distressing dreams in young children that may progress to nightmares of monsters, of rescuing others, or of threats to the self or others, or there may be frightening dreams without recognizable content. Young children, rather than reliving the trauma through repeated intrusive memories may reexperience the trauma through repetitive play (e.g., a child who was involved in a shooting may repeatedly reenact shootings with a toy gun).(3) Reminders of the trauma (people, places, activities, or situations that remind the child of the original traumatic event) may also lead to intense psychological or physiological distress that a child may struggle to verbalize.

To make the diagnosis, at least three symptoms are required from the avoidance cluster (efforts to avoid trauma reminders, including talking about the traumatic event or other trauma reminders; inability to recall an important aspect of the trauma; decreased interest or participation in previously enjoyed activities; detachment or estrangement from others; restricted affect; and sense of a foreshortened future). While there is a recognition in the *DSM-IV-TR* that young children may have difficulty verbalizing their internal thoughts and feelings, the Task Force on Research Diagnostic Criteria has recommended lowering the requirement in this cluster from three symptoms to one.(32) In addition, there may be omen formation (i.e., a belief in the ability to foresee future untoward events) and a diminished ability to report on psychosocial impairment (especially in younger children), and this needs to be borne in mind during evaluation.(3)

The last cluster, hyperarousal, requires at least two symptoms (difficulty falling or staying asleep, irritability or angry outbursts, difficulty concentrating, hypervigilance, and increased startle reactions). Hyperarousal may present with a variety of physical symptoms in young children, including headaches and stomachaches.(3)

All of the aforementioned symptoms cause marked distress and impairment (in at least one important life domain) and persist for at least 1 month following trauma. In the initial month after trauma, a diagnosis of acute stress disorder (ASD) should be considered. The major distinction between PTSD and ASD is the latter's emphasis on dissociative symptoms, with the *DSM-IV-TR* requiring the presence of at least three of five dissociative symptoms (reduced awareness of the surroundings, derealization, depersonalization, dissociative amnesia, and emotional numbing). (3) Several authors have proposed the concept of subthreshold or partial PTSD, which considers that a child/adolescent may present a number of symptoms below threshold for avoidance or hyperarousal criteria (subthreshold syndrome), or may even present without any symptom for one or more of the reexperiencing, avoidance, or hyperarousal criteria (partial syndrome). (33) In an investigation of children aged 7 to 19, with severe burns, who were compared with 30 nonburned subjects matched for age, sex, SES (socioeconomic status), and parents' marital status according to *DSM-III* criteria, Stoddard et al. (1989) documented that 6.7% of youth met criteria for PTSD,(34) with children almost three times that number meeting criteria for partial PTSD;(34) found that 50% of children exposed to community violence in an inner-city community met criteria for PTSD and another 21% met criteria for partial PTSD.

In addition to PTSD and ASD, studies among traumatized children and adolescents describe associations with a broad range of other psychopathological outcomes, in particular mood disorders, other anxiety disorders (e.g., generalized anxiety disorder, separation anxiety disorder), behavioral disorders (e.g., attention-deficit hyperactivity disorder, conduct disorder), and substance use disorders.(35) For example, in a 10–year longitudinal study using a representative population sample of children aged 9, 11, and 13 years, exposure to at least one traumatic event by age 16 was reported by 68% of youth, with 13.4% developing some posttraumatic stress symptoms.(36) Lifetime occurrence of other mood (12.1%), anxiety (9.8%), and disruptive behavior disorders (19.2% of youth who were exposed to trauma) was also high.(36)

COMORBIDITY

Adolescents with PTSD have a substantially higher risk of co-occurring disorders, both in their lifetime and during the past year.(36, 37) Giaconia and colleagues in a community study of older adolescents reported that four of five adolescents with PTSD met criteria for at least one additional disorder and more than two-fifths had two or more other lifetime disorders. Also, more than 40% of adolescents with PTSD, compared with fewer than 8% of their peers, met criteria for major depression by age 18, with PTSD usually preceding or occurring at the same age as depression for those adolescents with both disorders. In contrast, onset of alcohol dependence preceded onset of PTSD in about a half of cases.

Developmental mental health histories of adults with PTSD were documented across the first three decades of life in the longitudinal Dunedin Multidisciplinary Health and Development Study: 100% of those diagnosed with past-year PTSD and 93.5% of those with lifetime PTSD at age 26 had met criteria for another mental disorder between ages 11 and 21,(38) suggesting that as PTSD almost always develops in the context of other mental disorders, it is crucial that research examining the etiology of the disorder take into account lifetime developmental patterns of comorbidity. Adolescents with PTSD also face social, academic, cognitive, and emotional difficulties and are at an increased risk of suicidal thoughts and attempts.(36, 37)

NEUROBIOLOGY

Developmental differences in the neurobiological underpinnings of PTSD across the life cycle have also raised questions about whether PTSD is the same or different disorder in children compared with adults. The disorder is thought to be associated with a range of complex psychobiological disturbances, involving multiple neurotransmitter and neuroendocrine systems(see other chapters in this volume). Both the hypothalamic–pituitary–adrenal (HPA) axis and locus ceruleus/ norepinephrine/ sympathetic nervous system are critical in the physiological response to trauma. Neuroendocrine investigations in adults have yielded findings of low-, normal-, and even high-circulating plasma levels of cortisol and both high and low urinary cortisol levels.(39) A recent systematic review and meta-analysis of basal cortisol levels in adults with PTSD found no systematic difference in basal cortisol levels between people with PTSD and controls.(40) However, in subgroup analyses assessing plasma or serum, significantly lower levels were observed in people with PTSD than in controls not exposed to trauma. Lower levels were also found in people with PTSD when females were included, in studies on physical or sexual abuse, and in afternoon samples. The results of this meta-analysis suggest that low cortisol levels do not relate to PTSD in general but rather seem to mirror trauma exposure and PTSD subgroups. Similar to the findings in adults, studies of the psychobiological profile of PTSD in youth have produced mixed results. Methodological differences across studies, including differences in assessment of PTSD, differences in the age range and gender ratio, the length of time lapsed since the trauma, and timing and source (plasma versus urine) of cortisol measurement, may be contributory to these discrepancies.(39)

One of the best replicated neuroanatomical abnormalities in adults with PTSD is hippocampal volume reduction. The hippocampus, a structural component of the limbic system, has a key role in memory processing, and a growing body of work suggests that the secretion of glucocorticoids during traumatic stress can have neurotoxic effects on the hippocampus.(41, 42) Increased level of glucocorticoids have also been documented in children with histories of maltreatment and PTSD.(43, 44) Further, it has been hypothesized that the putative neurotoxic effects of glucocorticoids may vary according to a number of factors, namely, (i) the developmental stage of the hippocampus, (ii) the amount and sustainability of cortisol released, and (iii) the severity and/or the chronicity of the trauma/s.(45) However, pediatric studies have failed to document hippocampal volume reductions in children and adolescents (46–48) and have instead found either no differences in hippocampal volume between PTSD and controls or larger hippocampal volumes. This suggests that smaller hippocampal volumes may be the result of longstanding neurodevelopmental experiences of traumatic stress, such that chronic and/or cumulative exposure of stress during childhood may be necessary for hippocampal damage. This is in keeping with the developmental model of PTSD that De Bellis has proposed, namely, that childhood trauma may result in perturbations of biological stress response systems resulting initially in elevated corticotrophin-releasing hormone (CRH) release and increased secretion of cortisol. Over time, elevated levels of cortisol in the central nervous system can exert neurotoxic effects on the developing brain and possibly explain the hippocampal and other brain structural and functional abnormalities that occur in PTSD.(43) With enhanced negative feedback inhibition of the HPA axis, there is eventually a lowering of basal cortisol. Thus, the clinical features characteristic of PTSD may be attributed to cortisol dysregulation that, in turn, fails to shut down the catecholaminergic response in limbic structures. Resulting prolonged increases in noradrenergic activity could, in turn, lead to an overconsolidation of traumatic memories that underlie the intrusive and avoidance symptoms seen in PTSD.(49)

Consistent with the theory that volumetric abnormalities of the hippocampus may represent a biological marker of chronic stress, a small pilot longitudinal study of children with a history of maltreatment ($N = 15$) found that PTSD symptoms and cortisol levels at baseline were associated with changes in hippocampal volume over a 12–18-month period.(45) Several studies in children have also noted reductions in cerebellar (50) and corpus callosal (46, 47) volumes. Consistent with this finding, Jackowski et al. (51), using diffusion tensor imaging

(DTI; a relatively new technique that provides information on white matter coherence and myelination) in maltreated children with PTSD, found reduced fractional anisotropy (a measure of water diffusion) in medial and posterior corpus callosal regions. However, whether the corpus callosal disturbances are a function of the disorder (PTSD) or of the trauma per se (maltreatment) is questionable, as the study did not include matched trauma-exposed children without PTSD. Further investigation of the effects of trauma on corpus callosal and corticolimbic circuit abnormalities appears to be a promising avenue for better understanding the etiopathophysiology of pediatric PTSD.(51)

Relatively few studies in children have examined posttraumatic catecholamine secretion. In one prospective study of children and adolescents hospitalized for motor vehicle accidents, significantly elevated plasma noradrenaline concentrations were demonstrated in children with PTSD at 1 and 6 months after the accident compared to non-PTSD and control groups. In contrast, evening salivary cortisol concentrations normalized at 6 months, although these concentrations were elevated at the 1-month time point.(52) Moreover, the higher noradrenaline concentrations at 6 months were independent of severity in the PTSD group. The authors hypothesized that elevations in nordadrenaline at 6 months may reflect a persistence of PTSD rather than be a marker of severity. De Bellis et al. (43) in an investigation of catecholamine and cortisol levels in prepubertal children with PTSD secondary to past child maltreatment experiences found that children with PTSD had higher levels of urinary norepinephrine and dopamine levels than both children with overanxious disorder and controls, higher urinary epinephrine levels than children with overanxious disorder and higher cortisol levels than normal controls.

Of note, the majority of children with PTSD had comorbid psychopathology, including mood, anxiety, behavioral, and dissociative symptoms. The confounding biological effects of comorbidity in PTSD have, to date, received little attention and warrants further study. Preliminary investigations in adults have reported higher evening salivary cortisol levels in adults with PTSD comorbid with depression compared with those with only PTSD and only depression,(53) and higher norepinephrine levels in patients with PTSD and depression than in patients with only PTSD or normal controls.(54)

RISK AND RESILIENCE

As not all children who are trauma-exposed develop PTSD, there has been considerable emphasis in recent years on identifying mediating and moderating variables that interact in the onset and persistence of the disorder. Major questions in the field are, "What characteristics determine which children/adolescents will thrive in the face of trauma?" "What are the inherent characteristics that underpin the ability to cope with trauma?" The term resilience is widely used as an "umbrella" term in the trauma context and, in general, typifies those children and adolescents who experience trauma but who do not go on to develop PTSD. It is not possible to talk about resilience without talking about vulnerability or risk. Resilience is multidimensional and modifiable and is determined by a variety of neurobiologic, genetic, temperamental, and environmental factors that confer protection in the face of risk.(55) The first community-based prospective study to follow up children into adulthood and to examine the extent to which potentially malleable individual-level factors measured in childhood could account for the risk of exposure to traumatic events and the risk of PTSD development after exposure (56) found that youth with high levels of depressive and anxious feelings in first grade were 1.5 times more likely to experience PTSD once exposed to trauma, while those with high teacher ratings of aggressive/disruptive problems soon after entry into the first grade were more likely to experience traumatic events involving assaultive violence but not after other types of traumatic events.

A number of risk factors for childhood PTSD following trauma exposure have been identified. These include female gender, previous trauma exposure, the presence of a preexisting psychiatric disorder (particularly an anxiety disorder), parental psychopathology, and the lack of social support.(35) Girls have consistently been found to report more PTSD symptoms than boys following exposure to a wide variety of traumas and may, in fact, be up to six times more likely to meet criteria for PTSD than boys after major trauma.(6, 37, 57) It has been suggested that girls' higher risk of trauma exposure may, in part, be explained by the age at which trauma occurs, in that females have higher rates of PTSD after trauma exposure in childhood compared with exposure after the age of 15 years.(58) Other factors that may be contributory to females' higher risk for PTSD are the type of trauma (particularly sexual violence), differences in neuroendocrine responses to stress, and heightened peritrauma perceptions of threat or uncontrollability.(58) In terms of the traumatic event itself, level of exposure to dangerous events predicts risk for later PTSD, with this association found for almost all types of trauma. However, the nature and severity of injury have most often been found to be unrelated to both acute and persistent PTSD.(59) Heightened arousal (and increased noradrenergic activity) in the immediate aftermath of trauma, in the form of elevated heart rate, also appears to be related to later PTSD outcome in injured children.(58) In a study that investigated the extent to which heart rate levels soon after a traumatic event (as measured during emergency medical services transport) predicted PTSD symptom severity assessed at 6 weeks and 6 months later in child trauma victims, Nugent et al. (60) found that heart rate had the strongest relationship, among other factors, to subsequent PTSD symptoms.

Children who live in social situations characterized by a high degree of social disruption are at higher risk of developing PTSD. In contrast, "protective" factors such as social support, low levels of parental PTSD, and low levels of parental trauma-related distress have been shown to predict lower levels of PTSD symptoms in children. There is mounting evidence that parental PTSD is a risk factor for childhood PTSD. Children of Holocaust survivors with PTSD have a higher prevalence of PTSD and lower cortisol excretion than demographically matched control subjects.(61) A study that examined how parental responses following pediatric injury might influence children's posttraumatic stress responses found that parental posttraumatic stress symptoms (PTSS) significantly predicted symptomatology in the child.(60) Furthermore, there was an interaction between the child's initial physiological reactivity and parental symptoms of posttraumatic stress. High levels of parental PTSS were especially deleterious for children who excreted low levels of cortisol soon after their accident, whereas parental PTSS were less relevant for children with high levels of initial cortisol. Similarly, high parental PTSS were associated with greater child PTSS in children with low in-hospital heart rate (HR). Thus, these results suggest that children who are not identified on the basis of their initial biological responses as being at increased risk for developing PTSS may still develop PTSS, on the basis of their parents' response to the traumatic event. There is some indication that the effects of parental PTSD may stem from early *in utero* effects and fetal programming of the HPA axis in that data from a group of mothers and babies exposed to the September 11 attacks showed that both mothers and babies of mothers who developed PTSD in response to September 11 had lower cortisol levels compared with mothers and their babies who did not develop PTSD.(62)

Converging evidence from mainly twin and family studies supports the role of genetic influences in the vulnerability to PTSD. Molecular studies in adults, namely, candidate gene association studies, have now identified associations with genes involved in various neurotransmitter pathways, including dopamine (dopamine receptor -2 gene [DRD2], dopamine transporter gene [DAT]) and serotonin (serotonin transporter gene [SLC6A4]). However, these studies are limited by their cross-sectional nature and the relative paucity of information they yield regarding the underlying biological dysregulations in PTSD.(63) Of interest is a study in medically injured children that examined genetic polymorphisms in the FKBP5 gene, an HPA axis gene that regulates glucocorticoid receptor gene activity. The authors noted a significant association between two polymorphisms of FKBP5 and peritraumatic dissociation.(64) Very recently, four polymorphism of the same gene were found to interact with the severity of child abuse in a sample of adults as a predictor of adult PTSD symptoms. (65) Another promising approach to the identification of the genetic underpinnings of PTSD is gene expression profiling of peripheral blood mononuclear cells.(66) Preliminary findings in adults indicate that signature patterns of gene expression may enable early identification of trauma survivors who go on to develop PTSD. These results are encouraging and pave the way for further investigation of the predictive value of gene expression signatures in child trauma survivors.

ASSESSMENT

Accurate and thorough assessment of traumatized children and adolescents with PTSD is crucial for the implementation of any appropriate intervention. However, information relating to trauma exposure may not be spontaneously volunteered, and consequently, PTSD symptoms may easily be missed. Moreover, youth with PTSD often carry other diagnoses (e.g., major depression), making it difficult for clinicians to distinguish PTSD from overlapping symptoms. Distinguishing youth with exposure to single discrete traumatic events from those with exposure to chronic or pervasive trauma is also important, as youth with the former tend to present with less complex symptomatology and are usually more responsive to treatment. Exposure to repeated and pervasive trauma, also known as complex or developmental trauma, refers to the cumulative effect of simultaneous or sequential occurrence of different forms of abuse and/ or maltreatment (e.g., physical abuse, sexual abuse, emotional abuse and neglect, witnessing domestic violence).

Historically, measures and interviews designed for adults have been adapted for youth by simplifying language and concepts.(67) While many of these are in existence, few are based on *DSM-IV* criteria, standardized, and well validated. Arguably, with the exception of the Clinician-Administered PTSD Scale for Children and Adolescents (CAPS-CA), there is no widely accepted "gold" standard measure for making the diagnosis and/or assessing treatment effects. The American Academy of Child and Adolescent Psychiatry (1) advocates for a multiinformant approach to assessment. The level of agreement between child and parent (or guardian) may be poor for PTSD and for ASD;(68) however, informants other than the child may yield potentially valuable sources of information. In fact, Scheeringa et al. (69) found that combined parent–child reports yielded significantly more symptoms and higher rates for reexperiencing, avoidance, and hyperarousal criteria (almost a twofold increase) and for the overall diagnosis of PTSD (37.5%) than parent report alone (4.2%). The almost ninefold increase in diagnosis from combined reports suggests that the diagnostic rates for children who are unable to endorse symptoms themselves may greatly underestimate the true numbers.

In addition to enquiring about the presence of PTSD symptoms, both child and parent should be asked about symptom severity and functional impairment. Assessment should further focus on family factors, in particular the response of the parents to the trauma and the ability of the parents to communicate with the child and support and enhance coping, and the impact of the trauma on the functioning of the family unit.(70) There are several challenges to the assessment of PTSD in youth and these include the following:

(i)   Assessment of multiple trauma—many measures require the child/adolescent to report on a variety of traumatic events but only one traumatic event (either the most bothersome or the most recent) is used as a basis for assessing current PTSD symptoms;

(ii) Difficulty in determining the nature and extent of certain traumatic experiences (e.g., exposure to domestic violence);

(iii) Uncertainty about the suitability and utility of many of the assessment instruments across multinational and multiethnic settings;

(iv) Optimal integration of information from multiple informants (e.g., self-report measures may do well to capture internalizing symptoms; however, parents are often more reliable informants about behavior and externalizing symptomatology) and optimal integration of multimodal data points, namely, emotional, behavioral, physiological, genetics data.(67)

Measures for the assessment of trauma currently in use can be divided into four main domains:

(i)   Child/adolescent self-report measures that screen for a history of trauma exposure only (e.g., Childhood Trauma Questionnaire, Survey of Exposure to Community Violence);

(ii) Child/adolescent self-report measures that screen for PTSD symptoms (Children's Impact of Traumatic Events-Revised [IES-R]),(71) Trauma Symptom Checklist for Children (72), Child PTSD Symptom Scale (CPSS; 73), Child Post-Traumatic Stress Disorder Reaction Index (CPTSD-RI; 74);

(iii) Child and adolescent clinician-administered diagnostic interviews that screen for both trauma exposure and PTSD (Clinician-Administered PTSD Scale for Children and Adolescents [CAPS-CA]; (75)), Kiddie Schedule for Affective Disorders and Schizophrenia (K-SADS; (76)), Diagnostic Interview for Children and Adolescents- Revised (DICA-R; (77)). The CAPS-CA is a semistructured comprehensive clinical interview intended for children/adolescents aged 8 to 18 years . It is modeled on the adult CAPS, comprises 32 items, and evaluates trauma exposure, makes diagnoses of current and lifetime PTSD, and assesses symptom severity. The K-SADS is similarly a semistructured interview for children/adolescents aged 6 to 18 years that, in addition to assessing for present and life-time PTSD, provides diagnoses on a range of other psychiatric disorders;

(iv) Child/adolescent self-report measures that screen for associated symptoms, for example, dissociation and resilience (e.g., Adolescent Dissociative Experiences Scale [A-DES], (78); Connor-Davidson Resilience Scale [CD-RISC], (79)). The A-DES is a 30-item self-report measure of a variety of dissociative experiences for youths aged 12 to 18 years that may be useful in examining dissociative experiences and psychopathological dissociation in clinical and nonclinical samples of adolescents.(80) The CD-RISC, a 25-item self-report measure with sound psychometric properties may also be useful in clinical and research settings, as well as in investigations of the neurobiology of resilience and in the assessment of interventions to enhance resilience. However, there is limited data on its use in children and adolescents and on its use across different cultures.(55, 81)

No single measure is ideally suited to every child and situation. Self report measures usu-ally take a shorter time to administer than clinician-administered instruments. Instruments also differ with respect to the PTSD symptom "time frame" that they measure (i.e., 1 week, 1 month). Ultimately, the choice of instrument will depend on the context and the purpose for which it is being used (whether research or clinical), its psychometric properties and user friendliness, the age of the child being assessed, its validation across cultural settings, and cost and accessibility (for comprehensive reviews see (79, 82)). In very young children, elicitation of information could also be aided by a variety of verbal and nonverbal strategies, including storytelling, drawing, play, and the use of dolls and toys.(70)

Other psychiatric and medical conditions may mimic the symptoms of PTSD and these need to be ruled out. For example, avoidant symptoms (social withdrawal and emotional numbing) and hyperarousal symptoms (sleep difficulties, irritability) may mimic major depres-sive disorder. Similarly, PTSD can be mistaken for another anxiety disorder, including general-ized anxiety disorder, social anxiety disorder, or obsessive compulsive disorder, because of the overlap of symptoms such as irritability, physiological and psychological hyperarousal upon reexposure to feared stimuli, sleep problems, hypervigilance, increased startle reaction, and avoidance. PTSD can be misdiagnosed as an alcohol or drug use disorder, as alcohol and/or drugs may be used by youth as self-medication to produce affective dulling and as a means of avoiding trauma reminders. PTSD should also be differentiated from a psychotic disorder, which it can mimic through symptoms such as flashbacks, hypervigilance, paranoia, sleep difficulties, restricted affect, and/or social withdrawal. Lastly, a number of general medical conditions (e.g., asthma, epilepsy, migraine, hyperthyroidism) and medications (e.g., steroids, antiasthmatics, diet pills, antihistamines) may mimic some of the symptoms of PTSD.

TREATMENT

Practice parameters developed by the American Academy of Child and Adolescent Psychiatry (1), which are in the process of being revised, advocate for a multimodal prevention–intervention approach. This encompasses triage for trauma-exposed children by strengthening coping skills for any anticipated trauma responses and grief reactions and treatment of acute and chronic PTSD and other disorders that may develop in the aftermath of trauma. One of the first steps in management is education of the child and parent/s about the disorder. This should be done in consultation with the relevant primary care physician/s and school personnel. Inclusion of parents in treatment is important for symptom resolution and allows parents to monitor their child's symptoms, learn behavior management techniques, and work with their own emotional distress related to the trauma. The choice of treatment modality for a given child will depend on (i) symptom severity and associated impairment, (ii) presence of comorbid conditions and asso-ciated risk factors, (iii) developmental age and cognitive functioning of the child, (iv) treatment preference of the child/parents, and (v) availability and affordability issues. In the main, inter-ventions comprising psychotherapy (including trauma-focused cognitive–behavior therapy and family therapy) and pharmacotherapy are widely used. The AACAP guidelines (1) recommend that treatment of mild PTSD should begin with psychotherapy.

1. Psychotherapies

Trauma-Focused Cognitive–Behavior Therapy (CBT) and CBT

There are now several validated models of psychotherapy in use for childhood PTSD. Individual trauma-focused cognitive–behavior therapy (TF-CBT) has the best empirical evidence as a beneficial treatment for child and adolescent PTSD. Several rigorous controlled trials of TF-CBT and CBT have examined efficacy in children 3 to 17 years of age, in various trauma contexts (particularly in sexually abused children), with symptoms ranging from PTSD to other anxiety, mood, and behavioral disorders.(35) In general, TF-CBT interventions include the following components: psychoeducation, parenting skills, relaxation (e.g., progressive muscle relaxation, focused breathing), affect awareness and regulation (e.g., identification of emotions, positive self-talk), cognitive restructuring (recognizing the relationship between thoughts, feelings, and behaviors, correcting irrational thoughts), trauma narrative (developing a narrative of the traumatic events), *in vivo* graded exposure, conjoint child–parent sessions, and planning for future safety and development.

In a large multisite study, Cohen et al. (83) compared TF-CBT with child-centered therapy (CCT). Children aged 8 to 14 years and their primary caretakers were randomly assigned to either of the aforementioned treatments, which consisted of 12 weekly sessions of 45 minutes for the child individually and 45 minutes for the parent, although 3 of the weekly sessions involved 30 minutes of joint parent–child therapy. All of the children had significant symptoms of PTSD, with 89% meeting full PTSD criteria. Specific elements of TF-CBT included skills in emotional expression, training in coping skills, gradual exposure, cognitive processing of the trauma, some psychoeducation, joint parent–child sessions, and parent management skills.(83) CCT was supportive in nature, allowing the child or parent to guide the structure and content of their own treatment, whereby children were encouraged to formulate their own personal strategies for change. At treatment follow-up, children who received TF-CBT exhibited significantly greater improvements on measures of PTSD, depression, behavior problems, and associated symptoms (abuse-related attributions and shame) than those who received CCT.

King et al. (84) randomly assigned 36 sexually abused children and adolescents to individual CBT, family CBT, or a wait-list control condition and found that children in both active conditions had a significantly superior response in PTSD symptoms and self-reports of fear and anxiety compared with the wait-list condition. In a study to assess the durability of TF-CBT, 82 sexually abused children aged 8 to 15 years who were assigned to TF-CBT or nondirective supportive therapy (NST) delivered over 12 sessions were followed up over 12 months. Among the 49 treatment completers, children in the TF-CBT group had significantly greater improvement in PTSD, dissociative symptoms, depression, and social competence than children who received NST.(85) Similarly, Kolko (86) randomly assigned 55 physically abused or physically maltreated youth to one of three conditions: individual child and parent CBT, family therapy (FT), or routine community services (RCS). CBT was similar in format to TF-CBT used in other studies. CBT and FT were composed of twelve 1-hour sessions per week, while the total duration of RCS varied but involved more weekly therapist contact hours than the other two conditions. CBT produced significantly greater improvement than both FT and RCS on measures of externalizing symptoms, conflict, and global assessment of functioning.

At least two studies provide support for the efficacy of school-based CBT for children who are similarly exposed to traumatic events.(87, 88) In one of these, Stein et al. (2003) randomized sixth-grade students who were exposed to community violence and experiencing posttraumatic stress symptoms to either Group Cognitive-Behavioral Intervention (CBITS) or a 3-month wait-list control condition. Components of CBITS included psychoeducation, graded exposure (e.g., writing, drawing), cognitive and coping skills training (e.g., thought stopping, relaxation), and social skills training, with 10 weekly group session (5–8 students). CBITS compared with wait listing produced significant improvements in PTSD symptoms, depression, and psychosocial function. Treatment gains on all measures were maintained at the 6-month follow-up in CBITS-treated youth. In the first cluster randomized trial of a school-based intervention for children exposed to armed conflict in a low-income setting in Indonesia, 15 sessions of a manualized group intervention administered by paraprofessionals was compared with a wait-listed condition.(89) The intervention, over 5 weeks, integrated CBT techniques (trauma-processing activities) with cooperative play and creative-expressive exercises (drama, dance and music). Girls benefited more from the intervention than boys, with reductions in PTSD symptoms and improvements in hope and functioning.

Although data are few, there is some emerging evidence that TF-CBT may be efficacious in youth exposed to complex trauma. Feather and Ronan (90) assessed a manualized, 16-session TF-CBT in four youth aged 9 to13 years who were multiply traumatized (exposed to childhood physical abuse, childhood sexual abuse, emotional abuse, interpersonal violence, and domestic violence). All four children reported a decrease in PTSD symptoms and an increase in coping posttreatment.

In a meta-analysis of 21 psychosocial treatment studies for pediatric PTSD, TF-CBT met *well-established* criteria for efficacy; school-based CBT met criteria for *probably efficacious*, and other treatments (including CBT, EMDR, family therapy, and child–parent psychotherapy) met criteria for *possibly efficacious*.(91) Specifically cognitive–behavior grounded therapies were superior to non-cognitive behavior therapies in reducing posttraumatic stress symptoms, depression anxiety, and externalizing behavior problems. However, studies of the relative efficacy of different modalities (i.e., individual vs. group) and dismantling studies of the critical components of treatment (e.g., exposure vs. cognitive restructuring) are needed.(92) Treatment studies suggest that 12 sessions of TF-CBT is acceptable in children and adolescents with uncomplicated PTSD, although a small number of children and adolescents may require longer-term treatment. The child/adolescent's response to therapy will determine the timing and pacing of sessions. As far as possible, an integrated approach should be adopted in the treatment of any comorbid conditions (e.g., major depression, substance abuse).

Eye Movement Desensitization and Reprocessing (EMDR)

EMDR is possibly an efficacious treatment in children and adolescents with PTSD (91), although the majority of studies to date have had serious methodological shortcomings. A group of 6- to 16-year-old children ($N = 33$) with a *DSM-IV* diagnosis of PTSD were randomly assigned to 8 weekly EMDR sessions or to a wait list group. Posttreatment scores of the EMDR group were significantly lower than the wait-list group, with improvement in reexperiencing symptoms the most significant between-group difference over time (Ahmad et al. 2007). Relative efficacy of CBT and EMDR was compared in a study in 12-13-year-old sexually abused girls who were randomly assigned to receive up to 12 sessions of either treatment. Both treatments produced significant improvement in PTSD symptoms and general behavior although EMDR produced faster improvements. However, interpretation of these findings are limited by the small sample ($N = 14$). Another non-CBT study compared individual brief psychoanalytic therapy with group therapy that included a psychoeducational component.(93) The authors reported substantial improvements in both treatment groups, although the individual brief psychoanalytic condition led to a greater improvement in PTSD symptoms. However, as the individual therapy condition consisted of 30 weeks while the group treatment received 18 sessions, results may be confounded by the difference in treatment dose.

Prevention of PTSD and Early Identification of At-Risk Youth

Although widely used, the preventive benefits of single-session psychological interventions (e.g., psychological debriefing) in adults are controversial. Psychological debriefing may interfere with the natural course of adjustment and recovery by sensitizing the child to trauma reminders without providing ample opportunity to process the experience and, in so doing, produce negative outcomes.(94) Current evidence does not support the role of single-session debriefing as a routine early intervention for children of any age. Stallard et al. (95) compared single-session debriefing with supportive talk in children aged 7 to 18 years involved in motor vehicle accidents. Interventions were initiated within 2 weeks of the accident occurring. Although children in both groups made significant improvements on measures of PTSD severity, depression, and anxiety at the 8-month follow-up assessment, it was unclear whether the improvements were better or worse than what might have been expected from natural recovery rates. In contrast, TF-CBT has been shown to be an effective early intervention 1 to 6 months posttrauma for symptomatic children, although its beneficial effects as a very early intervention in the first 4 weeks posttrauma has yet to be demonstrated.(96) Coupled with this is the issue of early screening. Empirically supported triage for psychological referral and intervention in acute trauma settings is consistent with current thinking about prevention practices. For example, the STEPP (Screening Tool for Early Predictors of PTSD) is a triage screening tool that was developed for use in acute care settings to alert clinicians to injured children and their parents who are at high risk of posttraumatic stress. Its brevity (4 dichotomous questions asked each of the child and parent and 4 readily available pieces of information from medical records), simple scoring rule, and excellent psychometric properties make it suitable for administration in acute care settings.(97, 98)

2. Pharmacotherapies

Currently, little is known about the effectiveness of pharmacotherapeutic agents in pediatric PTSD, and there are few controlled studies to make firm pharmacological treatment recommendations. The NICE guidelines state that drug treatments should not be routinely prescribed for children and adolescents with PTSD as "at present there is too little evidence from RCTs (randomized controlled trials), open-label studies or case-control studies to recommend the use of any psychotropic medication to treat PTSD in children and young adults".(99) Many experts would agree that there is a lack of data to support the use of medication alone, in the absence of psychotherapy. Early open trials in children and adolescents with PTSD have reported benefits with propranolol,(100) clonidine,(101) guanfacine,(102) carbamazepine,(103) tricyclics (e.g., imipramine), novel antipsychotics (e.g., risperidone, olanzapine), opiates (e.g., morphine; 104), and citalopram,(105) among others. In a prospective double-blind, pilot study of acute stress disorder (ASD), 25 children (aged 2 to 19 years) who had sustained serious burns were randomly assigned to imipramine or chloral hydrate treatment.(106) Imipramine was significantly more effective than chloral hydrate in treating ASD symptoms. Saxe et al. (104, 107) conducted a naturalistic study to investigate the relationship between the dose of morphine administered during a child's hospitalization for acute burns and the course of posttraumatic stress disorder (PTSD) symptoms over the 6-month period following discharge from the hospital. Children who received higher doses of morphine had a greater reduction in PTSD symptoms over 6 months. The authors conducted pathway analyses to test the potential mediating roles of pain reduction, noradrenergic attenuation, and separation anxiety on the association between morphine and PTSD. Their results suggested that a reduction in separation anxiety may mediate the association between morphine administration and PTSD symptom reduction at the 3-month follow-up.(107) The first controlled trial of divalproex sodium (an antikindling agent with potential usefulness in reducing aggression in PTSD) in conduct-disordered youth with PTSD provides preliminary evidence for its short-term efficacy in PTSD.(108) Twelve participants were randomized into either a high-dose (500–1,500 mg per day or therapeutic plasma levels for seizure control between 50–120 ng/ml) or low dose (up to 250 mg/day) condition. At the end of 8 weeks of treatment, patients in the high-dose condition had significantly greater improvement and fewer core PTSD symptoms.

Clinicians have tended to rely on clinical experience and extrapolation of data from adult populations to inform their choice of medications in this population.(109) Based on an earlier survey of child psychiatrists by Cohen et al.(110), 95% of psychiatrists said that they had used pharmacotherapy to treat childhood and adolescent PTSD. Medications most frequently used were selective serotonin reuptake inhibitors and α-adrenergic agonists. Selective serotonin reuptake inhibitors (SSRIs) were rated by respondents as being most effective for treating overall PTSD symptoms, including reexperiencing symptoms and avoidance numbing symptoms. Alpha-adrenergic agonists were rated as most effective for hyperarousal symptoms. Seedat et al. (105) compared improvement in 24 child and adolescent subjects to 14 adult subjects provided with 20–40 mg/day of citalopram in an open-label study and demonstrated equivalent improvements between the groups. A Turkish open trial of fluoxetine also showed effectiveness in improving PTSD symptoms (earthquake-related) among 26 participants aged 7 to 17 years.(111) One study assessed the potential benefits of adding an SSRI, sertraline, versus placebo, to TF-CBT in a double-blind design to 10-to-17-year-olds (N-24) who had PTSD secondary to sexual abuse.(112) Both groups experienced significant improvement, but there was little benefit to adding sertraline to TF-CBT.

Selective serotonin reuptake inhibitors have been shown to be effective for children and adolescents with other anxiety disorders (e.g., social phobia, generalized anxiety disorder, separation anxiety disorder; 113) and a review of nine randomized double-blind studies on the efficacy of pharmacotherapy for generalized anxiety disorder, separation anxiety disorder, and social phobia found strong evidence for the efficacy of SSRIs for the treatment of these anxiety disorders with standardized effect sizes varying between medium and large.(114) Children and adolescents with PTSD who also have comorbid mood and anxiety disorders are likely to benefit from an SSRI.

Recently the use of the SSRIs in children and adolescents has come under scrutiny owing to concerns about the increased risk of suicidal ideation and behavior in youth treated for depression.(115, 116) This led to a reanalysis of published and unpublished studies by the US Food and Drug Administration and the UK's Medicines and Healthcare products Regulatory Agency (MHRA). A systematic review by Hetrick et al. (116) concluded that "it is unclear what the effect of SSRIs is on suicide completion. While untreated depression is associated with the risk of completed suicide and impacts on functioning, it is unclear whether SSRIs modify this risk in a clinically meaningful way." However, other data suggest that the SSRIs (e.g., fluoxetine, paroxetine, sertraline, and citalopram) exhibit both safety and efficacy in pediatric depression, with no evidence for increased suicidality after commencement of treatment.(117) While concerns regarding the use of SSRIs in pediatric depression may not apply to the treatment of PTSD, it is prudent that children and adolescents with PTSD who are commenced on SSRIs be carefully monitored, particularly in the initiation phase of treatment.

CONCLUSIONS

Pediatric PTSD is a prevalent and disabling disorder that is characterized by complex and unique neurobiological and developmental alterations. Although findings with respect to the directions of these alterations have been mixed, studies that have examined early biological predictors of PTSD in children and adolescents have been relatively consistent. Accurate assessment of PTSD in this population, and early identification of those children at risk, is crucial in order to target interventions appropriately. Despite the lack of randomized controlled studies to inform pharmacological management, the field is now in a better position to discriminate the effectiveness of specific treatment approaches in this age group. At the same time, more rigorous and larger-scale psychosocial and pharmacological trials that examine both treatment predictors and mediating and moderating elements are needed. Finally, studies that evaluate whether psychoeducation, CBT, and pharmacological manipulations (e.g., propranolol) may be usefully implemented in children and adolescents at very early time points, following exposure to traumatic events, would be of great importance.

REFERENCES

1. American Academy of Child and Adolescent Psychiatry. Practice parameters for the assessment and treatment of children and adolescents with posttraumatic stress disorder. J Am Acad Child Adolesc Psychiatry 1998; 37(Suppl): 4S–26S.
2. Perry BD, Azad I. Posttraumatic stress disorders in children and adolescents. Curr Opin Pediatr 1999; 11(4): 310–6.
3. American Psychiatric Association. Diagnostic and Statistical Manual of Mental Disorders 4th ed. text revision. American Psychiatric Association: Washington, DC; 2000.
4. American Psychiatric Association. Diagnostic and Statistical Manual of Mental Disorders 3rd ed. American Psychiatric Association: Washington, DC; 1980.
5. McFarlane A. Posttraumatic phenomena in a longitudinal study of children following a natural disaster. J Am Acad Child Adolesc Psychiatry 1987; 26(5): 764–9.
6. Cuffe SP, Addy CL, Garrison CZ et al. Prevalence of PTSD in a community sample of older adolescents. J Am Acad Child Adolesc Psychiatry 1998; 37(2): 147–54.
7. Carrion VG, Weems CF, Ray R, Reiss AL. Toward an empirical definition of pediatric PTSD: the phenomenology of PTSD in youth. J Am Acad Child Adolesc Psychiatry 2002a; 41(2): 166–73.
8. Scheeringa M, Zeanah C, Myers L, Putnam F. Predictive validity in a prospective follow-up of PTSD in preschool children. J Am Acad Child Adolesc Psychiatry 2005; 44(9): 899–906.
9. Scheeringa MS. Developmental considerations for diagnosing PTSD and acute stress disorder in preschool and school-age children. Am J Psychiatry 2008; 165(10): 1237–9.
10. Meiser-Stedman R, Smith P, Glucksman E, Yule W, Dalgleish T. The posttraumatic stress disorder diagnosis in preschool- and elementary school-age children exposed to motor vehicle accidents. Am J Psychiatry 2008; 165(10): 1326–37.

11. Scheeringa MS, Peebles CD, Cook CA, Zeanah CH. Toward establishing procedural criterion and discriminant validity for PTSD in early childhood. J Am Acad Child Adolesc Psychiatry. 2004; 40(1): 52–60.

12. Lavigne JV, Gibbons RD, Christoffel KK et al. Prevalence rates and correlates of psychiatric disorders among preschool children. J Am Acad Child Adolesc Psychiatry 1996; 35(2): 204–14.

13. Reinherz HZ, Giaconia RM, Lefkowitz ES, Pakiz B, Frost AK. Prevalence of psychiatric disorders in a community population of older adolescents. J Am Acad Child Adolesc Psychiatry 1993; 32(2): 369–77.

14. Saigh PA, Green BL, Korol M. The history and prevalence of post-traumatic stress disorder with special reference to children and adolescents. J Sch Psychol 1996; 34(2): 107–31.

15. McNally RJ. Assessment of posttraumatic stress disorder in children and adolescents. J Sch Psychol 1996; 3(2): 133–45.

16. Fletcher K. Childhood posttraumatic stress disorder. In: Mash EJ, Barkley RA, eds. Child Psychopathology, 2nd edn. Guilford Press: New York, 2003; 330–71.

17. McLeer SV, Deblinger E, Atkins MS, Foa EB, Ralphe DL. Posttraumatic stress disorder in sexually abused children. J Am Acad Child Adolesc Psychiatry 1988; 27: 650–4.

18. Kiser LJ, Ackerman BJ, Brown E et al. Posttraumatic stress disorder in young children: a reaction to purported sexual abuse. J Am Acad Child Adolesc Psychiatry 1988; 27:645–9.

19. Schwarz ED, Kowalski JM. Posttraumatic stress disorder after a school shooting: effects of symptom threshold selection and diagnosis by DSM-III, DSM-III-R, or proposed DSM-IV. Am J Psychiatry 1991; 148: 592–7.

20. Terr LC. Chowchilla revisited: the effects of psychic trauma four years after a school bus kidnapping. Am J Psychiatry 1983; 140: 1543–50.

21. Arroyo W, Eth S. Children traumatized by Central American Warfare. In: Eth S, Pynoos RS, eds. Posttraumatic stress disorder in children. Washington, DC: American Psychiatric Association, 1985; 101–20.

22. Saigh PA. On the development of posttraumatic stress disorder pursuant to different modes of traumatization. Behav Res Ther 1991; 29: 213–6.

23. Handford HA, Mayes SD, Matterson RE et al. Child and parent reaction to the three mile island nuclear accident. J Am Acad Child Adolesc Psychiatry 1986; 25: 346–56.

24. Earls F, Smith E, Reich W, Jung KG. Investigating psychopathological consequences of a disaster in children: a pilot study incorporating a structured diagnostic interview. J Am Acad Child Adolesc Psychiatry 1988; 27: 90–95.

25. Shannon MP, Lonigan CJ, Finch Jr AJ, Taylor CM. Children exposed to disaster: I. Epidemiology of posttraumatic stress symptoms and symptom profiles. J Am Acad Child Adolesc Psychiatry 1994; 33: 80–93.

26. Lonigan CJ, Shannon MP, Taylor CM, Finch AJ, Sallee FR. Children exposed to disaster: risk factors for the development of posttraumatic symptomatology. J Am Acad Child Adolesc Psychiatry 1994; 33: 94–105.

27. Bryant RA. Early predictors of posttraumatic stress disorder. Biol Psychiatry 2003; 53(9): 789–95.

28. Kassam-Adams N, Winston FK. Predicting child PTSD: The relationship between acute stress disorder and PTSD in injured children. J Am Acad Child Adolesc Psychiatry 2004, 43: 403–11.

29. Meiser-Stedman R, Yule W, Smith P, Glucksman E, Dalgleish T. Acute stress disorder and posttraumatic stress disorder in children and adolescents involved in assaults or motor vehicle accidents. Am J Psychiatry 2005; 162: 1381–3.

30. Dalgleish T, Meiser-Stedman R, Kassam-Adams N et al. Predictive validity of acute stress disorder in children and adolescents. Br J Psychiatry 2008; 192(5): 392–3.

31. Bryant RA, Salmon K, Sinclair E, Davidson P. The relationship between acute stress disorder and posttraumatic stress disorder in injured children. J Trauma Stress 2007; 20(6): 1075–9.

32. Task Force on Research Diagnostic Criteria- Infancy and Preschool: Research diagnostic criteria for infants and preschool children: the process and empirical support. J Am Acad Child Adolesc Psychiatry 2003; 42: 1504–12.

33. Mylle J, Maes M. Partial posttraumatic stress disorder revisited. J Affect Disord 2004; 78(1): 37–48.

34. Horowitz K, McKay M, Marshall R. Community violence and urban families: experiences, effects, and directions for intervention. Am J Orthopsychiatry 2005; 75(3): 356–68.

35. Pine DS, Cohen JA. Trauma in children and adolescents: risk and treatment of psychiatric sequelae. Biol Psychiatry 2002; 51(7): 519–31.

36. Copeland WE, Keeler G, Angold A, Costello EJ. Traumatic events and posttraumatic stress in childhood. Arch Gen Psychiatry 2007; 64(5): 577–84.

37. Giaconia RM, Reinherz HZ, Silverman AB et al. Traumas and posttraumatic stress disorder in a community population of older adolescents. J Am Acad Child Adolesc Psychiatry 1995; 34(10): 1369–80.

38. Koenen KC, Moffitt TE, Caspi A et al. The developmental mental-disorder histories of adults with posttraumatic stress disorder: a prospective longitudinal birth cohort study. J Abnorm Psychol 2008; 117(2): 460–6.

39. Pervanidou P. Biology of post-traumatic stress disorder in childhood and adolescence. J Neuroendocrinol 2008; 20(5): 632–8.
40. Meewisse ML, Reitsma JB, de Vries GJ, Gersons BP, Olff M. Cortisol and post-traumatic stress disorder in adults: systematic review and meta-analysis. Br J Psychiatry 2007; 191: 387–92.
41. Sapolsky RM, Uno H, Rebert CS, Finch CE. Hippocampal damage associated with prolonged glucocorticoid exposure in primates. J Neurosci 1990; 10(9): 2897–902.
42. Gould E, Tanapat P. Stress and hippocampal neurogenesis. Biol Psychiatry 1999; 46(11): 1472–9.
43. De Bellis MD, Baum AS, Birmaher B et al. Developmental traumatology. Part I: Biological stress systems. Biol Psychiatry 1999a; 45(10): 1259–70.
44. Carrion VG, Weems CF, Ray RD et al. Diurnal salivary cortisol in pediatric posttraumatic stress disorder. Biol Psychiatry 2002b; 51(7): 575–82.
45. Carrion VG, Weems CF, Reiss AL. Stress predicts brain changes in children: a pilot longitudinal study on youth stress, posttraumatic stress disorder, and the hippocampus. Pediatrics 2007; 119(3): 509–16.
46. De Bellis MD, Keshavan MS, Clark DB et al. Developmental traumatology. Part II: Brain development. Biol Psychiatry 1999b; 45(10): 1271–84.
47. De Bellis MD, Keshavan MS, Shifflett II et al. Brain structures in pediatric maltreatment-related posttraumatic stress disorder: a sociodemographically matched study. Biol Psychiatry 2002; 52(11): 1066–78.
48. Carrion VG, Weems CF, Eliez S et al. Attenuation of frontal asymmetry in pediatric posttraumatic stress disorder. Biol Psychiatry 2001; 50(12): 943–51.
49. Delahanty DL, Nugent NR. Predicting PTSD prospectively based on prior trauma history and immediate biological responses. Ann N Y Acad Sci 2006; 1071: 27–40.
50. De Bellis MD, Kuchibhatla M. Cerebellar volumes in pediatric maltreatment-related posttraumatic stress disorder. Biol Psychiatry 2006; 60(7): 697–703.
51. Jackowski AP, Douglas-Palumberi H, Jackowski M et al. Corpus callosum in maltreated children with posttraumatic stress disorder: a diffusion tensor imaging study. Psychiatry Res 2008; 162(3): 256–61.
52. Pervanidou P, Kolaitis G, Charitaki S et al. The natural history of neuroendocrine changes in pediatric posttraumatic stress disorder (PTSD) after motor vehicle accidents: progressive divergence of noradrenaline and cortisol concentrations over time. Biol Psychiatry 2007; 62(10): 1095–102.
53. Young EA, Breslau N. Cortisol and catecholamines in posttraumatic stress disorder: an epidemiologic community study. Arch Gen Psychiatry 2004; 61(4): 394–401.
54. Yehuda R, Siever LJ, Teicher MH et al. Plasma norepinephrine and 3-methoxy-4-hydroxyphenylglycol concentrations and severity of depression in combat posttraumatic stress disorder and major depressive disorder. Biol Psychiatry 1998; 44(1): 56–63.
55. Connor KM, Zhang W. Recent advances in the understanding and treatment of anxiety disorders. Resilience: determinants, measurement, and treatment responsiveness. CNS Spectr 2006; 11(10 Suppl 12): 5–12.
56. Storr CL, Ialongo NS, Anthony JC, Breslau N. Childhood antecedents of exposure to traumatic events and posttraumatic stress disorder. Am J Psychiatry 2007; 164(1): 119–25.
57. Singer MI, Anglin TM, Song LY, Lunghofer L. Adolescents' exposure to violence and associated symptoms of psychological trauma. JAMA 1995; 273(6): 477–82.
58. Olff M, Langeland W, Draijer N, Gersons BP. Gender differences in posttraumatic stress disorder. Psychol Bull 2007; 133(2): 183–204.
59. Langeland W, Olff M. Psychobiology of posttraumatic stress disorder in pediatric injury patients: a review of the literature. Neurosci Biobehav Rev 2008; 32(1): 161–74.
60. Nugent NR, Christopher NC, Delahanty DL. Emergency medical service and in-hospital vital signs as predictors of subsequent PTSD symptom severity in pediatric injury patients. J Child Psychol Psychiatry 2006; 47(9): 919–26.
61. Yehuda R, Halligan SL, Bierer LM. Cortisol levels in adult offspring of Holocaust survivors: relation to PTSD symptom severity in the parent and child. Psychoneuroendocrinology 2002; 27(1–2): 171–80.
62. Yehuda R, Engel SM, Brand SR et al. Transgenerational effects of posttraumatic stress disorder in babies of mothers exposed to the World Trade Center attacks during pregnancy. J Clin Endocrinol Metab 2005; 90(7): 4115–8.
63. Nugent NR, Amstadter AB, Koenen KC. Genetics of post-traumatic stress disorder: informing clinical conceptualizations and promoting future research. Am J Med Genet C Semin Med Genet 2008; 148C(2): 127–32.
64. Koenen KC, Saxe G, Purcell S et al. Polymorphisms in FKBP5 are associated with peritraumatic dissociation in medically injured children. Mol Psychiatry 2005; 10(12): 1058–9.
65. Binder EB, Bradley RG, Liu W et al. Association of FKBP5 polymorphisms and childhood abuse with risk of posttraumatic stress disorder symptoms in adults. JAMA 2008; 299(11): 1291–305.
66. Segman RH, Shefi N, Goltser-Dubner T et al. Peripheral blood mononuclear cell gene expression profiles identify emergent post-traumatic stress disorder among trauma survivors. Mol Psychiatry 2005; 10(5): 500–13, 425. Erratum in: Mol Psychiatry 2005; 10(5): 514.

67. Hawkins SS, Radcliffe J. Current measures of PTSD for children and adolescents. J Pediatr Psychol 2006; 31(4): 420–30.

68. Meiser-Stedman R, Smith P, Glucksman E, Yule W, Dalgleish T. Parent and child agreement for acute stress disorder, post-traumatic stress disorder and other psychopathology in a prospective study of children and adolescents exposed to single-event trauma. J Abnorm Child Psychol 2007; 35(2): 191–201.

69. Scheeringa MS, Wright MJ, Hunt JP, Zeanah CH. Factors affecting the diagnosis and prediction of PTSD symptomatology in children and adolescents. Am J Psychiatry 2006; 163(4): 644–51.

70. Salmon K. Remembering and reporting by children: the influence of cues and props. Clin Psychol Rev 2001; 21(2): 267–300.

71. Weiss DS, Marmar CR. The impact of events scale-revised. In: Wilson JP, Keane T, eds. Assessing Psychological Trauma and PTSD. Guilford Press: New York; 1987.

72. Briere J. Trauma Symptom Checklist for Children (TSCC). Odessa, FL: Psychological Assessment Resources; 1996.

73. Foa EB, Riggs DS, Dancu DV, Rothbaum BO. Reliability and validity of a brief instrument for assessing post-traumatic stress disorder. J Trauma Stress 1993; 6: 459–73.

74. Pynoos RS, Frederick C, Nader K et al. Life threat and posttraumatic stress in school-age children. Arch Gen Psychiatry 1987; 44: 1057–63.

75. Newman E, Weathers FW, Nader K et al. Clinician-Administered PTSD Scale for Children and Adolescents (CAPS-CA). Los Angeles: Western Psychological Services; 2004.

76. King NJ, Tonge BJ, Mullen P et al. Treating sexually abused children with posttraumatic stress symptoms: a randomized clinical trial. J Am Acad Child Adolesc Psychiatry 2000; 39(11): 1347–55.

77. Reich W, Leacock N, Shanfield C. Diagnostic Interview for Children and Adolescents-Revised (DICA-R). St. Louis, MO: Washington University; 1994.

78. Armstrong JG, Putnam FW, Carlson EB, Libero DZ, Smith SR. Development and validation of a measure of adolescent dissociation: the adolescent dissociative experiences scale. J Nerv Ment Dis 1997; 185(8): 491–7.

79. Connor KM, Davidson JR. Development of a new resilience scale: the Connor-Davidson Resilience Scale (CD-RISC). Depress Anxiety 2003; 18: 76–82.

80. Ohan JL, Myers K, Collett BR. Ten-year review of rating scales. IV: scales assessing trauma and its effects. J Am Acad Child Adolesc Psychiatry 2002; 41(12): 1401–22.

81. Jørgensen IE, Seedat S. Factor structure of the Connor-Davidson resilience scale in South African adolescents. Int J Adolesc Med Health 2008; 20(1): 23–32.

82. Strand VC, Sarmiento TL, Pasquale LE. Assessment and screening tools for trauma in children and adolescents: a review. Trauma Violence Abuse 2005; 6(1): 55–78.

83. Cohen JA, Deblinger E, Mannarino AP, Steer RA. A multisite, randomized controlled trial for children with sexual abuse-related PTSD symptoms. J Am Acad Child Adolesc Psychiatry 2004; 43(4): 393–402.

84. Kaufman J, Birmaher B, Brent D et al. Schedule for affective disorder and schizophrenia for school-age children-present and lifetime version (K-SADS-PL): Initial reliability and validity data. J Am Acad Child Adolesc Psychiatry 1997; 36: 980–8.

85. Cohen JA, Mannarino AP, Knudsen K. Treating sexually abused children: 1 year follow-up of a randomized controlled trial. Child Abuse Negl 2005; 29(2): 135–45.

86. Kolko DJ. Individual cognitive behavioral treatment and family treatment and family therapy for physically abused children and their offending parents: A comparison of clinical outcomes. Child Maltreatment 1996; 1: 322–42.

87. Kataoka SH, Stein BD, Jaycox LH et al. A school-based mental health program for traumatized Latino immigrant children. J Am Acad Child Adolesc Psychiatry 2003; 42(3): 311–8.

88. Stein BD, Jaycox LH, Kataoka SH et al. A mental health intervention for school children exposed to violence: a randomized controlled trial. JAMA 2003; 290(5): 603–11.

89. Tol WA, Komproe IH, Susanty D et al. School-based mental health intervention for children affected by political violence in Indonesia: a cluster randomized trial. JAMA 2008; 300(6): 655–62.

90. Feather JS, Ronan KR. Trauma-focused cognitive-behavior therapy for abused children with posttraumatic stress disorder: a pilot study. NZ J Psychol 2006; 35: 132–45.

91. Silverman WK, Ortiz CD, Viswesvaran C et al. Evidence-based psychosocial treatments for children and adolescents exposed to traumatic events. J Clin Child Adolesc Psychol 2008; 37(1): 156–83.

92. Nikulina V, Hergenrother JM, Brown EJ et al. From efficacy to effectiveness: the trajectory of the treatment literature for children with PTSD. Expert Rev Neurother 2008; 8(8): 1233–46.

93. Trowell J, Kolvin I, Weeramanthri T et al. Psychotherapy for sexually abused girls: psychopathological outcome findings and patterns of change. Br J Psychiatry 2002; 180: 234–47.

94. Rose S, Bisson J, Wessely S. A systematic review of single-session psychological interventions ('debriefing') following trauma. Psychother Psychosom 2003; 72(4): 176–84.

95. Stallard P, Velleman R, Salter E et al. A randomised controlled trial to determine the effectiveness of an early psychological intervention with children involved in road traffic accidents. J Child Psychol Psychiatry 2006; 47(2): 127–34.

96. Cohen JA. Treating acute posttraumatic reactions in children and adolescents. Biol Psychiatry 2003; 53(9): 827–33.

97. Ward-Begnoche WL, Aitken ME, Liggin R et al. Emergency department screening for risk for post-traumatic stress disorder among injured children. Inj Prev 2006; 12(5): 323–6.

98. Winston FK, Kassam-Adams N, Garcia-España F, Ittenbach R, Cnaan A. Screening for risk of persistent posttraumatic stress in injured children and their parents. JAMA 2003; 290(5): 643–9.

99. NICE. National Institute for Clinical Excellence: Post-traumatic Stress Disorder. The management of PTSD in adults and children in primary and secondary care. Royal College of Psyhiatrists. Cromwell Press Limited, Trowbridge, Wiltshire, 2005.

100. Famularo R, Kinscherff R, Fenton T. Propranolol treatment for childhood posttraumatic stress disorder, acute type: a pilot study. Am J Dis Child 1988; 142(11): 1244–7.

101. Harmon RJ, Riggs PD. Clinical perspectives: clonidine for posttraumatic stress disorder in preschool children. J Am Acad Child Adolesc Psychiatry 1996; 35(9): 1247–9.

102. Horrigan JP, Barnhill LJ. Risperidone and PTSD in boys. J Neuropsychiatry Clin Neurosci 1999; 11: 126–7.

103. Looff D, Grimley P, Kuller F, Martin A, Shonfield L. Carbamzepine and PTSD. J Am Acad Child Adolesc Psychiatry 1995; 34(6): 703–4.

104. Saxe G, Stoddard F, Courtney D et al. Relationship between acute morphine and the course of PTSD in children with burns. J Am Acad Child Adolesc Psychiatry 2001; 40(10): 915–21.

105. Seedat S, Stein DJ, Ziervogel C et al. Comparison of response to selective serotonin reuptake inhibitor in children, adolescents, and adults with PTSD. J Child Adolesc Psychopharmacol 2002; 12(1): 37–46.

106. Robert R, Blakeney PE, Villarreal C, Rosenberg L, Meyer WJ 3rd. Imipramine treatment in pediatric burn patients with symptoms of acute stress disorder: a pilot study. J Am Acad Child Adolesc Psychiatry 1999; 38(7): 873–880.

107. Saxe G, Geary M, Bedard K et al. Separation anxiety as a mediator between acute morphine administration and PTSD symptoms in injured children. Ann N Y Acad Sci 2006; 1071: 41–5.

108. Steiner H, Saxena KS, Carrion V, et al. Divalproex sodium for the treatment of PTSD and conduct disordered youth: a pilot randomized controlled clinical trial. Child Psychiatry Hum Dev 2007; 38(3): 183–93.

109. Stein DJ, Ipser JC, Seedat S. Pharmacotherapy for post traumatic stress disorder (PTSD). Cochrane Database Syst Rev 2006; 1: CD002795.

110. Cohen J, Mannarino A, Rogal S. Treatment practices for childhood posttraumatic stress disorder. Child Abuse Negl 2001; 25: 123–35.

111. Yorbik O, Dikkatli S, Cansever A, Sohmen T. The efficacy of fluoxetine treatment in children and adolescents with posttraumatic stress disorder symptoms (Turkish). Klinik Psikofarmakoloji Bulteni 2001; 11: 251–6.

112. Cohen JA, Mannarino AP, Perel JM, Staron V. A pilot randomized trial of combined trauma-focused CBT and sertraline for childhood PTSD symptoms. J Am Acad Child Adolesc Psychiatry 2007; 46(7): 811–9.

113. Research Unit on Pediatric Psychopharmacology Anxiety Study Group. Fluvoxamine for the treatment of anxiety disorders in children and adolescents. N Engl J Med 2001; 344(17): 1279–85.

114. Dieleman GC, Ferdinand RF. Pharmacotherapy for social phobia, generalised anxiety disorder and separation anxiety disorder in children and adolescents: an overview. Tijdschr Psychiatr 2008; 50(1): 43–53.

115. Scahill L, Hamrin V, Pachler ME. The use of selective serotonin reuptake inhibitors in children and adolescents with major depression. J Child Adolesc Psychiatr Nurs 2005; 18(2): 86–9.

116. Hetrick S, Merry S, McKenzie J, Sindahl P, Proctor M. Selective serotonin reuptake inhibitors (SSRIs) for depressive disorders in children and adolescents. Cochrane Database Syst Rev 2007; 18(3): CD004851.

117. Sharp SC, Hellings JA. Efficacy and safety of selective serotonin reuptake inhibitors in the treatment of depression in children and adolescents: practitioner review. Clin Drug Investig 2006; 26(5): 247–55.

12 | Ethnocultural issues

Alexander McFarlane and Devon Hinton

There is an objective truth—which she might call historical fact as opposed to historical interpretation. And you have to reach for it . . . the most important thing any human being can do is to be as objective as possible about the past, that is the only thing on which a secure identity—individual or society—can be based. And linked to this is the feeling that doing it is a virtual impossibility. Because the moment you try, all the forces of delusion, self-aggrandizement, guilt, brain-washing by public perceptions, conspire to distort the past almost as soon as it has happened.

(Interview with Pat Barker, *The Guardian*, October 1998) (1)

INTRODUCTION

Posttraumatic stress disorder (PTSD) is a unique disorder because it conveys how the environment and the process of adjustment to severe traumatic stress can be extremely detrimental to an individual's adaptation. The process of interaction between internal and social resources brings into focus how individuals' experience and the meaning that they assign to an event play a critical role in psychological outcome. The attribution of meaning involves looking at the individuals' personal relationships in the context of society and culture. This embeddedness of experience implies that PTSD is not an illness implicit to the individual alone as it also involves an interaction with the sociocultural environment over time.(2) The belief that individuals can control their own destiny is only a relatively recent notion and is one of the dimensions in which cultural expectations define the impact of experience on psychological well-being. Religion and the prevailing cultural norms about restitution and dealing with grief are cultural domains where resources can mitigate the impact of trauma.(3)

This chapter will discuss these issues while accepting the importance of the role of neurobiology and the universality of the psychological stress response.(4) These form the stage on which ethnic and cultural factors are played out. Perhaps most important to this process is the dimension of intrusion and avoidance in the traumatic stress response.(5) These axes of reaction are manifest in both individuals' cognitive and affective domains and the way that society at large contains and relives trauma.(6) The critical aspect of this process is the subtle manner in which the past often comes to be played out in the future and moulds the shape and affect of current reactions and attitudes without the roots being recognized.

The role of culture is easy to lose in the world of objectivity and statistically based research with the current ascendancy of biological observations. The stated importance of an ethnocultural perspective can be dismissed as platitudinous in the world of reductionism because of few facts and many assertions. The contributions that it makes do not have the same focused objective dimensions as does research into changes in specific domains of neurotransmitter systems, for example. However, there is a great need to look at the relevance of more empirically based observations about trauma to the lives of traumatized people and the meaning they ascribe to their suffering.(7, 8)

DEFINITION OF CULTURE

Culture is a phenomenon that has several dimensions: It is the distinctive practices and beliefs as well as a development or improvement of the intellect or behavior due to education, training, or experience. The idea that it is a process that involves active development and change is implicit in the use of the word to describe the act of processing of cultivated land, animals, and so on.(9) The definitions of culture are as many and varied as cultures that exist. One of the primary characteristics of a culture is that it provides a context for survival. Rappaport (10) has described a complex set of relationships between quite divergent variables in a society comparing it to an ecosystem where the culture is defined as the system which is evolved to ensure the survival of the population in the context of the resources available. Thus, culture has a regulatory function that is experienced as an ideology by the population, whereas its contribution to survival is latent and unconscious among the members of the culture.(11)

Culture contributes divergent tensions, not the least of which comes from the human need for dependence; therefore, its loss becomes traumatic.(3) Individuals who are strongly identified with a culture and its values are protected and buffered by the support and sense of identity that it provides, particularly at times of trauma.(3) The power of culture lies in the fact that it is a protector, integrator, and security system.(12) This protection is at a cost because it limits individuality and freedom of expression and the loss leaves a deep sense of disorientation.

Culture provides a frame of belief that assists in dealing with illness and traumatic events as well as their causes. This function has a dimension that persists and does not disappear with treatment or the reconstruction of the damage after a disaster. Traumatic events do have predictable consequences that are unavoidable, although they can be minimized through preparation, training, and risk appraisal. Distress, loss, and sickness must, therefore, be managed and adapted to by both individuals and groups. Culture is the vehicle that embodies the values enriching these processes and the rituals contributing to healing.(13, 14) Suffering and illness are profound personal experiences as well as communications to the group.(3)

The traumatic stress field is one that is especially influenced by these forces. The nature of a traumatic experience is partly defined by cultural expectations about risk. Fatalistic cultures are accepting of the existence of traumatic events because they have external and unmodifiable risks and that these must be constantly faced. However, this belief system can undermine the potential for successful mitigation of risk, although it provides a useful set of beliefs and constructs for dealing with tragedy when it arises. The social system also provides valuable models for how to adapt once the trauma has arisen.(15) The models of intervention that we propose in the face of disaster, such as debriefing, are in part social movements that mobilize belief systems and support networks and give cultural permission to emote and seek help.(16) These belief systems help overcome the natural resistance to asking for help and the cultural tradition of not showing pain or distress. The advocacy for particular treatment approaches also comes from subcultural beliefs about the benefits and superiority of one treatment over another in the context of competing tribes of therapist. This internecine battle is often disguised with the language of science, which emphasizes the differences between approaches rather than the nonspecific aspects of treatment and the common origins of many competing approaches.

There are also often major cultural gulfs between clinicians and their patients. This divide is summarized in this quote about the inability of the welfare professionals to document and intervene in child abuse until recent times.

> In England, a different factor was at work during those years, and that a mind-set prevailed which allowed damage and abuse to go unrecognized. They were the years of scrupulous professional regard for what was thought of as "working class culture." In their numbing desire to be "non-judgemental," educated people in the welfare trade did not "talk down" to the economically disadvantaged nor teach them how to live their lives. So the dysfunctional became a model, and their expectations for their clients—of stability and routine in childcare, for example—were low. They had every bit of jargon at their fingertips, and liberal clichés bubbled on their lips; it was just in practical observation that they were deficient. (17)

Most discussion of culture and trauma focus on the comparison between different societies and the way that they adapt and create meaning in response to particular types of experience or the phenomenology of the stress response in culturally distinct groups. Victims' status itself creates a distinct cultural group and behavioral expectations. This latter dimension of the forces and influence of culture is possibly of most significance to clinicians.

THE CULTURAL DETERMINATION OF MEANING

The personal meaning of traumatic experience of the individual is influenced by the social context in which it occurs. Victims and the significant people in their surroundings may have different and fluctuating assessments both of the reality of what has happened and of the extent of their suffering.(18) As a result, victims and witnesses may have strongly conflicting agendas in the need for repair: heal, forget, or take revenge. At the individual level, this dynamic can be seen as one of the forces that is played out in the repressed memory debate, where the accused have used scientific argument to alienate and deny the traumatic reality of the victims. These conflicts between a trauma's meaning to victims and witnesses create an environment for the trauma to be perpetuated. When it comes to the conflict of nations, soon, not the trauma itself but the allocation of blame and responsibility may become the central issue.

Many personal testimonies of trauma survivors describe the absence of support by the people on whom they counted and being blamed for bringing horrendous experiences upon themselves, which left deeper scars than the actual traumatic events themselves.(19) Similarly, victims often feel ashamed and disgusted by their own failure to prevent what has happened. (14) Thus, for many victims a violation of their self and social ideals becomes part of the traumatic experience. This is also true for nations who have been beaten in war. This sense of self-betrayal is particularly acute if a nation was unprepared and did not anticipate the intentions or strength of their enemy. Members of that nation may find it difficult to respect those who fought or the leaders who played a part in the loss of national pride. The liberators and the resistance fighters can become powerful reminders of this shame.

Once the period of a trauma is over there can be a dramatic shift in attitudes. Ironically, both a victim of PTSD, and the larger society that may be expected to respond with compassion, forbearance, or financial sacrifices have a stake in believing that the trauma is not really the cause of the individual's suffering. Society becomes resentful about having its illusions of safety and predictability disturbed by people who remind them of how fragile security can be. One of the reasons for this failure of empathy is the gulf between the experience of the victim and their ability to express it in language that provokes empathy in those who do not know the experience.

THE CONFLICT BETWEEN THE INDIVIDUAL AND SOCIAL NEED

External validation of the reality of a traumatic experience in a safe and supportive context is a vital aspect of preventing and treating posttraumatic stress. However, the creation of such a context for recovery can become very complicated when the psychological needs of victims are in conflict with their social network.(20) When victims' helplessness persists, as in chronic PTSD, or when the meaning of the trauma is secret, forbidden, or unacceptable, such as occurs in intrafamilial abuse, or state violence, the trauma fails to elicit donation of resources, restitution, or metering out of justice. In the restoration of government at the end of a war, there may be a conflict between the resistance leadership and the established holders of power who went into the safety of exile. Validation of bravery of the resistance fighters may threaten a non-democratic government that was installed at liberation because this enhances their legitimate political profile. Lack of validation and support is likely to perpetuate the haunting traumatic memories that evoke a sense of victimization and social alienation.

One of the paradoxes about the predicament of survivors (whether they be soldiers or civilian victims) is that the larger social group often lacks any realistic understanding of their predicament. Primo Levi, who was an Italian chemist who survived the death camps of Nazi Germany, wrote passionately about the changed perception of the victims of this terrible incarceration. In the years immediately following the war he described how: "I encountered people who didn't want to know anything, because the Italians, too, had suffered, after all, even those who didn't go to the camps! They used to say, 'For heaven's sakes, it's all over,' and so I remained quiet for a long time."(21)

In 1955 Levi noted that it had become "indelicate" to speak of the camps—"One risks being accused of setting up as a victim, or of indecent exposure." Thus was confirmed the terrible, anticipatory dream of the victims, during and after the camps: that no one would listen, and if they listened they wouldn't believe. Once people did start to listen, and believe, the other obsession of the survivor began to eat away at Levi—the shame, and guilt, of survival itself, made worse in his case by the embarrassment of fame. Why should he, Levi, have survived? Had he made compromises that others had refused? Had others died in his place? His only resource to ward off the enemies of memory was words. But "the trade of clothing facts in words," he wrote, "is bound by its very nature to fail."

The importance of language, that we can communicate and we must communicate, that language is vital to humanity, and that the deprivation of language is the first step of destruction of a man, was enforced within the camp (words were replaced by blows—"that was how we knew we were no longer men"). (22)"

For the victims of individual and hidden traumas such as child abuse and domestic violence, the recurrence of the victimization and denial by the immediate social network is far more insidious and hence harder to identify.(23) Due to the social stigma attached to these forms of trauma, their occurrence is kept hidden, which means that there is very little chance of any realistic social awareness emerging. This was also the lot of the "comfort women" enslaved by the Japanese army.(24) The women's movement has been the voice for these concerns and has greatly contributed to the breaking down the social dismissal of sexual violence. This collective advocacy has challenged the minimization of the dark and silent world of familial abuse that shatters the advocated social ideals of modern conservative politicians.

Victims of trauma often become subjects of passionate concern from those around them, concern that may have no direct reflection on their actual well-being. Often voiceless about their innermost fears and becoming accustomed to passive acquiesce, victims of trauma are a means for a variety of political and social ends, both for good and ill; they can be nurtured or idealized, and just as easily spurned, stigmatized, and rejected. Between 1947 and 1982, Israeli society moved from the latter to the former position in regards to its attitude toward Holocaust survivors, without ever resting in the middle of the pendulum by treating them as fellow human beings who had been exposed to the unspeakable.(25) Bloom (26) has described how the field of traumatic stress emerged out of a political process advocating compassion for the Vietnam veterans. They were seen as the victims of government policy and the resultant terror of collective violence.

THE PROBLEM AND THE NATURE OF TRAUMATIC MEMORY

The most dramatic achievement of human culture is language. It has no innate or independent existence, yet it has driven an enormous amount of human evolution.(27) Language also defines and binds cultures. It is challenging to consider that before the existence of the gramophone, language could only be understood as a collective social memory. It is a phenomenon that can only exist between individuals. As the sophistication of societies increases it becomes the pervasive glue that creates the ties between groups and defines the boundaries that are more or less permeable between cultures.

The limitation of language becomes apparent when experiences occur so infrequently between individuals that there is no collective way of expressing the nature and consequences of that event.(28) By definition these experiences have the capacity to fall outside the world of the spoken culture. Hence, the expression of traumatic experience is a much more complex task than appears at first hand. War is the greatest collective human trauma and the need to write history and develop military tactics has necessitated its exploration. There is a variety of data that suggest there is an immense difficulty in constructing a true representation of war.

Janet (29) highlighted that another of the critical dimensions of traumatic experience is the difficulty of creating a representation of it in narrative memory. The event becomes trapped in the primary sensory memories rather than developing a transformed and more symbolic structure that has a linguistic base. Hence, the very nature of traumatic experience is its propensity to bypass linguistic representation.(30) Perhaps one way of conceptualizing this phenomenon is to consider that traumatic experiences are defined by their capacity to disrupt the use of language. Creative expression does not naturally emerge to convey these events. One of the most boring jobs for the officers in the world War II was censoring the letters of the men, who seemed to have enormous difficulty capturing the nature of terror and the chaos of combat.(31) Siegfried Sassoon reflected the social consequences of this problem, conveying their experience in his peace statement that was published in *The Times* and read out in the House of Commons (32).

> I have seen and endured the sufferings of the troops, and I can no longer be a party to prolong these sufferings for ends which I believe to be evil and unjust. I am not protesting against the conduct of the War, but against the political errors and insincerities for which the fighting men are being sacrificed. On behalf of those who are suffering now I make this protest against the deception which is being practised on them; also I believe that I may help to destroy the callous complacency with which the majority of those at home regard the continuance of agonies which they do not share, and which they have not sufficient imagination to realize. (p. 218) (33)

Grasping the nature of the trauma, therefore, requires a great deal of imagination and empathy if the truth is not to be avoided. The listener or interpreter has to compensate for the fact that most victims have impaired capacity to translate the intense emotions and perceptions related to the trauma into communicable language. Not being able to give a coherent account of the trauma to others, or even to oneself, without feeling traumatized all over again, makes it difficult for a culture to create representations of these experiences. The combination of the wish of the bystander not to be disturbed by the raw emotions of injured people and the problems of victims articulating what they feel and need makes it extremely difficult to stay focused on working through the impact of the trauma. Instead of clear-cut statements that convey the reality of what has happened, traumatic memories start leading a life of their own as disturbing symptoms.(33)

When the memories of the trauma remain unprocessed, traumatized individuals tend to become like Pavlov's dogs: subtle reminders become conditional stimuli to reexperience frightening feelings and perceptions belonging to the past. Hence social and cultural rituals that do not process the experience have the capacity to sustain the trauma and inflict pain by touching the wound that has not healed. This emphasizes that cultures should ideally provide some symbolic transformation of an experience. To facilitate social healing they should provide hope in the recall of horror. They must tell the story of suffering while not wounding the bereaved by adding the dread of their memories of the dead. They must encourage reconciliation rather than driving retribution and motivating a further cycle of violence by creating a universal image of suffering where no one is spared the agony of violence. The message is to heal but not through the romanticization of victors or the humiliation of those who were routed.

The awareness in a society of the memories that drive its values and the roots of its culture are critical to healthy identifications and preventing an acting out of old wounds in social prejudices and victimizations. Grossman (34) has highlighted how the increasing distance we have from birth and death in developed societies means that we have lost the experiences that teach respect for life and death. Increasingly, Western cultural ideas are subject to distortions through the media, which feasts on trauma and suffering, and the aggression depicted in the cinema and video games. This portrays a far more aggressive and ruthless world than reality demonstrates historically, as there have been tremendous prohibitions to killing even in war. The identification of youth with this Hollywood culture and its implicit messages may explain the spate of violent crime being committed by youth across the Western world. Previously, the importance of submission as a strategy and an understanding that much aggression was a threatening posture rather than a desire to kill was implicit cultural knowledge. The danger of living in a media-driven culture is that it both misrepresents long-standing inhibitions against violence and also destroys the cultural diversity that has been the core of the survival of social groups.

CROSS-CULTURAL STUDIES

There are a variety of case reports that have examined the trauma response in particular minority groups.(11) These reports often convey unique and stark cultural comparisons, but the perspective of the heightened sensitivity to difference in the outside observer is what drives these comparisons. When these perceived distinctions are subjected to scientific observation, what is striking is the relative lack of data suggesting cultural specificity in the trauma response, although the healing rituals vary greatly.(35) A sensitivity to this variance is an important issue for the development of humanitarian aid to Third World disasters and civil wars. The problems of ethnic conflict and the refugee crisis that often follows are going to be a growing international problem emphasizing the importance of this body of knowledge.(36) The other groups who have been of particular interest are refugees who have been resettled in new host countries (37) and victims of torture (4) and gross human rights violations.(38) A critical step in studying these populations has been the development of cross-cultural instruments such as the Harvard trauma questionnaire.(1)

The large epidemiological studies of Vietnam veterans provide a particular insight into outcome of minorities in response to one category of event. The National Vietnam Veterans' Readjustment Study (NVVRS) (39) used several minority sample groups and found that in contrast to the PTSD prevalence rate of 13.7% among Whites, Blacks had a rate of 20.6%, and Hispanics 27.6%. There was also a suggestion that when they became ill there was a greater degree of disability and social maladjustment. However, the increased rate of disorder in the Blacks was accounted for by an increased combat exposure. These were analogous findings to those of Laufer et al. (40) who similarly found greater impact of combat on Blacks. Similar observations were made about Maori soldiers in the New Zealand army who served in Vietnam where combat exposure level, rank, and combat role accounted for the greater morbidity.(41) These findings are not representative of the general population. In the National Comorbidity Study, Kessler et al. (42) found that Whites had the higher rates of traumatization and PTSD. The most important cultural finding in this study was that for the same trauma, women had double the rate of PTSD of men. The embeddedness of women in their culture and attachments is one explanation for this vulnerability.(3) Trauma involves the carrying of the pain of those around one, which is particularly costly if individuals have strong attachments.

Case studies have exemplified some dimensions of war having specific effects on minorities.(43, 44) For example, Asian Americans fighting in the Vietnam War were more closely identified with the Viet Cong, which created many points of confusion in separating the self from the victim.(45) This is the reverse of the phenomenon observed in Southeast Asian refugees in the United States (46, 47), where the lack of social integration was an important stressor. Studies of refugee populations that make prevalence estimates (7) are difficult to interpret because the representativeness of the sample is often hard to determine, but they do demonstrate the extreme traumatization of these people and the need for humanitarian concerns not to be lost within the walls of cultural and geographical isolation.(48)

Natural disasters created by far the greatest devastation in Third World countries (49) because of the lack of risk management and the poor quality of building materials and construction standards (97.5% of disaster victims are in developing countries, (50)). The 2005 Indian Ocean Tsunami and its devastation are a potent reminder of the capacity of these events for devastation. Yet these events have been given little attention in epidemiological research because of the imperatives of survival in these economies.(51) The prevalence studies that have been conducted are generally difficult to interpret because of the nonrepresentative samples studied (e.g., the 1989 Mexico earthquake (52); the Amero mudslide (50)). Some important exceptions exist, including the study of the Armenian earthquake and the Puerto Rico floods and mudslides that had been previously sampled in the Epidemiological Catchment Area (ECA) study.(53) There are also a series of more recent events that have been studied but few of the data have found their way into the Western literature. The Kobe earthquake in Japan that killed thousands of people has been extensively examined and demonstrated some of the methodological issues about underreporting symptoms due to the cultural tradition of *bushido* where there is great shame associated with inappropriate displays of emotion.(11) The Iraqi occupation of Kuwait has also been studied using a strict epidemiological approach and demonstrated the similarities of response in a Moslem and Western culture and that gender stereotyping seemed to have little impact.(54)

The similarities of the trauma response across cultures presents significant support for the integrity of PTSD as a distinct diagnosis. A study of Khmer adolescent refugees suggested that PTSD as a result of war trauma surmounted the barriers of culture and language.(55) Implicit in PTSD is the notion that relatively independent of the nature of the traumatic stressor, the context, and the culture, there is a similar phenomenology and epidemiology.(2) This observation supports the idea of trauma as a unifying concept in contrast to the imperative of focusing on individual groups of victims. What cross-cultural studies have identified is the impact of culture on the road to care and the nature of treatment that is acceptable to the patient. For example, treatment-seeking Iranian torture victims living in Germany had poorer knowledge of German.(56) A useful strategy is to work in collaboration with traditional healers who address the health beliefs of the victims.(57) It appears the racial origin does not influence the response to treatment in a Veterans Affairs system.(58) This is an example that should also be followed in the context of Western society, where there is often a significant divide between the health beliefs of the patient and the professional.(59) Studies of the mental health literacy of populations demonstrates major divergences in the beliefs within a culture about the effectiveness and appropriateness of different treatments.(60)

THE WAY CULTURE INFLUENCES THE PRESENTATION OF SYMPTOMS

Studies of refugee populations have highlighted the propensity to somatization of PTSD in non-Western groups.(61–63) The irony is that the majority of patients in First World settings also present with these concerns, but the doctor's apostolic role persuades the patient to avoid this method of complaint and focus on the cognitive and affective symptoms.(64) The history of trauma-related syndromes has focused on the role of somatization.(65) In the 1890s there was a major focus on the investigation of hysteria and its multiple manifestations. During World Wars I and II there were epidemics of conversion disorders, especially in battle situations where the soldiers were given little opportunity for the expression of their fear through action. The description of the phenomenology of these reactions did not unravel the importance of the expression of the trauma in the symptoms. Latterly, following the Vietnam War, there was the belief that the multiple ailments of the servicemen were due to their exposure to the herbicide Agent Orange.(66) Predictably, following the 1990 War against Iraq, the Gulf War syndrome rather than PTSD has emerged as the critical health issue where the somatic distress of the servicemen is the critical concern.

The other force at work in these situations is the role of compensation and the impact that litigation has on symptoms and their presentation. The suspicion of exaggeration and malingered distress is one of the cultural stigmas that haunt the trauma victim. There are two competing narratives in the legal arena that demonstrate how distress can be modified by the context and the listener. The counsel for the defense has little compunction in voicing suspicion and derision about the victim's complaints in contrast to the plaintiff's counsel who will subtly encourage and seek out real and imagined complaints. The impact of the culture of the law on the definition of the field and the public debate surrounding victims is a major social force. The critic Robert Hughes in the *Culture of Complaint* (67) discussed the issue that how society conceptualizes personal responsibility is dramatically influenced by the adversarial tradition. In its extremes, these tensions become manifest in the false memory debate and concerns about alien abduction and satanic ritual abuse. The multiple opinions that can be expressed about victims demonstrate the depth of divergence within a dominant culture

THE IMPACT OF TRAUMA ON CULTURE

The 20th century was marked by major international conflicts and unprecedented loss of life in war. World War I was a cataclysm that partly occurred because of the failure of military tactics to deal with the consequences of the new weapons and their destructive power. This conflict challenged conventional forms of expression and the abstract art movement was strongly influenced by a recognition that realism had failed to prepare people for what transpired.(68) The uncertainty and the emergence of new forms of disaster such as the atomic bomb, AIDS, and environmental degradation have left a pall of uncertainty and threat hanging over the world. (69) The world of art and philosophy has tried to grapple with this new reality of chance. In this way the threat of loss and the awareness of the brutality of the world have come to change art and culture in dramatic ways. Perhaps the most dramatic shifts occurred in the social dislocation and rebellion against authority at the time of the Vietnam War. Trauma is an abiding theme of the 20th century and has dominated our attempts to find cultural and political identity. Trauma is the constant concern of the media and, as a major social preoccupation, becomes a powerful organizing force. The need remains to develop a cultural narrative for traumatic situations that allows more effective organization to prevent the cycles of violence that we see being played out in places such as Yugoslavia. The misrepresentation of conflict and its consequences in romanticism and nationalism are major threats to peace and survival.

This indicates that the effect of trauma on culture is a bidirectional phenomenon. Just as culture provides a social vehicle for healing, cultures are changed and subcultures arise in an attempt to accommodate the effects of disasters, perceived social threats, and wars. Culture represents the need that people have for stories to heal suffering. Scientifically proved treatments are insufficient. There is a need for rituals to assist in healing. The rituals of bereavement and the narratives that are used to contend with death take on many different forms, all serve the same purpose—to integrate a person's experience into the stream of social adaptation.

Thus, there are a series of ways in which culture can assist in the understanding of suffering and the healing of these wounds.(11)

1. The comparison of different cultures can assist in understanding the nature of trauma and the ways of dealing with and resolving these traumas.
2. Studying groups who belong to minority cultures embedded in a larger social group can assist in understanding the impact of belonging to one culture while being embedded in a different host culture.(70)
3. The impact of a minority culture being overrun by an exogenous group can be a specific type of trauma in its own right that can disrupt the normal healing rituals of the minority culture and leave the entire group highly vulnerable to trauma.

To conclude this chapter, we would like to present some of the key questions that need to be addressed when trying to understand the presentation of trauma-related disorder in cross-cultural perspective and when attempting to develop culturally sensitive treatments:

TRAUMA-RELATED DISORDER IN CROSS-CULTURAL PERSPECTIVE: SOME KEY QUESTIONS

1. *Do traumatized members of other cultural groups meet the diagnostic criteria for posttraumatic stress disorder (PTSD) as specified in the most current version of the DSM-IV?*

It does seem that *DSM-IV*-defined PTSD symptoms occur in various cultural groups as a consequence of trauma, for example, among Cambodian refugees (7) and among Xhosa-speaking South African political detainees.(8)

2. *Across cultural groups, do the salience of DSM-IV-defined PTSD symptoms and symptom clusters (e.g., hyperarousal symptoms) vary?*

Increased salience of *DSM-IV*-defined PTSD symptoms may result from any or all of the following three causes: (a) the group's cultural interpretation of the symptom as being particularly dangerous or as being indicative of serious bodily, psychological, or spiritual problems; (b) the nature of the trauma, as in prolonged exposure to traumas and situations of stress leading to prominent hyperarousal; or (c) the fact that the group lacks institutionalized means, as in healing practices, to decrease those symptoms.

As an example, though two groups may initially have a similar severity of startle following a trauma, the two groups may have radically different interpretation of that symptom: Among Cambodian refugees, startle is considered to be an indicator of a "weak heart," (9) and generates multiple fears—worry that the "soul" may be displaced. Among trauma survivors in Mozambique, trauma-related dreams receive elaborate cultural explanation and lead to specific ritual action (10); likewise, among Cambodian survivors of the Pol Pot period, trauma-related nightmares are given elaborate interpretation, are considered an indicator of the physical and spiritual strength of the dreamer (11)—a bad dream results in feelings of vulnerability and increased anxiety and panic.

Studies have shown psychopathological dimensions to vary across cultural groups. For example, hyperarousal symptoms seem to be more prominent among elderly so-called Whites than among African Americans (12), and avoidance symptoms seem to be far less prominent among Kalahari Bushmen compared to previously studied groups.(13) The reasons for these differences have yet to be investigated.

3. *Are the rates of certain DSM-IV disorders, for instance, major depressive disorder or panic disorder, greater in certain traumatized groups?*

This would seem to be the case: Among Cambodian refugees (14), panic disorder is a very prominent aspect of the reaction to trauma. Their high rate of panic disorder appears to result from the severity of catastrophic cognitions about somatic and psychological symptoms, as well as prominent trauma associations to autonomic arousal.

4. *Across cultures, do the symptoms of non-PTSD disorders found in the DSM-IV have varying saliency among trauma victims, or do differences only emerge when more extensive lists are used that tap those constructs.*

For example, trauma victims in two different cultures may have the same rate and severity of major depressive disorder, but the frequency of the actual symptoms of major depressive disorder may vary, for example, there being more weight loss in one group and more negative affect in another. These differences may only emerge if symptom lists are used that separately assess symptoms clustered together for one criteria (e.g., insomnia and hypersomnia in the major depressive disorder criteria). Or differences may only emerge if symptoms characteristic of that construct, but not assessed in any of the criteria for that disorder, are assessed: tinnitus among patients with panic-disorder-type panic attacks.

5. *In other cultures, do certain symptoms and psychopathological dimensions not assessed in the DSM-IV attain greater salience in trauma victims?*

In various cultures, certain somatic symptoms seem to have more salience among persons with trauma-related disorder—for example, dizziness among Chinese populations (15), tinnitus among Cambodian refugees (16), gastrointestinal upset among Rwandan genocide survivors.(17) Or to give an example of nonsomatic symptom, the rate of sleep paralysis in trauma-related disorder appears to be very high among Cambodian refugees.(11)

Yet still, psychopathological dimensions not specifically addressed (or minimally addressed) in *DSM-IV* may be more prominent among trauma victims in certain cultural contexts, such as somatization, panic attacks, low self-esteem, low cultural-esteem, impaired psychological flexibility. To give another example, survival guilt is extremely salient among Rwandan genocide owing to cultural beliefs about the need to bury the dead in a set period of time according to traditional rites to assure the deceased's transformation into a benevolent ancestor.(18, 19)

6. *What is the local interpretation of trauma-caused symptoms? Are trauma-caused symptoms attributed to local cultural syndromes or spiritual causes? Do those cultural syndromes and spiritual explanations of trauma-caused symptoms shape the local experience of trauma-related disorder?*

One must investigate the local understanding of trauma-caused symptoms and psychopathological dimensions, that is, how those symptoms and psychopathological dimensions are thought to be generated in the culture in question. One must investigate local ways of talking about—and experiencing—trauma-related disorder. As a result of these cultural frames, a patient will interpret trauma symptoms in certain ways and will survey the body for evidence of having certain cultural syndromes after being traumatized, of having certain spiritual-based problems.

Among Mozambique war victims, trauma-related disorder is frequently expressed in terms of spirit possession.(20) In many cultures, certain somatic-type cultural syndromes are an important part of trauma-related disorder: Among Spanish-speaking populations of the Caribbean, *ataque de nervios* (21, 22); among Central Americans, a feeling of inner heat (23); and among civil war victims in Sierra Leone, a "hypertension" (haypatensi) syndrome.(24) Among Cambodian and Vietnamese refugees, weak heart is common way of understanding trauma-related symptoms. In these two cultures, weak heart is thought to cause a wide spectrum of symptoms: a feeling of energy depletion, startle, uncontrollable worry. Weak heart also causes fear of death from bodily dysfunction, especially cardiac arrest.(9, 25, 26) Among Cambodian refugees, various culturally specific panic attacks are prominent among trauma victims: orthostatic panic, "hit-by-the-wind" panic, neck-focused panic.(25–31) These panic attacks arise in large part due to local catastrophic cognitions and misconceptions about the body's physiology.

7. *Does the factor structure of symptoms resulting from trauma vary across cultures?*

In certain cultures, it may be that if you make an extensive list of symptoms—characteristic of PTSD, somatization, and other disorders—and then run a factor analysis, the clustering will radically vary across cultures. This clustering may result from the nature of the trauma and from the cultural interpretation of symptoms. For example, the Cambodian syndrome of weak heart will tend to cause panic symptoms, palpitations, and startle to be a prominent part of one factor. The structure of such factors will be clearer if the cultural syndrome, such as weak heart, are also listed.

8. *How do local cultural traditions aid in the recovery from trauma?*

Studies document that certain cultural institutions may play a key role in recovering from trauma: meditation among Cambodian refugees (32); ritual drumming in central Mozambique (10); sweat lodge rituals among certain American Indian groups (for a review, see (33)); and the transformation of iglata talk (drunken and boastful talk with peers) to waktoglaka talk (sober, sometimes tearful talk about war experiences in ceremonial settings) among Northern Plains Vietnam veterans, which is considered part of the process of "coming home."(34)

9. *How can state-of-the-art trauma treatments be adapted for patients in other cultural contexts?*

For a treatment to be culturally acceptable and effective for a particular cultural group, it should address prominent PTSD symptoms and dimensions (e.g., hyperarousal), comorbid *DSM-IV* conditions (e.g., panic disorder), psychopathological dimensions (e.g., low self-esteem), and symptoms (e.g., sleep paralysis). And the treatment should specifically address cultural syndromes prominent in trauma victims in that context, for example, *ataque de nervios* among Puerto Rican groups, "wind overload," neck-focused panic, and weak heart among Cambodian refugees. Those syndromes may involve various pyschopathological dimensions: depression, panic, anger. And for a treatment to be culturally acceptable and effective for a particular cultural group, it may be that healing traditions of the culture in question should be incorporated into treatment: Buddhist techniques for certain Asian populations.(32) Such treatments may not only promote acceptability and increase personal and cultural self-esteem but may also have important effects on specific dimensions of psychopathology.

CONCLUSION

In considering the effect of culture following traumatic events and describing its impact, there are a series of potential misinterpretations that can occur. Kleinman (35) uses the term *category fallacy* to refer to the mistake of assuming that our diagnostic categories will necessarily apply to other groups, for instance, that the *DSM-IV*-defined PTSD adequately depicts the response to traumatic events in other cultural groups. To avoid a category fallacy when studying trauma-related disorder in another context, one must consider the questions we outlined above.

We use the term *abstraction error* to describe the error of assuming that if the members of a cultural group are diagnosable as having PTSD then the relative prominence of *DSM-IV* symptoms and their meaning is the same. Finding that a group is diagnosable as having PTSD is just the beginning and not the end of the analysis.

We use the term *content error* to describe the mistake of assuming that the *DSM-IV* PTSD symptoms adequately describe the full spectrum of trauma-caused symptoms in a certain culture. To attain "content validity" (36) in the conceptualization of trauma-related disorder for a particular group, one needs to describe the full spectrum of trauma-related symptoms—and syndromes—for that group. For example, dizziness and the cultural syndrome of weak heart may be very prominent in certain cultural group and should be evaluated when assessing trauma-related disorder (and treatment outcomes) for that group.

We suggest the term *symptom fallacy* to refer to the mistake of assuming that the meanings associated with a certain symptom do not vary across groups, that the symptom meanings for a person from a particular social, economic, and cultural position will apply exactly to a person from a different social, economic, and cultural position. The identification of the presence of a trauma-related symptom, such as anger, is just the beginning of the analysis; in addition, one must identify the metaphors associated with the symptoms label (in the language in question), trauma associations, the local understanding of the symptom, associated ethnophysiology, and specific triggers (e.g., the acting-out behaviors of a gang-involved child).

REFERENCES

1. Barker P. 1998 (cited in Annan G). Ghosts, in New York Review; 1999.
2. Bronfenbrenner U, Ceci SJ. Nature-nurture reconceptualized in developmental perspective: a bioecological model. Psychol Rev 1994; 101(4): 568–86.

3. deVries. Trauma in cultural perspective, in traumatic stress: the effects of overwhelming experience on mind, body and society, van der Kolk BA, McFarlane, AC, Wesiaeth L, ed. Guilford: New York, 1996: 398–413.

4. Yehuda R, McFarlane AC. Conflict between current knowledge about posttraumatic stress disorder and its original conceptual basis. Am J Psychiatry 1995; 152(12): 1705–13.

5. American Psychiatric Association. Diagnostic and statistical manual of mental disorders. 4th ed. Washington DC; 1994.

6. Hinton DE, Chhean D, Pich V et al. Assessment of posttraumatic stress disorder in Cambodian refugees using the Clinician-Administered PTSD Scale: psychometric properties and symptom severity. J Trauma Stress 2006; 19(3): 405–9.

7. Wilson EO. Consilience: The Unity of Knowledge. Boston: Little, Brown; 1998.

8. Norris FH, Weisshaar DL, Conrad ML et al. A qualitative analysis of posttraumatic stress among Mexican victims of disaster. J Trauma Stress 2001; 14(4): 741–56.

9. Heinemann Australian Dictionary. 4th ed. Victoria: Heinemann Educational Australia; 1992.

10. Rappaport RA. Ritual ecology and systems. New Haven, CT: Yale University Press, 1984: 1–7.

11. Chemtob CM. Posttraumatic stress disorder, trauma and culture, in International Review of Psychiatry. Mak FL, Nadelson CC, ed. American Psychiatric Press: Washington DC, 1996; 257–92.

12. Brown GW, Prudo R. Psychiatric disorders in a rural and an urban population: Vol 1. Aetiology of depression. Psychol Med 1981; 11: 581–99.

13. McCall GJ, Resick PA. A pilot study of PTSD symptoms among Kalahari Bushmen. J Trauma Stress 2003; 16(5): 445–50.

14. Devon H, Phalnarith BA, Sonith P; Khin UM. Panic disorder among Cambodian refugees attending a psychiatric clinic. Prevalence and subtypes. Gen Hosp Psychiatry 2000; 22(6): 437–44.

15. Mainous AG 3rd, Smith DW, Acierno R, Geesey ME. Differences in posttraumatic stress disorder symptoms between elderly non-Hispanic Whites and African Americans. J Natl Med Assoc 2005; 97(4): 546–9.

16. Raphael B, Meldrum L, McFarlane, Alexander C. Does debriefing after psychological trauma work? Br Med J 1995; 310: 1479–80.

17. Mantel H. Killer Children. New York Rev Books, 1999: 4–5.

18. Winter J. Sites of Memory. Sites of Mourning. The Great War in European Cultural History. Cambridge: Cambridge University Press; 1995.

19. Lifton RJ. Home from the War. New York: Basic Books; 1973.

20. Guarnaccia PJ, Canino G, Rubio-Stipec M, Bravo M. The prevalence of ataques de nervios in the Puerto Rico disaster study. The role of culture in psychiatric epidemiology. J Nerv Ment Dis, 1993; 181(3): 157–65.

21. Caracciolo N ed. Uncertain refuge: Italy and the Jews during the holocaust. University of Illinois: Illinois; 1995.

22. Judt T. The courage of the elementary. New York Rev Books, 1999: 31–8.

23. Herman J. Trauma and recovery. New York: Basic Books; 1992.

24. Buruma I. The wages of guilt: Memories of war in Germany and Japan. New York: Meridian Press; 1995.

25. Solomon Z. From denial to recognition: attitudes toward Holocaust survivors from World War II to the present. J Trauma Stress 1995; 8(2): 215–28.

26. Bloom SL ed. Our hearts and our hopes are turned to peace: Origins of the International Society for Traumatic Stress Studies. International Handbook of Human Response to Trauma, ed. Shalev AY, Yehuda R, McFarlane AC. Kluwer/Plenum: New York, 2000; 27–50.

27. Deacon TW. The Symbolic Species. The Co-evolution of Language and the Brain. New York: WW Norton; 1997.

28. American Psychiatric Association. Diagnostic and Statistical Manual of Mental Disorders. 3rd ed. Washington, DC: American Psychiatric Association; 1980.

29. Janet P. Les Medications Psychologiques. Paris: Felix Alcan; 1919.

30. Van Der Kolk BA, Burbridge JA, Suzuki J. The psychobiology of traumatic memory. Clinical implications of neuroimaging studies. Ann N Y Acad Sci 1997; 821: 99–113.

31. Fussell P. The Great War and Modern Memory. London: Oxford University Press; 1975.

32. Sassoon S. Memoirs of an Infantry Officer. London: Faber and Faber; 1930.

33. Langer LL. Holocaust Testimonies: The Ruins of Memory. New Haven CT: Yale University Press; 1991.

34. Grossman D. On Killing: the psychological cost of learning to kill in war and society. Boston: Little, Brown; 1997.

35. Frueh BC, Brady KL, de Arellano MA. Racial differences in combat-related PTSD: empirical findings and conceptual issues. Clin Psychol Rev 1998; 18(3): 287–305.

36. de Girolamo G McFarlane AC, ed. Epidemiology of victims of international violence: a review of the literature. Int Rev Psychiatry, ed. Mak FL, Nadelson CC. American Psychiatric Press: Washington DC, 1996; 2: 93–119.

37. Hinton DE, Pich V, Chhean D, Pollack MH. 'The ghost pushes you down': sleep paralysis-type panic attacks in a Khmer refugee population. Transcult Psychiatry 2005; 42(1): 46–77.
38. Silove D ed. Torture and refugee trauma; implications for nosology and treatment of posttraumatic syndromes. International Review of Psychiatry, ed. Mak FL, Nadelson CC. American Psychiatric Press: Washington DC, 1996; 211–32.
39. Kulka RA, Schlenger WE, Fairbank JA et al. Trauma and the Vietnam War Generation: Report of Findings from the National Vietnam Veterans Readjustment Study. New York: Brunner/Mazel; 1990.
40. Laufer KS, Yager T, Frey-Wouters E et al. Comparative Adjustments of Veterans and their Peers, Vol 3. Post-war Trauma: Social and Psychological Problems of Vietnam Veterans in the Aftermath of the Vietnam War. New York: Center for Policy Research; 1981.
41. MacDonald C, Chamberlain K, Long N. Race, combat, and PTSD in a community sample of New Zealand Vietnam War veterans. J Trauma Stress 1997; 10(1): 117–24.
42. Kessler RC, Sonnega A, Bromet E, Hughes M, Nelson CB. Posttraumatic stress disorder in the National Comorbidity Survey. Arch Gen Psychiatry 1995; 52(12): 1048–60.
43. Loo LM. An integrative-sequential treatment model for posttraumatic stress disorder: a case study of the Japanese-American internment and redress. Clin Psychol Rev 1993; 13: 89–117.
44. Hamada, R, Chemtob CM, Sautner R, Sato R. Ethnic identity and Vietnam: a Japanese-American Vietnam veteran with PTSD. Hawaii Med J 1988; 47(3): 100–2, 105–6, 109.
45. Loo CM, Karam S, Ray S, Bill K. Race-related stress among Asian American veterans: a model to enhance diagnosis and treatment. Cult Divers Ment Health 1998; 4(2): 75–90.
46. Kinzie JD, Boehnlein JK, Leung PK et al. The prevalence of posttraumatic stress disorder and its clinical significance among Southeast Asian refugees. Am J Psychiatry 1990; 147(7): 913–7.
47. Mattson S. Mental health of southeast Asian refugee women: an overview. Health Care Women Int 1993; 14: 155–65.
48. Kagee A. Do South African former detainees experience post-traumatic stress? Circumventing the demand characteristics of psychological assessment. Transcult Psychiatry 2004; 41(3): 323–36.
49. Green BL ed. Cross-national and ethnocultural issues in disaster research. Ethnocultural aspects of posttraumatic stress disorder: issues, research and clinical applications, ed. Marsella AJ, Friedman MJ, Gerrity ET, Scurfield RM. American Psychological Applications: Washington DC, 1996: 341–61.
50. Lima BR, Pai S, Santacruz H. Psychiatric disorders in primary health care clinics one year after a major Latin American disaster. Stress Medicine 1991; 7: 25–32.
51. Igreja V. 'Why are there so many drums playing until dawn?' Exploring the role of Gamba spirits and healers in the post-war recovery period in Gorongosa, Central Mozambique. Transcult Psychiatry 2003; 40(4): 459–87.
52. de la Puente R. The mental health consequences of the 1985 earthquakes in Mexico. Int J Ment Health 1990; 19: 21–9.
53. Soloman SD, Canino GJ. Appropriateness of DSM-III-R criteria for posttraumatic stress disorder. Compr Psych 1990; 31: 227–37.
54. McFarlane AC, van der Kolk BA. The long-term effect of psychological trauma: a public health issue in Kuwait. Med Principles Pract 1996; 5: 59–75.
55. Sack WH, Seeley JR, Clarke GN. Does PTSD transcend cultural barriers? A study from the Khmer Adolescent Refugee Project. J Am Acad Child Adolesc Psychiatry 1997; 36(1): 49–54.
56. Priebe S, Esmaili S. Long-term mental sequelae of torture in Iran--who seeks treatment? J Nerv Ment Dis 1997; 185(2): 74–7.
57. Scurfield RM. Healing the warrior: admission of two American Indian war-veteran cohort groups to a specialized inpatient PTSD unit. Am Indian Alsk Native Ment Health Res 1995; 6(3): 1–22.
58. Rosenheck R, Fontana A. Race and outcome of treatment for veterans suffering from PTSD. J Trauma Stress 1996; 9(2): 343–51.
59. Schreiber S. Migration, traumatic bereavement and transcultural aspects of psychological healing: loss and grief of a refugee woman from Begameder country in Ethiopia. Br J Med Psychol 1995; 68: 135–42.
60. Jorm AF, Korten AE, Jacomb PA et al. "Mental health literacy": a survey of the public's ability to recognise mental disorders and their beliefs about the effectiveness of treatment. Med J Aust 1997; 166(4): 182–6.
61. Cheung P. Somatisation as a presentation in depression and post-traumatic stress disorder among Cambodian refugees. Aust N Z J Psychiatry 1993; 27(3): 422–8.
62. Kirmayer LJ. ed. Confusion of the senses: implications of ethnocultural variations in somatoform and dissociative disorders for PTSD. Ethnocultural aspects of posttraumatic stress disorder: issues, research and clinical applications ed. Marsella AJ, Friedman MJ, Gerrity ET, Scurfield RM. American Psychological Association: Washington DC, 1996; 131–63.
63. Uwanyiligira E. La Souffrance Psychologique des Survivants des Massacres au Rwanda: Approches Therapeutique. Nouvelle Revue d'Ethnopsychiatrie, 1997; 34: 87–104.
64. Balint M. The Doctor, his Patient and the Illness. London: Pitman; 1957.

65. Showalter E. Hysterical Epidemics and Modern Culture. London: Picador; 1997.

66. Hall W. The Agent Orange controversy after the Evatt Royal Commission. Med J Aust 1986; 145(5): 219–25.

67. Hughes R. Culture of Complaint: The Fraying of America. New York: Oxford University Press; 1993.

68. Conrad P. Modern Times: Modern Places. Life and Art in the 20th Century. London: Thames and Hudson; 1998.

69. Bagilishya D. Mourning and Recovery from Trauma; in Rwanda, Tears Flow Within. Transcult Psychiatry 2000; 37: 337–53.

70. Hinton DE, Chhean D, Pich V, Hofmann SG, Barlow DH. Tinnitus among Cambodian refugees: relationship to PTSD severity. J Trauma Stress 2006; 19(4): 541–6.

13 | Posttraumatic stress disorder after disasters

Andrea R Maxwell and Sandro Galea

INTRODUCTION

In a national study of the U.S. population, 15% of women and 19% of men reported exposure to a natural disaster during their lifetime.(1) Although a range of psychopathologies can occur after these events (2, 3), posttraumatic stress disorder (PTSD) is the most commonly studied and likely the sentinel psychopathology after exposure to a disaster.(3–6) In this chapter we present (a) an overview of the current evidence in the field regarding PTSD and disasters, (b) the challenges of postdisaster research with consideration of how these may influence our understanding of the consequences of disasters, and (c) future research directions to strengthen the field of PTSD and disasters. Before we embark on the chapter, we note two limitations. First, we do not intend this chapter to be a comprehensive review of all current evidence in the field of PTSD and disasters; instead, we provide a summary of some of this evidence, largely drawing from previous reviews in the field.(3–6). Second, substantial debate exists in the peer-reviewed literature as to what constitutes a disaster. We refer the reader to other work that has considered this question in greater detail.(7) In the context of this chapter, we consider disasters to be unexpected and acute events that can be human made, technological, or natural.(3, 7)

SUMMARY OF EVIDENCE REGARDING PTSD AFTER DISASTERS

We first consider the prevalence of PTSD after disasters among specific groups that are largely defined by their type and intensity of exposure: survivors, rescue workers, the general population, and children. This is followed by evidence from the literature regarding various sociodemographic covariates of PTSD after disasters—gender, social support, age, socioeconomic status, and race or ethnicity. We also note—reflecting the predominant analytic mode of most disaster literature—that we use the term *prevalence* rather than incidence to document the burden of PTSD after disasters because very few studies have ensured predisaster PTSD was absent in their participants. This convention is consistent with previous reviews in the literature.(4, 5)

Studies of human-made and technological disasters

In general, a high prevalence of PTSD has been documented among survivors of human-made or technological disasters, ranging from approximately 20% to 75%.(4, 5) For example, a study of the 1993 religious uprisings in Sivas, Turkey, found that the prevalence of PTSD 1 month postdisaster was 20.3% among survivors.(8) At the other extreme, by retrospectively assessing survivors of the 1998 Piper Alpha oil rig disaster 10 years postdisaster, Hull and colleagues showed that the prevalence of PTSD was 73% among survivors 3 months postdisaster.(9) Another study that assessed PTSD around 6 months after the 1995 Oklahoma City bombing found that 34.3% of survivors had PTSD (10); a similar burden of PTSD was found 1 month after the 1991 mass shooting in Killeen, Texas (11), 6 months after the 1992 Biljermeer plane crash (12), and 13 months after the 1998 Lockerbie plane crash.(13)

A substantial burden of PTSD has also been found among rescue workers after disasters. For instance, a substantial proportion of police officers were found to exhibit PTSD symptoms 1 to 2 years after the 1989 Hillsborough football stadium disaster in Sheffield, UK—44.3% exhibited severe symptoms, while an additional 41.4% exhibited moderate symptoms.(14) Studies of rescue workers after the September 11 terrorist attacks in New York City found that the prevalence of PTSD ranged from 22.5% at 2 weeks (15) to 20% 10 to 15 months after exposure.(16) After the 1989 USS *Iowa* gun turret explosion, 11% of volunteer disaster workers suffered from PTSD 1 month postdisaster.(17) Potentially complicating cross-study comparability of these results, the percent of rescue workers with PTSD may differ depending on the type of work performed. A study that assessed the prevalence of PTSD among rescue workers 2 to 3 years after the September 11 terrorists attacks in New York City found that the overall prevalence of PTSD was 12.4% but that of unaffiliated volunteers and construction/engineer workers was especially high—21.2% and 17.8%, respectively.(18)

Studies that have assessed the psychological burden of disasters among the general population have generally found, not surprisingly, a lower prevalence of PTSD than that of survivors or rescue workers.(4) After the Los Angeles civil disturbances, Hanson and colleagues estimated that the prevalence of PTSD 6 to 8 months after these disturbances was 4.1% in the general population.(19) Subsequent work of general populations collected within 12 months of disasters such as the September 11 terrorist attacks in New York City (20–22), the 1989 *Exxon Valdez* oil spill (23), and the 2004 train bombings in Madrid (24), found a similar burden of PTSD in relevant areas.

Because only a small number of studies have evaluated the prevalence of PTSD among children, few conclusions can be drawn as to the effect of disasters on them. After the 2001 chemical factory explosion in Toulouse, France, Godeau and colleagues found that 44.6% of directly exposed children aged 11 to 13 years and 28.5% of directly exposed children aged 15 to 17 years had symptoms consistent with PTSD.(25) In addition, the prevalence of PTSD among children was documented to be 38.4% 1 month after the 1984 school sniper attack in Los Angeles (26); 27% 3 months after the 1993 World Trace Center Bombing (27); 11.9% 9 months after the 1991 industrial fire in Hamlet, North Carolina, (28); and 18.4% 6 months after the September 11 attacks in New York City.(29) For a comprehensive review of the literature surrounding children and human-made disasters, see a review by Pfefferbuam and colleagues (30).

Although a wide range of correlates of PTSD after disasters have been examined, some factors have been studied repeatedly in the literature and merit brief comment. First, it is clear from the body of postdisaster research that the single central predictor of PTSD after disasters is the degree of exposure to the event.(2) As noted in our above summary of prevalences, the groups with the greatest direct exposure to disasters are also those that have a greater likelihood of developing PTSD. Similarly, within each exposure group, those with the most disaster-related traumatic events are the persons who have the greatest risk of developing PTSD. In terms of sociodemographic correlates, female gender has consistently been shown to be a risk factor for postdisaster PTSD.(23, 28, 31–34) In fact, most studies suggest that women have a nearly a twofold greater risk than men of PTSD, given comparable disaster-related exposure.(4) Some studies have also shown that social support is protective after disasters.(35, 36) In contrast, the evidence as to the effect of age (37–39), socioeconomic differences, such as the level of education (40–42), and race or ethnicity (20, 28, 43, 44) on the prevalence of PTSD after disasters has been inconsistent.

Studies of natural disasters

Many of the observations that can be drawn from natural disasters are similar to those drawn from technological and human-made disasters. For example, the prevalence of PTSD among highly exposed survivors was 24% 3 months after a 2000 Icelandic earthquake (45), 18.3% 6 months after the 1989 Newcastle earthquake (46), and 23% 14 months after the 1999 earthquake in Turkey.(47) After the 1988 Armenian earthquakes, a much higher prevalence (92%) was found among a nonrepresentative sample of survivors 2.5 years after exposure.(48)

Few studies have evaluated PTSD among rescue workers postdisaster, but in general, those conducted have documented a high prevalence. For example, 7 to 13 weeks after the Hurricane Katrina in 2005, 22% of firefighters and 19% of police officers in New Orleans met PTSD diagnostic criterion. (49) A comparable prevalence of PTSD was found among rescue workers both after the 2003 Bingol, Turkey earthquake—23% 2 months postdisaster (50) and after the 1999 Taiwan earthquake—21.4% 5 months postdisaster.(51)

Among the general population, the prevalence is largely lower than that of survivors or rescue workers. After the 2003 bushfires in Australia, 5% of young adults met criterion for PTSD 5 to 18 months postdisaster (52); correspondingly, 3.7% of a community affected by the 1985 Puerto Rican floods suffered from PTSD 2 years postdisaster.(53) In a community 100 km away from the epicenter of the 1999 Turkey earthquake, the prevalence of PTSD was 14% 14 months postdisaster (47); a similar prevalence was found in affected communities 6 months after the 1999 Mexican floods (54) and 2 months after the 2004 tsunami in Asia.(55)

A number of studies have assessed the impact of natural disasters on children and have largely showed a substantial burden of PTSD among this population. Six months after Hurricane Mitch in 1998, the prevalence of PTSD among adolescents ranged from 14% to 90%, dependent on the dose of exposure (56); another study found that the prevalence of PTSD ranged from 26% to 95% in different communities 1.5 years after the 1988 earthquake in Armenia, with the prevalence again dependent on the level of exposure.(57) In addition, 56% of school-aged children had moderate to very severe symptoms of PTSD 3 months after Hurricane Andrew in 1992 (58), results that were comparable to a study conducted 6 months after Hurricane Floyd.(59)

Analogous to the evidence for technological and human-made disasters, women are more likely than men to suffer from PTSD after disasters.(46, 60–63) Low social support may also contribute to greater PTSD symptomatology.(64–66) However, the evidence regarding age (63, 67), socioeconomic status (67–69), and race or ethnicity (61, 70, 71) remains inconclusive.

METHODOLOGICAL CHALLENGES OF POSTDISASTER RESEARCH

The challenges of postdisaster research are many and greatly influence our understanding of the mental health consequences of disasters. In examining some of these challenges, we start with a discussion of how the aftermath of a disaster affects development of the research plan and researchers themselves. We then turn our attention to issues surrounding sampling of the affected community, defining and finding the population of interest and garnering participation. This is followed by a consideration of how exposure and PTSD are characterized in individual studies and the effect of these characterizations on cross-study comparability. We end with a discussion of the difficulties inherent in measuring and analyzing covariates and health indicators.

Research plans and researchers

By their nature, disasters are largely unanticipated and disruptive. The aftermath of a disaster can be chaotic, with concurrent interruption of infrastructure ranging from telephone service to hospitals. These are hardly optimal conditions under which to initiate a research study. Research is typically long planned, completed under highly controlled circumstances, and supported by a wide spectrum of resources—all characteristics that may not be possible in a postdisaster setting. The effect of disasters on researchers themselves can also be complex. Oftentimes researchers may effectively function as the first wave of responders in postdisaster circumstances—an unfamiliar position for many that leads to complications. For example, anecdotal evidence in the field suggests that researchers—especially mental health clinicians—may identify with research participants affected by the disaster (57, 72), potentially limiting their objectivity and compromising their research.

Sampling the affected community

The difficulty of launching a research plan after a disaster has led to a preponderance of convenience sampling in the field.(3, 6) In cases where no other sampling method was feasible, convenience samples have contributed to the field and illuminated areas for further research. (18, 73) Overall, though, the conclusions that can be drawn from such studies are limited. In addition, the challenge of procuring a representative sample in postdisaster circumstances has greatly limited cross-study comparability in the field.(4) Here we discuss three aspects of recruiting a representative sample: defining the population of interest, finding this population, and acquiring participants.

In the process of defining a population for study, not only must the level and type of exposure—the "affected"—be delineated but also what constitutes the "who." For example, many studies have considered how disaster circumstances affect rescue workers, but who is included in this definition? Many studies have exclusively focused on police workers and firefighters, but Perrin and colleagues recently showed that unaffiliated volunteers, construction workers, and engineers were affected more than their traditional counterparts.(18)

Finding a population can also be difficult in postdisaster circumstances, as persons may be displaced and/or mobile after a disaster. A study that assessed the mental health of the affected population after Hurricane Katrina had difficulties tracking participants due to their mobility.(74) In addition, after Hurricane Katrina, many undocumented migrant workers left the area; as a result, studies that assessed the mental health burden after this event likely under-counted these persons.(75)

Even after a population is defined and found, the difficulties in enrolling participants can be considerable. Persons affected by the disaster may be hesitant to enroll in research not related to service utilization; in some communities this may be compounded by a mistrust of the medical and research field.(76) However, research has shown that those who do participate make favorable cost–benefits appraisals of their participation (77), and the majority are not adversely affected by research participation.(78, 79) Language and cultural barriers may also limit the ability of researchers to reach a community. For example, after the Marmara earthquake in Turkey, the refusal rate of potential female participants was higher when the interviewees were male as opposed to female.(47) All of these factors may limit the ability of researchers to adequately sample a population and elicit the relevant information from these communities.

Characterization of exposure and PTSD

Due to the heterogeneous nature of disasters, the resulting exposure after a particular disaster is likely unique. Assuming that the nature of exposure is related to broad categories of disasters such as "natural disasters" may even be problematic, as one natural disaster may differ greatly from another. Instead, specific dimensions such as duration and intensity may be more relevant for characterization of the exposure. For example, a disaster that unfolds slowly over time such as the Chernobyl disaster (80) may be characterized by prolonged exposure, while the exposure after a mass shooting—a "point" event—may be characterized as acute.(81) Because of the unique nature of exposure, drawing generalizations across studies in the literature must be performed carefully with consideration of these limitations.

The changing definitions of PTSD over the years may also affect the ability to compare results among studies in the field of PTSD and disasters. As is documented elsewhere in this book, the definition of PTSD has changed since its introduction under the auspices of *DSM-III* in 1980.(82) Meaningful differences have been introduced in the revised edition of the *DSM-III* (DSM-III-R) published in 1987 (83) and in the *DSM-IV* criterion, introduced in 1994.(84) While this changing definition of PTSD is a challenge to all PTSD research, it is particularly important in the context of disaster-related research where only a handful of studies may be conducted after any given disaster. This results in comparisons across *DSM* eras being near inevitable in the field for the purposes of drawing generalizable inference.

Covariate assessment

The challenges associated with assessing covariates that may influence the central associations of interest are not unique to postdisaster research but are greatly heightened by the scarcity of research after any particular disaster. The covariates assessed frequently differ from study to study, limiting the ability to determine the covariates most important for predicting psychopathology and to compare studies both within disasters and across disasters. Certain covariates like gender are regularly measured by postdisaster studies (68, 85), but others like perievent emotional reactions are not.(86) Effects of additional covariates such as socioeconomic status, social support, racial identity, and other demographical characteristics remain to be illuminated. In addition, studies frequently use different models to assess the relationship between covariates and psychopathology; because of this, their association is often obscured.(4, 5, 87) For example, Weismann and colleagues found that it was not gender itself but rather the underlying social and economic circumstances that explained the relationship between gender and PTSD observed in most studies.(88) Clearly, much more work needs to be carried out to aid our understanding of correlates for PTSD. In nondisaster research, the abundance of studies often overcomes these limitations, but studies of disasters are limited in number, accentuating these difficulties.

Assessing incident disorders

One of the central difficulties in assessing psychopathology after disasters is demonstrating that the case is a "new"—or incident—case. Due to the unpredictability of disasters, predisaster measures of mental disorders such as PTSD are rarely available. Some exceptions exist (89, 90), but these are largely where preexisting studies were in place. For a case to be potentially caused by a disaster, its onset must occur after the event; unfortunately, most disaster studies have limited access to the timeline of disease onset due to the lack of preexisting data. For a further discussion of the problems of postonly studies and approaches to address them, we refer the reader to other resources.(91)

Another challenge to measuring health indicators after disasters is characterizing the full breadth of psychopathology that may occur. While PTSD is likely the sentinel disaster psychopathology (92) and the focus of most postdisaster research, (3, 6) it may often manifest with concurrent comorbidity.(93) Studies of disasters increasingly need to consider these comorbidities to fully assess the mental health burden after disasters and the patterns of PTSD manifestation postdisaster. For example, a number of studies have found a higher prevalence of depression among those affected by postdisaster PTSD as compared to controls.(10, 47, 57, 94–96) Some studies have also shown postdisaster PTSD to be associated with anxiety disorders (94–96), substance abuse (31, 97), somatization (98), and functional impairment.(10, 99, 100) However, most of this evidence remains inconclusive due to the limited number of comparable studies.

Lastly, postdisaster studies are increasingly incorporating biological measures into their measurements to elucidate the relationship between mental disorders and the underlying biochemical and genetic factors.(101, 102) Including these measures creates another dimension of issues for disaster research, such as the reliability of these measures and their feasibility in postdisaster circumstances. This area of research will likely become increasingly important in the coming years.

RESEARCH DIRECTIONS

We suggest that there are four central directions for future research in the field: (a) comprehensive research for comorbid disorders, (b) studies concerned with the nature of disaster exposure, (c) inquiry about the course of PTSD, and (d) interventional studies and the need to determine effective treatments of PTSD after disasters.

Comorbid disorders

As shown earlier, PTSD may manifest with concurrent comorbid disorders such as depression, substance abuse, and anxiety disorder. However, studies have yet to fully characterize what these comorbid disorders may be and the longitudinal course of them in conjunction with PTSD. In addition, the long-term physical consequences of PTSD need to be examined to fully assess the burden of the disease. For example, a recent study showed that PTSD might increase the risk of cardiovascular disease.(103) Further studies similar to this need to be conducted, to confirm this finding and explore other potential physical manifestations of PTSD.

Exposure

As we note in this review, overall, evidence from the literature and reviews of this evidence show that a higher disaster-related exposure is associated with a higher prevalence of PTSD.(4, 5, 21, 22, 25, 47, 55, 80, 104) For instance, those closest to the site of the disaster have been documented to have a higher prevalence of PTSD than those further away.(22, 25, 47, 80) In addition, as seen above, the prevalence of PTSD is typically highest among survivors, followed by rescue workers, with the general population having the lowest prevalence of PTSD. These three types of samples represent the heterogeneous nature of exposure among the affected population. For example, survivors directly experienced the attack itself, while rescue workers directly experienced the aftermath of the attack. In contrast, the exposure for the general population is typically indirect: Some people may have lost a friend or family member, suffered a poor outcome from the disaster such as displacement or employment loss, or experienced the disaster through the media.

Whether indirect exposure is sufficient for causing psychopathology in the general population is currently in debate in the literature. In a study of primary care patients, Neria and colleagues found that indirect exposure was not related to the risk of PTSD.(44) However, studies of national populations after September 11 (22, 105) and population in an area far from the Oklahoma City bombing (106) indicate that a relation may exist between the two. Models that have been suggested to mediate this relation include widespread media exposure to mediums such as television (107, 108) and perceived threat and relative risk appraisal.(109) Future work that examines the relation between PTSD and indirect exposure, as well as potential mechanisms that mediate this relation, is well indicated.

In addition, the concept of indirect exposure raises important considerations about the burden of PTSD after disasters. Because a greater number of people are indirectly exposed to disasters rather than directly exposed, the overall health burden may be weighted toward those who are indirectly exposed and show signs of partial PTSD rather than survivors who have full PTSD.(4, 5) This may have important implications for public health policies after disasters.

Course of PTSD and longitudinal studies

The uncertainty surrounding the exact trajectory of PTSD after disasters reveals the need for more longitudinal studies in the field, as the risk factors for persistent PTSD and the course of delayed-onset PTSD have yet to be determined. Typically, postdisaster studies have relied on cross-sectional studies (6) that provide an illustration of a population at one point in time, thereby estimating the burden of mental health, which is useful to both researchers and public health officials.(110) However, establishing how this burden evolves over time is very difficult with this type of study.

In general, researchers have found that the prevalence of PTSD decreases over time.(5) A study of survivors of a mass shooting found that the prevalence of PTSD decreased from 28% 1 to 2 months after the incident to 17% 1 year later.(81) A similar decline was found in studies of the NYC population after the September 11 attacks (111), a community affected by the 1988 Lockerbie disaster (13), survivors of the 2004 Asian earthquake and tsunamis (55), and survivors of the 1989 Newcastle earthquake.(112) Among children, La Greca and colleagues found that 3 months after Hurricane Andrew, 29.8% experienced severe to very severe symptoms of PTSD; this declined to 18.1% at 7 months and 12.5% at 10 months.(65) A similar decrease was found by a study that assessed the functioning of children after the 1993 World Trade Center attacks.(27) Studies of rescue workers after the 1988 Piper Alpha oil rig disaster (90) and the USS Iowa gun turret explosion (17) have also documented a decline in the prevalence of PTSD over time. Furthermore, a study of the general U.S. population after the September 11 attacks showed a decrease in PTSD from 17% at 2 months to 5.8% at 6 months, indicating that the prevalence of PTSD may also decrease among indirectly exposed persons.(105)

However, the persistence of PTSD in some populations has yet to be fully characterized. Norris and colleagues found that the prevalence of PTSD among survivors of Hurricane Andrew slightly increased from 26% at 6 month to 29% 30 months postdisaster.(113) Similarly, a study after a 1998 earthquake in Northern China found that the prevalence of PTSD increased between 3 and 9 months in 2 affected villages.(114) Delayed-onset PTSD may also complicate the projected course of PTSD, as McFarlane found in a study of firefighters after the 1983 Australian bush fire.(115) Future work may fruitfully examine the course of PTSD and correlates of persistent PTSD.

Interventional studies

We address the topic of interventional studies for postdisaster treatment of PTSD briefly, referring the interested reader to a more complete review of interventional treatments.(116) Most research to date has considered survivors of traumatic events in general, rather than focusing on survivors of disasters. Even drawing from this wider arena of research, the evidence is inconsistent. In fact, a recent meta-analysis showed that single-session critical-incident debriefing—once a commonly used clinical intervention—may actually be harmful.(117) Overall, cognitive–behavioral therapy (CBT) may currently be the most promising psychosocial intervention, as indicated by research.(116) Studies have shown that CBT initiated within the first month after a trauma may prevent psychological sequelae as compared to other interventional methods such as supportive counseling or repeated assessments.(118–120) For pharmacotherapy, SSRIs are often used as the first-line medications for the treatment of PTSD.(121)

The evidence regarding effective treatments, specifically after disasters, is sparse, as few studies have been conducted in postdisaster circumstances.(122, 123, 124) Many therapies, ranging from psychological to pharmacological, have yet to be evaluated in the postdisaster context, thereby limiting the ability of communities and governments to mitigate the mental health consequences of disasters.

CONCLUSION

Many methodological challenges are inherent in the study of postdisaster mental health consequences. Because of these challenges, several aspects of postdisaster PTSD remain largely underdeveloped in the literature. For example, the prevalence of PTSD after disasters has been well characterized in some populations; however, in others such as children or those of low socioeconomic status, further work needs to be conducted. More important, while the course of PTSD after disasters is still a nascent area of research, more longitudinal studies of representative populations could greatly assist in the determination of trajectories of PTSD such as the occurrence of delayed-onset PTSD. Furthermore, the field has yet to fully determine the effect of comorbid disorders and indirect exposure on the burden of PTSD. Future work also needs to explore the role of different interventions in mitigating PTSD after disasters. These subjects represent integral areas of inquiry for the improvement of both the postdisaster research field and postdisaster public health practice.

REFERENCES

1. Kessler RC, Sonnega A, Bromet E, Hughes M, Nelson CB. Posttraumatic stress disorder in the national comorbidity survey, Arch Gen Psychiatry 1995; 52: 1048–60.
2. Neria Y, Gross R, Marhsall R eds. 9/11: Mental Health in the Wake of Terrorist Attacks. Cambridge University Press: New York; 2006.
3. Norris FH, Elrod CL. Psychosocial consequences of disaster: a review of past research. In: Norris FH, Galea S, Friedman MJ, Watson PJ, eds. Methods for Disaster Mental Health Research. The Guilford Press: New York, 2006: 20–42.
4. Galea S, Nandi A, Vlahov D. The epidemiology of post-traumatic stress disorder after disasters. Epidemiol Rev 2005; 27: 78–91.
5. Neria Y, Nandi A, Galea S. Post-traumatic stress disorder following disasters: a systematic review, Psychol Med 2008; 38: 467–80.
6. Norris FH, Friedman MJ, Watson PJ. 60,000 disaster victims speak: Part I, An empirical review of the empirical literature, 1981–2001, Psychiatry 2002; 65: 207–39.
7. McFarlane AC, Norris FH. Definitions and concepts in disaster research. In: Norris FH, Galea S, Friedman MJ, Watson PJ, eds. Methods for Disaster Mental Health Research. The Guilford Press: New York, 2006; 3–19.
8. Sungur M, Kaya B. The onset and longitudinal course of a man-made post-traumatic morbidity: survivors of the Sivas disaster. Int J Psychiatry Clin Pract 2001; 5: 195–202.
9. Hull AM, Alexander DA, Klein S. Survivors of the Piper Alpha oil platform disaster: long-term follow-up study. Br J Psychiatry 2002; 181: 433–8.
10. North CS, Nixon SJ, Shariat S et al. Psychiatric disorders among survivors of the Oklahoma City bombing. JAMA 1999; 282: 755–62.
11. North CS, Smith EM, Spitznagel EL. Posttraumatic stress disorder in survivors of a mass shooting. Am J Psychiatry 1994; 151: 82–8.
12. Carlier IV, Gersons BP. Stress reactions in disaster victims following the Bijlmermeer plane crash. J Trauma Stress 1997; 10: 329–35.
13. Scott RB, Brooks N, McKinlay W. Post-traumatic morbidity in a civilian community of litigants: a follow-up at 3 years. J Trauma Stress 1995; 8: 403–17.
14. Sims A, Sims D. The phenomenology of post-traumatic stress disorder. A symptomatic study of 70 victims of psychological trauma. Psychopathology 1998; 31: 96–112.
15. Fullerton CS, Ursano RJ, Reeves J, Shigemura J, Grieger T. Perceived safety in disaster workers following 9/11, J Nerv Ment Dis 2006; 194: 61–3.
16. Centers for Disease Control and Prevention, Mental health status of World Trade Center rescue and recovery workers and volunteers - New York City, July 2002-August 2004, MMWR Morb Mortal Wkly Rep 2004; 53: 812–5.
17. Ursano RJ, Fullerton CS, Kao TC, Bhartiya VR. Longitudinal assessment of posttraumatic stress disorder and depression after exposure to traumatic death. J Nerv Ment Dis 1995; 183: 36–42.
18. Perrin MA, DiGrande L, Wheeler K et al. Differences in PTSD prevalence and associated risk factors among World Trade Center disaster rescue and recovery workers, Am J Psychiatry 2007; 164: 1385–94.
19. Hanson RF, Kilpatrick DG, Freedy JR, Saunders BE. Los Angeles County after the 1992 civil disturbances: degree of exposure and impact on mental health. J Consult Clin Psychol 1995; 63: 987–96.
20. Adams RE, Boscarino JA. Differences in mental health outcomes among Whites, African Americans, and Hispanics following a community disaster. Psychiatry 2005; 68: 250–65.

21. Galea S, Ahern J, Resnick H et al. Psychological sequelae of the September 11 terrorist attacks in New York City. N Engl J Med 2002; 346: 982–7.
22. Schlenger WE, Caddell JM, Ebert L et al. Psychological reactions to terrorist attacks: findings from the national study of Americans' reactions to September 11. JAMA 2002; 288: 581–8.
23. Palinkas LA, Petterson JS, Russell J, Downs MA. Community patterns of psychiatric disorders after the Exxon Valdez oil spill. Am J Psychiatry 1993; 150: 1517–23.
24. Miguel-Tobal JJ, Cano-Vindel A, Gonzalez-Ordi H et al. PTSD and depression after the Madrid March 11 train bombings. J Trauma Stress 2006; 19: 69–80.
25. Godeau E, Vignes C, Navarro F et al. Effects of a large-scale industrial disaster on rates of symptoms consistent with posttraumatic stress disorders among schoolchildren in Toulouse. Arch Pediatr Adolesc Med 2005; 159: 579–84.
26. Pynoos RS, Frederick C, Nader K et al. Life threat and posttraumatic stress in school-age children. Arch Gen Psychiatry 1987; 44: 1057–63.
27. Koplewicz HS, Vogel JM, Solanto MV et al. Child and parent response to the 1993 World Trade Center bombing. J Trauma Stress 2002; 15: 77–85.
28. March JS, Amaya-Jackson L, Terry R. Posttraumatic symptomatology in children and adolescents after an industrial fire. J Am Acad Child Adolesc Psychiatry 1997; 36: 1080–8.
29. Hoven CW, Duarte CS, Lucas CP et al. Psychopathology among New York city public school children 6 months after September 11. Arch Gen Psychiatry 2005; 62: 545–52.
30. Pfefferbaum B, Pfefferbaum RL, Gurwitch RH et al. Children's response to terrorism: a critical review of the literature. Curr Psychiatry Rep 2003; 5: 95–100.
31. Grieger TA, Fullerton CS, Ursano RJ. Posttraumatic stress disorder, alcohol use, and perceived safety after the terrorist attack on the pentagon. Psychiatr Serv 2003; 54: 1380–2.
32. Pulcino T, Galea S, Ahern J. Posttraumatic stress in women after the September 11 terrorist attacks in New York City, J Womens Health (Larchmt) 2003; 12: 809–20.
33. Schuster MA, Stein BD, Jaycox L et al. A national survey of stress reactions after the September 11, 2001, terrorist attacks. N Engl J Med 2001; 345: 1507–12.
34. Green BL, Korol M, Grace MC et al. Children and disaster: age, gender, and parental effects on PTSD symptoms. J Am Acad Child Adolesc Psychiatry 1991; 30: 945–51.
35. Dalgleish T, Joseph S, Thrasher S, Tranah T, Yule W. Crisis support following the Herald of Free-Enterprise disaster: a longitudinal perspective. J Trauma Stress 1996; 9: 833–45.
36. McCarroll JE, Fullerton CS, Ursano RJ, Hermsen JM. Posttraumatic stress symptoms following forensic dental identification: Mt. Carmel, Waco, Texas. Am J Psychiatry 1996; 153: 778–82.
37. Gregg W, Medley I, Fowler-Dixon R et al. Psychological consequences of the Kegworth air disaster. Br J Psychiatry 1995; 167: 812–7.
38. Luce A, Firth-Cozens J. Effects of the Omagh bombing on medical staff working in the local NHS trust: a longitudinal survey. Hosp Med 2002; 63: 44–47.
39. Trautman R, Tucker P, Pfefferbaum B et al. Effects of prior trauma and age on posttraumatic stress symptoms in Asian and Middle Eastern immigrants after terrorism in the community. Community Ment Health J 2002; 38: 459–74.
40. Cardenas J, Williams K, Wilson JP, Fanouraki G, Singh A. PSTD, major depressive symptoms, and substance abuse following September 11, 2001, in a midwestern university population. Int J Emerg Ment Health 2003; 5: 15–28.
41. Johnson SD, North CS, Smith EM. Psychiatric disorders among victims of a courthouse shooting spree: a three-year follow-up study. Community Ment Health J 2002; 38: 181–94.
42. Epstein RS, Fullerton CS, Ursano RJ. Posttraumatic stress disorder following an air disaster: a prospective study. Am J Psychiatry 1998; 155: 934–8.
43. Galea S, Vlahov D, Tracy M et al. Hispanic ethnicity and post-traumatic stress disorder after a disaster: evidence from a general population survey after September 11, 2001. Ann Epidemiol 2004; 14: 520–31.
44. Neria Y, Gross R, Olfson M et al. Posttraumatic stress disorder in primary care one year after the 9/11 attacks. Gen Hosp Psychiatry 2006; 28: 213–22.
45. Bodvarsdottir I, Elklit A. Psychological reactions in Icelandic earthquake survivors. Scand J Psychol 2004; 45: 3–13.
46. Carr VJ, Lewin TJ, Webster RA et al. Psychosocial sequelae of the 1989 Newcastle earthquake: I, Community disaster experiences and psychological morbidity 6 months post-disaster. Psychol Med 1995; 25: 539–55.
47. Basoglu M, Kilic C, Salcioglu E, Livanou M. Prevalence of posttraumatic stress disorder and comorbid depression in earthquake survivors in Turkey: an epidemiological study. J Trauma Stress 2004; 17: 133–41.
48. Najarian LM, Goenjian AK, Pelcovitz D, Mandel F, Najarian B. The effect of relocation after a natural disaster. J Trauma Stress 2001; 14: 511–26.
49. Centers for Disease Control and Prevention (CDC). Health hazard evaluation of police officers and firefighters after Hurricane Katrina--New Orleans, Louisiana, October 17–28 and November 30-December 5, 2005. MMWR Morb Mortal Wkly Rep 2006; 55: 456–8.

50. Ozen S, Sir A. Frequency of PTSD in a group of search and rescue workers two months after 2003 Bingol (Turkey) earthquake. J Nerv Ment Dis 2004; 192: 573–5.

51. Chang CM, Lee LC, Connor KM et al. Posttraumatic distress and coping strategies among rescue workers after an earthquake. J Nerv Ment Dis 2003; 191: 391–8.

52. Parslow RA, Jorm AF, Christensen H. Associations of pre-trauma attributes and trauma exposure with screening positive for PTSD: analysis of a community-based study of 2,085 young adults. Psychol Med 2006; 36: 387–95.

53. Canino G, Bravo M, Rubio-Stipec M, Woodbury M. The impact of disaster on mental health: prospective and retrospective analyses. Int J Ment Health 1990; 19: 51–69.

54. Norris FH, Murphy AD, Baker CK, Perilla JL. Postdisaster PTSD over four waves of a panel study of Mexico's 1999 flood. J Trauma Stress 2004; 17: 283–92.

55. van Griensven F, Chakkraband ML, Thienkrua W et al. Mental health problems among adults in tsunami-affected areas in southern Thailand. JAMA 2006; 296: 537–48.

56. Goenjian AK, Molina L, Steinberg AM et al. Posttraumatic stress and depressive reactions among Nicaraguan adolescents after Hurricane Mitch. Am J Psychiatry 2001; 158: 788–94.

57. Goenjian AK, Pynoos RS, Steinberg AM et al. Psychiatric comorbidity in children after the 1988 earthquake in Armenia. J Am Acad Child Adolesc Psychiatry 1995; 34: 1174–84.

58. Vernberg EM, Silverman WK, La Greca AM, Prinstein MJ. Prediction of posttraumatic stress symptoms in children after Hurricane Andrew. J Abnorm Psychol 1996; 105: 237–48.

59. Russoniello CV, Skalko TK, O'Brien K et al. Childhood posttraumatic stress disorder and efforts to cope after Hurricane Floyd. Behav Med 2002; 28: 61–71.

60. Shannon MP, Lonigan CJ, Finch AJ Jr, Taylor CM. Children exposed to disaster: I, Epidemiology of post-traumatic symptoms and symptom profiles, J Am Acad Child Adolesc Psychiatry 1994; 33: 80–93.

61. Garrison CZ, Bryant ES, Addy CL et al. Posttraumatic stress disorder in adolescents after Hurricane Andrew. J Am Acad Child Adolesc Psychiatry 1995; 34: 1193–201.

62. Caldera T, Palma L, Penayo U, Kullgren G. Psychological impact of the Hurricane Mitch in Nicaragua in a one-year perspective. Soc Psychiatry Psychiatr Epidemiol 2001; 36: 108–14.

63. Durkin ME. Major depression and post-traumatic stress disorder following the Coalinga and Chile earthquakes: a cross-cultural comparison. J Soc Behav Pers 1993; 8: 405–20.

64. Norris FH, Kaniasty K. Received and perceived social support in times of stress: a test of the social support deterioration deterrence model. J Pers Soc Psychol 1996; 71: 498–511.

65. La Greca A, Silverman WK, Vernberg EM, Prinstein MJ. Symptoms of posttraumatic stress in children after Hurricane Andrew: a prospective study. J Consult Clin Psychol 1996; 64: 712–23.

66. Weiss DS, Marmar CR, Metzler TJ, Ronfeldt HM. Predicting symptomatic distress in emergency services personnel. J Consult Clin Psychol 1995; 63: 361–8.

67. Norris FH, Kaniasty K, Conrad ML, Inman GL, Murphy AD. Placing age differences in cultural context: a comparison of the effects of age on PTSD after disaster in the United States, Mexico, and Poland. J Clinical Geropsychology 2002; 8: 153–73.

68. Catapano F, Malafronte R, Lepre F et al. Psychological consequences of the 1998 landslide in Sarno, Italy: a community study. Acta Psychiatr Scand 2001; 104: 438–42.

69. Kilic C, Ulusoy M. Psychological effects of the November 1999 earthquake in Turkey: an epidemiological study. Acta Psychiatr Scand 2003; 108: 232–8.

70. La Greca AM, Silverman WK, Wasserstein SB. Children's predisaster functioning as a predictor of posttraumatic stress following Hurricane Andrew. J Consult Clin Psychol 1998; 66: 883–92.

71. Perilla JL, Norris FH, Lavizzo EA. Ethnicity, culture and disaster response: identifying and explaining ethnic differences in PTSD six months after Hurricane Andrew. J Soc Clin Psychol 2002; 21: 20–45.

72. Steinberg AM, Brymer MJ, Steinberg JR, Pfefferbaum B. Conducting research on children and adolescents after disaster. In: Norris FH, Galea S, Friedman MJ, Watson PJ, eds. Methods for Disaster Mental Health Research. The Guilford Press: New York, 2006: 243–53.

73. North CS, Pfefferbaum B, Narayanan P et al. Comparison of post-disaster psychiatric disorders after terrorist bombings in Nairobi and Oklahoma City. Br J Psychiatry 2005; 186: 487–93.

74. Kessler RC, Galea S, Jones RT, Parker HA. Hurricane Katrina Community Advisory Group, Mental illness and suicidality after Hurricane Katrina. Bull World Health Organ 2006; 84: 930–9.

75. Galea S, Brewin CR, Gruber M et al. Exposure to hurricane-related stressors and mental illness after Hurricane Katrina. Arch Gen Psychiatry 2007; 64: 1427–34.

76. Corbie-Smith G, Thomas SB, St George DM. Distrust, race, and research. Arch Intern Med 2002; 162: 2458–63.

77. Newman E, Kaloupek DG. The risks and benefits of participating in trauma-focused research studies. J Trauma Stress 2004; 17: 383–94.

78. Newman E, Walker EA, Gefland A. Assessing the ethical costs and benefits of trauma-focused research. Gen Hosp Psychiatry 1999; 21: 187–96.

79. Galea S, Nandi A, Stuber J et al. Participant reactions to survey research in the general population after terrorist attacks. J Trauma Stress 2005; 18: 461–5.

80. Havenaar JM, Rumyantzeva GM, van den Brink W et al. Long-term mental health effects of the Chernobyl disaster: an epidemiologic survey in two former Soviet regions. Am J Psychiatry 1997; 154: 1605–7.
81. North CS, Smith EM, Spitznagel EL. One-year follow-up of survivors of a mass shooting. Am J Psychiatry 1997; 154: 1696–702.
82. American Psychiatric Association, Diagnostic and Statistical Manual of Mental Disorders, 3rd edn. American Psychiatric Association: Washington, DC; 1980.
83. American Psychiatric Association, Diagnostic and Statistical Manual of Mental Disorders, 3rd edn, revised. American Psychiatric Association: Washington, DC; 1987.
84. American Psychiatric Association, Diagnostic and Statistical Manual of Mental Disorders, 4th edn. American Psychiatric Association: Washington, DC; 1994.
85. Stuber J, Resnick H, Galea S. Gender disparities in posttraumatic stress disorder after mass trauma. Gend Med 2006; 3: 54–67.
86. Pfefferbaum B, Stuber J, Galea S, Fairbrother G. Panic reactions to terrorist attacks and probable posttraumatic stress disorder in adolescents. J Trauma Stress 2006; 19: 217–28.
87. Galea S, Ahern J. Invited commentary: considerations about specificity of associations, causal pathways, and heterogeneity in multilevel thinking. Am J Epidemiol 2006; 163: 1079–82.
88. Weissman MM, Neria Y, Das A et al. Gender differences in posttraumatic stress disorder among primary care patients after the World Trade Center attack of September 11, 2001. Gend Med 2005; 2: 76–87.
89. Asarnow J, Glynn S, Pynoos RS et al. When the earth stops shaking: earthquake sequelae among children diagnosed for pre-earthquake psychopathology. J Am Acad Child Adolesc Psychiatry 1999; 38: 1016–23.
90. Alexander DA. Stress among police body handlers, a long-term follow-up. Br J Psychiatry 1993; 163: 806–8.
91. Galea S, Maxwell AR. Methodological challenges in studying the mental health consequences of disasters, In: Neria Y, Galea S, Norris FH, eds. Mental Health Consequences of Disasters. Cambridge University Press, in press.
92. Brunello N, Davidson JR, Deahl M et al. Posttraumatic stress disorder: diagnosis and epidemiology, comorbidity and social consequences, biology and treatment. Neuropsychobiology 2001; 43: 150–62.
93. Breslau N, Chase GA, Anthony JC. The uniqueness of the DSM definition of post-traumatic stress disorder: implications for research. Psychol Med 2002; 32: 573–6.
94. Brooks N, McKinlay W. Mental health consequences of the Lockerbie disaster. J Trauma Stress 1992; 5: 527–43.
95. Green BL, Lindy JD, Grace MC, Leonard AC. Chronic posttraumatic stress disorder and diagnostic comorbidity in a disaster sample. J Nerv Ment Dis 1992; 180: 760–6.
96. McFarlane AC, Papay P. Multiple diagnoses in posttraumatic stress disorder in the victims of a natural disaster. J Nerv Ment Dis 1992; 180: 498–504.
97. Stewart SH, Mitchell TL, Wright KD, Loba P. The relations of PTSD symptoms to alcohol use and coping drinking in volunteers who responded to the Swissair Flight 111 airline disaster. J Anxiety Disord 2004; 18: 51–68.
98. Foa EB, Stein DJ, McFarlane AC. Symptomatology and psychopathology of mental health problems after disaster. J Clin Psychiatry 2006; 67(2): 15–25.
99. Pfefferbaum B, North CS, Doughty DE et al. Posttraumatic stress and functional impairment in Kenyan children following the 1998 American Embassy bombing. Am J Orthopsychiatry 2003; 73: 133–40.
100. North CS, Tivis L, McMillen JC et al. Coping, functioning, and adjustment of rescue workers after the Oklahoma City bombing. J Trauma Stress 2002; 15: 171–5.
101. Galea S, Acierno R, Ruggiero K et al. Social context and the psychobiology of posttraumatic stress. Ann NY Acad Sci 2006; 1071: 231–41.
102. Kilpatrick DG, Koenen KC, Ruggiero KJ et al. The serotonin transporter genotype and social support and moderation of posttraumatic stress disorder and depression in hurricane-exposed adults. Am J Psychiatry 2007; 164: 1693–9.
103. Kubzansky LD, Koenen KC, Spiro A 3rd, Vokonas PS, Sparrow D. Prospective study of posttraumatic stress disorder symptoms and coronary heart disease in the Normative Aging Study. Arch Gen Psychiatry 2007; 64: 109–16.
104. Tucker P, Pfefferbaum B, Nixon SJ, Dickson W. Predictors of post-traumatic stress symptoms in Oklahoma City: exposure, social support, peri-traumatic responses. J Behav Health Serv Res 2000; 27: 406–16.
105. Silver RC, Holman EA, McIntosh DN, Poulin M, Gil-Rivas V. Nationwide longitudinal study of psychological responses to September 11, JAMA 2002; 288: 1235–44.
106. Pfefferbaum B, Seale TW, McDonald NB et al. Posttraumatic stress two years after the Oklahoma City bombing in youths geographically distant from the explosion. Psychiatry 2000; 63: 358–70.

107. Ahern J, Galea S, Resnick H, Vlahov D. Television images and probable posttraumatic stress disorder after September 11: the role of background characteristics, event exposures, and perievent panic, J Nerv Ment Dis 2004; 192: 217–26.

108. Ahern J, Galea S, Resnick H, Kilpatrick D, Bucuvalas M. Television images and psychological symptoms after the September 11 terrorist attacks, Psychiatry 2002; 65: 289–300.

109. Marshall RD, Bryant RA, Amsel L et al. The psychology of ongoing threat: relative risk appraisal, the September 11 attacks, and terrorism-related fears, Am Psychol 2007; 62: 304–16.

110. Verger P, Dab W, Lamping DL et al. The psychological impact of terrorism: an epidemiologic study of posttraumatic stress disorder and associated factors in victims of the 1995–1996 bombings in France. Am J Psychiatry 2004; 161: 1384–9.

111. Galea S, Vlahov D, Resnick H et al. Trends of probable post-traumatic stress disorder in New York City after the September 11 terrorist attacks. Am J Epidemiol 2003; 158: 514–24.

112. Carr VJ, Lewin TJ, Webster RA et al. Psychosocial sequelae of the 1989 Newcastle earthquake: II, Exposure and morbidity profiles during the first 2 years post-disaster. Psychol Med 1997; 27: 167–78.

113. Norris FH, Perilla JL, Riad JK, Kaniasty K, Lavizzo EA. Stability and change in stress, resources, and psychological distress following natural disaster: findings from hurricane andrew. Anxiety Stress Coping 1999; 12: 363–96.

114. Wang X, Gao L, Shinfuku N et al. Longitudinal study of earthquake-related PTSD in a randomly selected community sample in north China. Am J Psychiatry 2000; 157: 1260–6.

115. McFarlane AC. The longitudinal course of posttraumatic morbidity. The range of outcomes and their predictors. J Nerv Ment Dis 1988; 176: 30–9.

116. Gibson LE, Hamblen JL, Zvolensky MJ, Vujanovic AA. Evidence-based treatments for traumatic stress: an overview of the research with an emphasis on disaster settings, In: Norris FH, Galea S, Friedman MJ, Watson PJ, eds. The Guilford Press: New York, 2006: 208–25.

117. van Emmerik AA, Kamphuis JH, Hulsbosch AM, Emmelkamp PM. Single session debriefing after psychological trauma: a meta-analysis. Lancet 2002; 360: 766–71.

118. Bryant RA, Moulds ML, Nixon RV. Cognitive behaviour therapy of acute stress disorder: a four-year follow-up. Behav Res Ther 2003; 41: 489–94.

119. Bryant RA, Harvey AG, Dang ST, Sackville T, Basten C. Treatment of acute stress disorder: a comparison of cognitive-behavioral therapy and supportive counseling. J Consult Clin Psychol 1998; 66: 862–6.

120. Ehlers A, Clark DM, Hackmann A et al. A randomized controlled trial of cognitive therapy, a self-help booklet, and repeated assessments as early interventions for posttraumatic stress disorder. Arch Gen Psychiatry 2003; 60: 1024–32.

121. Davis LL, Frazier EC, Williford RB, Newell JM. Long-term pharmacotherapy for post-traumatic stress disorder. CNS Drugs 2006; 20: 465–76.

122. Basoglu M, Salcioglu E, Livanou M. A randomized controlled study of single-session behavioural treatment of earthquake-related post-traumatic stress disorder using an earthquake simulator. Psychol Med 2007; 37: 203–13.

123. Chemtob CM, Nakashima J, Carlson JG. Brief treatment for elementary school children with disaster-related posttraumatic stress disorder: a field study, J Clin Psychol 2002; 58: 99–112.

124. Gillespie K, Duffy M, Hackmann A, Clark DM. Community based cognitive therapy in the treatment of posttraumatic stress disorder following the Omagh bomb. Behav Res Ther 2002; 40: 345–57.

14 | Symptom exaggeration in posttraumatic stress disorder

Alzbeta Juven-Wetzler, Rachel Sonnino, Danit Bar-Ziv, and Joseph Zohar

INTRODUCTION

Posttraumatic stress disorder (PTSD) is unique among psychiatric disorders as, per definition, the trigger is known; the *critical* event is part of the core diagnosis. Because there is an external event, in many cases PTSD is linked to compensation; for example, in case of car accidents compensation is sought from the insurance company, while in other cases (such as war-related PTSD) the address is the Ministry of Defense, and so on.

As in most of the cases the compensation, level of disability, and subsequently the financial gain, is based on a combination of symptom severity and functioning, the patient might have an inherent incentive to exacerbate the symptoms. Moreover, as the patients often feel as though they are a victim, they also feel justified in using this approach ("They are responsible for this, they need to pay for it").

The authors are by no means suggesting that PTSD is merely a "compensation neurosis," rather they propose to face the uniqueness of PTSD described above and to examine the monitoring of PTSD through a prism aimed to illuminate the issue of symptom exacerbation.

Cofactoring with an "exacerbation index" is important not only for getting an accurate clinical picture of the actual (factual) status of a given patient but it is also important in order to increase the validity of the diagnosis of PTSD. Mingling intentional exacerbation with genuine PTSD may prevent proper diagnosis and treatment of patients who really suffer from PTSD and for whom it may be hard to pass the barriers of disbelief rooted by cases of intentional exacerbation. If ways can be found to better identify this fraction of patients with symptom exaggeration, who are often quite vocal and demanding, and to separate them from cases of genuine PTSD, it would boost the validity and confidence in the diagnosis of PTSD.

MALINGERING VS. EXAGGERATION

Noting the Diagnostic and Statistical Manual of Mental Disorders (DSM), 4th edition definition of *malingering* as "the intentional production of false or grossly exaggerated physical or psychological symptoms, motivated by external incentives" (1, p. 683), we prefer to use the term *exaggerators* rather than *malingerers*, in order to include those whose exaggeration is not consciously intentional. As we shall see in the following sections, the distinction between *intentional* and *nonintentional* is less pertinent when considering the implications of symptom exaggeration, although it does come into play when discussing how to recognize cases of exaggeration and how to deal with them once identified.

CLINICAL AND SOCIAL IMPLICATIONS OF SYMPTOM EXAGGERATION

The severity of PTSD has been monitored initially for two primary purposes—clinical and research purposes. Clinical monitoring of severity is intended to quantify the patient's status and to help the clinician get a more accurate impression of how a particular patient responds to a given treatment. For research purposes, a severity score is sometimes used as a stricter inclusion criterion than the diagnostic threshold, and repeated measures allow statistical comparison of different treatment trials and control groups.

However, the severity of PTSD has another, financial, implication—that of disability support and/or compensation. Monetary benefits available to PTSD patients include various welfare-based disability allowances to compensate for the patient's inability to function normally in his or her everyday lives—inability to hold a job, to continue social activities, and so on.(2) These benefits depend heavily on the severity of the PTSD symptoms as assessed by a psychiatrist. The monetary implication of the severity of PTSD (as assessed by a clinician) is rooted in the very characteristic that makes PTSD unique among psychiatric disorders—that the disorder is triggered by an external event in a defined time. If a certain party can be held responsible for the traumatic event, and the resulting impaired function can be confirmed by a mental health professional, litigation is possible for compensation from the relevant organization.

In addition, a further repercussion of a PTSD diagnosis rated at a given severity level is that of the "social reaction" to the disorder. The social benefits of assuming a sick role may provide sympathy, care, and attention otherwise not forthcoming from family members and friends. Depending on the nature of the triggering traumatic event, the associated stigma of a mental health problem may be outweighed by the accompanying "hero" role that can be assumed by having survived certain ordeals, especially with growing public awareness and acceptance of this disorder.

One might assume that for clinical or research purposes patients would have no vested interest in influencing the severity score of their PTSD symptoms. However, the monetary and social incentives described above are unfortunately entwined in the process, as the severity of PTSD as outlined by the clinician or the researcher may be quoted and relied on in applications for monetary benefits/legal actions.

The desire to have their PTSD assessed as more severe than it actually is may prompt some individuals to misreport their symptoms in order to portray them as harsher and more disabling. As the diagnosis of posttraumatic stress disorder (PTSD), like most but not all psychiatric disorders, is based in large part on the patient's report of subjective symptoms; this is possible in a way that would not be the case in some physical diseases, where objective testing (e.g., EMR for a patient complaining of muscle weakness) would refute unfounded claims of illness and would help to give a complementary evaluation of the severity of the symptoms.

THE EPIDEMIOLOGICAL AND RESEARCH IMPACT OF SYMPTOM EXAGGERATION

Determining the prevalence of PTSD is difficult because any baseline sample screened for the "true" rate of PTSD is itself potentially tainted with exaggerators. However, large epidemiological studies, in which the sample was not chosen following exposure to traumatic events, and participants were anonymous, (and, therefore, can be expected to have been more honest about symptoms) are most likely to attain accurate prevalence rates, with the least contamination from exaggerator data. One such study, the U.S. National Comorbidity Study (3) found PTSD to have a prevalence of 7.8%.

The financial loss caused by symptom exaggeration in PTSD is perhaps the most prominent of consequences when examined from a public interest point of view, but the effect exaggeration has on research must also be considered. Patients who expect the severity of their PTSD as measured in clinical research to serve other purposes, whether monetary or social, or even those who have a specific reason for wanting to be included in a particular study (either to access an otherwise unavailable or expensive treatment or to sidestep a lengthy waiting list in regular treatment clinics), may give inflated descriptions of symptoms, and the implications for PTSD research are manifold. First, prevalence rates of PTSD, if they include exaggerators, may be grossly inflated. Rosen (4) points out high prevalence of PTSD in studies where malingering was not ruled out, in comparison with epidemiological data (where exaggeration can be assumed minimal), and Summerfield (5) points out that these inflated prevalence rates, if published as accurate, can then mislead others. In fact, a vicious circle can ensue, whereby an initially exaggeration-tainted sample gives rise to escalated prevalence rates, which in turn lure subsequent researchers into a false sense of security regarding the purity of their samples (given that the prevalence rate matches the prevalence found in previous research), and these results, if published, merely serve to strengthen the notion that finding a prevalence such as this does not require further investigation of the possibility of exaggeration. In addition to elevated prevalence figures, as most research stipulates a certain level of PTSD severity as an inclusion criterion, exaggeration in the screening process would result in less severe cases entering the sample, skewing subsequent biological and clinical measures and analyses (e.g., in a study looking at a biological parameter that is specific to PTSD, including non-PTSD or mild cases of PTSD might hamper the interpretation of the biological results). Furthermore, in the majority of studies examining potential or current treatments for PTSD, severity is used as a measure of the treatment's success. Any participant who exaggerates symptoms at the baseline measurement in such a study would be expected to do the same at the follow-up phase, thus creating a flat effect of no response, data contamination, and a blurring of the clinical signal.

WHY DOES SYMPTOM EXAGGERATION IN PTSD GO UNNOTICED?

Since the diagnosis of PTSD was introduced into the *DSM* (6), concerns have been voiced that the symptoms of the disorder were relatively easy to simulate.(7–10) Concerns such as these led to the addition of a note regarding malingering in the discussion of PTSD in *DSM-IV* (1): "Malingering should be ruled out in those situations in which financial renumeration, benefit eligibility, and forensic determinations play a role" (p. 467). A study performed in 2002 demonstrated how difficult it can be to recognize symptom fabrication by professional actors.(11) This makes the more subtle task of identifying exaggeration, cases in which genuine symptoms are reported as more severe than truly experienced, seem even more daunting. Not only is the difference between the experience and presentation more subtle but some cases involve "amateur dramatics" as well, as in the case of survivors of the sinking of the Aleutian Enterprise (12), who later admitted being advised by their attorneys regarding symptoms they may have, presumably in an attempt to manipulate diagnosis or severity rating of PTSD. Particularly telling is the case of one fisherman survivor who wanted to go back to work but was told by his attorney that it would "look better" if he did not.

In the face of such obstacles, it is not surprising that the possibility of exaggeration (or malingering, as required by *DSM-IV*) is at best discussed in general terms with regard to the entire sample and very rarely examined in detail. This is despite the fact that studies specifically investigating PTSD in the context of compensation claims and lawyer involvement have found connections between these and PTSD severity.(13, 14) However, although the findings arouse suspicion, these studies do not actually imply that the litigation status influences patients to portray their symptoms as more disruptive and disturbing, rather than the symptom severity being the cause of the litigation. Indeed, several studies have failed to demonstrate an "improvement" in PTSD symptoms, following finalization of compensation claims.(13, 15, 16) Yet this lack of improvement does not necessarily mean all cases were genuine and can be interpreted in two other ways. One possibility is that the patients are still suspicious and refrain from admitting that they have a deliberate exacerbation. The other possibility is that the process of symptom exaggeration in itself is not harm free, and the long time that patients present themselves with certain symptoms might have resulted in "adapting" or "imprinting" of these symptoms (something along the lines of disuse atrophy—if an arm is not used for several weeks—let alone months or even years—then it is very difficult, if not impossible, to bring it back to full function). Hence, the possibility of exaggeration in cases with such large financial rewards at stake needs to be ruled out carefully and certainly should not be swept under the carpet.

IDENTIFICATION OF SYMPTOM EXAGGERATORS

The identification of PTSD patients suspected of exaggerating their symptoms in order to attain secondary benefits is a difficult task. One interesting study took advantage of changes in Croatian legislation regarding compensation for veterans in 2001.(17) This group observed a change in symptom reports of compensation-seeking veterans, following reforms of the national regulations for compensation criteria in Croatia. Distribution of diagnoses (based on reported symptoms) changed between the years 2000 and 2002 in a manner tending toward the better compensation rates awarded to certain PTSD-related diagnoses by the 2001 reform. This would imply some level of reporting bias on the part of compensation seekers, be it conscious or not.

However, such a method can be applied only in unique circumstances, where changes in the legislation governing compensation rights offer an opportunity to examine patients before and after the reform. Furthermore, it gives a picture from a prevalence point of view, but still no answer regarding individual patients. For specific, everyday purposes, a simpler method is needed. We will review here techniques examined and proposed for detecting symptom exaggeration, including the use of clinical interview, psychological scales, cognitive testing, and physiological measures.

Identifying a suspected malingerer/exaggerator is possible in several ways.(18, 19) Some of these methods are more suitable for conscious malingerers who are deliberately trying to pull the wool over the eyes of the clinician, whereas others are appropriate for more subtle cases, where symptom exaggeration is suspected, and where it is uncertain whether the patient is even aware himself of embellishing the description of his symptoms.

The exact methods used to identify suspected cases of symptom exaggeration are usually kept confidential to a great extent, as knowledge of how the techniques work can give deliberate exaggerators an opportunity to prepare in advance and possibly alter their performance so as to evade detection.

CLINICAL INTERVIEW AND CORROBORATION OF DATA

Although we will briefly review psychological, cognitive, and physiological methods for detecting symptom exaggeration in PTSD, one should not overlook the classical basic approach, that is, comprehensive clinical interview in which inconsistencies and atypical presentation might direct us to focus and carefully investigate overreporting.

The clinician should not show open signs of suspicion or incredulity (which risks arousing an exaggerator's suspicion, thus increasing his efforts to appear sincere), yet symptom reports should not be taken at face value. Given the high success rates for PTSD-naive subjects in feigning PTSD symptoms using a symptom checklist (8, 9), the use of open-ended questions, at least initially, is prudent (18), and the patient's responses can then be explored in more detail. Examples of instances in which a particular symptom was manifest should be requested and, where possible, corroborated with reports from family members and friends or other sources.

The clinical interview can also serve as an opportunity to observe the patient, which can provide insights as to the veracity of the symptoms reported (e.g., a patient claiming lack of concentration who does not display any difficulty concentrating during the interview or a claim of extreme irritability that is not evident in the patient's behavior). However, given the subjectivity of both administering and interpreting the clinical interview, it is a good idea to combine it with more standardized testing for symptom exaggeration for a fuller picture.

SCALES TO IDENTIFY SYMPTOM EXAGGERATION

There are no specific scales formulated for the detection of malingering or symptom overreporting in PTSD alone. General scales attempting to detect symptom exaggeration usually include questions about both genuine and improbable symptoms, under the premise that those who are fabricating or overreporting their symptoms will be more suggestible to the decoy items than patients who respond accurately and according to their actual experience.(20)

The Minnesota Multiphasic Personality Inventory (MMPI-2) has been used to detect symptom feigning in a range of disorders, including PTSD. The D and F-K scales are often used to detect malingering in general, and, less commonly, the PK and PS scales for combat-PTSD specifically. Detection methods in MMPI-2, as with scales in general, tend to focus on overendorsement of symptoms, with a suspiciously high number of symptoms overall or of rare symptoms. An additional focus is on certain more subtle symptoms that may be missed by an exaggerator not sufficiently knowledgeable about the intricacies of the disorder's symptoms.(21) The advantage of the MMPI-2 scale in identifying symptom overreporting is that the length (it is estimated to take 1-2 hours to complete) makes it difficult for individuals attempting to portray an untrue presentation to keep up the pretense in a convincing way. Studies using the MMPI-2 in PTSD populations have uncovered high rates of symptom exaggeration, particularly in individuals involved in compensation claims/litigation.(22) However, its immense length is one of the MMPI-2's downfalls as well. Not every situation is conducive to administering such a lengthy test, and the results are not easily interpreted (only a trained individual can score and interpret the results). This kind of investment of time and effort may be worthwhile in individual cases, perhaps in forensic and legal settings, and although not foolproof, could contribute to the overall picture of whether a supposed PTSD patient is indeed such. However, for a clinician with a hunch that something is amiss with a particular patient's description of PTSD symptoms, or for use in clinical trials that seek to ensure that all participants do indeed suffer from the necessary severity of PTSD, more specific as well as shorter and simpler methods are needed.

The Structured Interview of Reported Symptoms (SIRS, 20) consists of 172 items and looks at trends such as endorsement of rare or absurd symptoms, or improbable symptom combinations. It also includes items that lean toward detection of feigned cognitive dysfunction.

The SIRS was found to successfully distinguish between simulators and genuine PTSD patients in a study examining the feigning of a number of disorders.(20) A study looking at the effectiveness of the SIRS in detecting feigned symptoms in PTSD compensation and disability claimants also found it effective.(23)

The Miller Forensic Assessment of Symptoms (M-FAST) is relatively short (takes 10 to 15 minutes to administer), measuring endorsement of rare symptom combinations, atypical symptoms, and excessive reporting. It has been successful at differentiating nonpatients provided with diagnostic information from a clinical sample of PTSD patients.(24)

The Trauma Symptom Inventory (TSI) was not developed as a tool for detecting malingering but rather as an assessment of the sequelae of traumatic events. However, it comprises three subscales that point toward possible symptom exaggeration and have been found effective in detecting coached feigners of PTSD.(25)

COGNITIVE TESTING AND SYMPTOM EXAGGERATION

There is no conclusive evidence to suggest that PTSD patients demonstrate deficits in most cognitive functions.(26, 27) First, it is unclear whether deficits found reflect a preexisting vulnerability to PTSD or a deficit brought about by the disorder itself.(28) In addition, any cognitive deficits observed could stem not from the PTSD but rather from a comorbid disorder, such as depression, which is commonly comorbid with PTSD.(29)

Whether or not PTSD patients actually suffer a decline in cognitive function and whether this is caused directly by PTSD or by a comorbid disorder, cognitive testing can potentially be used to detect symptom exaggeration in PTSD, particularly in cases where a decline in cognitive function is reported. No cognitive dysfunction should result in an individual performing worse than if he were to guess the answers on a particular test. Several cognitive tests have been used to identify individuals who are "working hard" to appear to have low cognitive abilities. For instance, in forced choice questions (where the subject is asked to choose the answer to each question from two or more options, only one of which is correct), even a patient who is unable to work out the answer to the question should attain a score comparable to the guess rate, determined by the number of options for each question. Improbable patterns of performance can also be identified as a person trying to "fake bad." The detection of a probable case of symptom exaggeration by this method was described by Rosen and Powel (30) in their case description of a patient who, claiming to suffer memory deficits as part of his PTSD symptomatology, completed a forced choice memory test with an accuracy of only 31%, where the two-choice design set the chance rate at 50%. Through the use of this test it was apparent that the patient was making a concerted effort to perform badly rather than that he had genuine memory deficits.

Despite the potential use of cognitive testing in detecting symptom exaggeration for patients claiming cognitive deficits, a paradoxical finding in a neuropsychological study is that issuing a warning prior to the test, that they should complete the test honestly because the testers are able to identify malingering, actually hampers the test's ability to detect feigning, as patients seeking to mislead do so in a less pronounced way, making it harder to detect the effect.(31, 32) This can be expected in PTSD patients as well, implying that attempts to identify exaggerators should not be made known to the patient.

Other cognitive phenomena can be utilized in detecting patients who are exaggerating their symptom severity. For instance, the primacy and recency effects observed in intact memory performance (the tendency to remember more words from the beginning and end of a list than from the middle) are also present in memory-deficient patients, yet these effects are hard to emulate by individuals who are reporting less than they truly recall from what they were asked to remember.(33)

PHYSIOLOGICAL MEASURES AND SYMPTOM EXAGGERATION

The idea of being able to use physiological measures to confirm a patient's symptom descriptions is very interesting. Just as a blood test can help us to measure physiological attributes, a person's physiological measures might be harnessed to help us to answer as to whether a particular individual has PTSD. Several studies have attempted to find such a measure, examining heart rate, blood pressure, skin conductance, and so on, both at baseline and after traumatic stressors; however, Gerardi et al. (34) found that only diastolic blood pressure differentiated PTSD from a control group trying to fake PTSD symptoms. Thus, it appears that physiological measures that were examined so far were not particularly effective in differentiating between genuine and faked PTSD.

A further issue with the use of some of the physiological measures is related to their specificity and validity. For instance, in a 6-year follow-up of survivors of the Oklahoma City bombing, although exposed individuals were found to have a more pronounced autonomic response to trauma reminders than nonexposed individuals, this pronounced autonomic response was not correlated to whether or not they had developed PTSD.(35) Thus, it would appear that physiological measures used here (heart rate and blood pressure) were not discriminative enough to differentiate between trauma survivors with and without PTSD, implying that the current measures available would not be effective in identifying cases of symptom exaggeration. Rare cases of individuals claiming to have PTSD when in fact they did not even experience the trauma they claim to have suffered might perhaps offer a further physiological measure as a potential additional diagnostic reliner, but the subtlety of overreporting appears to require a less direct approach.

CONCLUSION

Because per definition there is an external and known trigger, PTSD is linked to compensation proportionally more than other psychiatric disorders. Although PTSD should not be reduced to a compensation neurosis, the issue of symptom exaggeration need not be swept under the carpet. The search for differentiating individuals with genuine PTSD vs. those who are intentionally or nonintentionally exacerbating their symptoms is important in clinical practice as well as in clinical research, as the participants who fake PTSD are weakening the validity and the confidence of the diagnosis in PTSD.

There is a fine line that clinicians should walk when exploring the various ways to identify symptom overreporting. An individual who is intentionally pretending to have developed PTSD should be neither diagnosed, treated, nor granted benefits. On the other hand, handling of overreporters needs to be much more delicate, as it might include a group of genuine PTSD sufferers who are, for whatever reason, and at different levels of consciousness, exaggerating or embellishing their symptoms. Even for those who are deliberately doing this, the diagnosis of PTSD may still be valid based on their genuine symptoms and they have a right to be treated and to receive compensation in line with the severity of their true symptoms.

Reviewing the current literature suggests three major avenues that were explored in order to aid the clinician in identifying overreporting. The methods that have been examined were scales (such as MMPI-2 and SIRS), cognitive tests (such as forced-choice and free-recall memory tests), and physiological measures (which include heart rate, blood pressure, GSR, etc.). Unfortunately, all of these methods were not found to have either the specificity or the validity required from a respected diagnostic test.

As the awareness of PTSD is growing and subsequently there is a parallel growth in the compensation related to PTSD, the need to find appropriate tools to aid the clinician in differential diagnosis of symptom exacerbation in PTSD is growing.

The authors believe that modern technologies (like brain imaging) and better cognitive solutions will be instrumental in developing the appropriate tools to differentiate between symptom exacerbation and genuine PTSD.

REFERENCES

1. American Psychiatric Association. *Diagnostic and statistical manual of mental disorders* (4th ed.). Washington, DC: Author; 1994
2. Kessler RC. Posttraumatic stress disorder: the burden to the individual and to society. J Clin Psychiatry 2000; 61 (5):4–12.
3. Kessler RC, Sonnega A, Bromet E, Hughes M, Nelson CB. Posttraumatic stress disorder in the National Comorbidity Survey. Arch Gen Psychiatry 1995; 52(12):1048–60.
4. Rosen GM. DSM's cautionary guideline to rule out malingering can protect the PTSD data base. Anxiety Disorders 2006; 20: 530–535.
5. Summerfield D. A critique of seven assumptions behind psychological trauma programmes in war–affected areas. Social Science and Medicine 1999; 48: 1449–1462.
6. American Psychiatric Association. *Diagnostic and statistical manual of mental disorders* (3rd ed.). Washington, DC: Author; 1980.
7. Eldridge G. Contextual issues in the assessment of posttraumatic stress disorder. Journal of Traumatic Stress 1991; 4: 7–23.
8. Lees–Haley P, Dunn J. The ability of naïve subjects to report symptoms of mild brain injury, post–traumatic stress disorder, major depression, and generalized anxiety disorder. Journal of Clinical Psychology 1994; 50: 253–256.
9. Burges C, McMillan T. The ability of naïve participants to report symptoms of post–traumatic stress disorder. British Journal of Clinical Psychology 2001; 40(2): 209–214.
10. McNally R. Progress and controversy in the study of posttraumatic stress disorder. Annual Review of Psychology 2003; 54:229–252.
11. Hickling EJ, Blanchard EB, Mundy E, Galovski TE. Detection of malingered MVA related posttraumatic stress disorder: An investigation of the ability to detect professional actors by experienced clinicians, psychological tests and psychophysiological assessment. Journal of Forensic Psychology Practice 2002; 2: 33–54.
12. Rosen GM. The *Aleutian Enterprise* sinking and posttraumatic stress disorder: Misdiagnosis in clinical and forensic settings. Professional Psychology: Research and Practice 1995; 1: 82–87.
13. Blanchard EB, Hickling EJ, Taylor AE et al. Effects of litigation settlements on posttraumatic stress symptoms in motor vehicle accident victims. Journal of Traumatic Stress 1998; 11(2): 337–354.
14. Ehlers A, Mayou RA, Bryant B. Psychological predictors of chronic posttraumatic stress disorder after motor vehicle accidents. Journal of Abnormal Psychiatry 1998; 107(3):508–19.
15. Sayer NA, Spoont M, Nelson DB, Clothier B, Murdoch M. Changes in psychiatric status and service use associated with continued compensation seeking after claim determinations for posttraumatic stress disorder. Journal of Traumatic Stress 2008; 21(1): 40–48.
16. Fontana A, Rosenheck R. Effects of compensation–seeking on treatment outcomes among veterans with posttraumatic stress disorder. Journal of Nervous and Mental Disease 1998; 186(4): 223–230.
17. Kozarić-Kovačić D, Bajs M, Vidošić S et al. Change of diagnosis of posttraumatic stress disorder related to compensation–seeking. Croatian Medical Journal 2004; 45(4): 427–433.
18. Knoll J, Resnick PJ. The detection of malingered post–traumatic stress disorder. Psychiatric Clinics of North America 2006; 29: 629–647.
19. Resnick PJ. My favorite tips for detecting malingering and violence risk. Psychiatric Clinics of North America 2007; 30: 227–232.
20. Rogers R, Kropp PR, Bagby RM, Dickens SE. Faking specific disorders: a study of the Structured Interview of Reported Symptoms (SIRS). Journal of Clinical Psychology 1992; 48(5):643–8.
21. Rogers R, Sewell KW, Martin MA, Vitacco MJ. Detection of feigned mental disorders: A meta–analysis of the MMPI–2 and malingering. Assessment 2003; 10(2): 160–177.
22. Gold PB, Frueh BC. Compensation–seeking and extreme exaggeration of psychopathology among combat veterans evaluated for posttraumatic stress disorder. Journal of Nervous and Mental Disease 1999; 187(11):680–684.
23. Rogers R, Payne JW, Berry DTR, Granacher RP Jr. Use of the SIRS in compensation cases: an examination of its validity and generalizability. Law Hum Behav. 2009; 33(3):213–24.
24. Guy LS, Kwartner PP, Miller HA. Investigating the M–FAST: psychometric properties and utility to detect diagnostic specific malingering. Behavioral Sciences & the Law 2006; 24(5): 687–702.
25. Guriel J, Yanez T, Fremouw W et al. Impact of coaching on malingered posttraumatic stress symptoms on the M–FAST and the TSI. Journal of Forensic Psychology Practice 2004; 4(2): 37–56.

26. Moore SA. Cognitive abnormalities in posttraumatic stress disorder. Current Opinion in Psychiatry 2008; 22:19–24.

27. Elsesser K, Sartory G. Memory performance and dysfunctional cognitions in recent trauma victims and patients with posttraumatic stress disorder. Clinical Psychology and Psychotherapy 2007; 14:464–474.

28. Parslow RA, Jorm AF. Pretrauma and posttrauma neurocognitive functioning and PTSD symptoms in a community sample of young adults. American Journal of Psychiatry 2007; 164: 509–515.

29. Johnsen GE, Kanagaratnam P, Asbjornsen AE. Memory impairments in posttraumatic stress disorder are related to depression. Journal of Anxiety Disorders 2008; 22:464–474.

30. Rosen GM, Powel JE. Use of a symptom validity test in the forensic assessment of posttraumatic stress disorder. Anxiety Disorders 2003; 17: 361–367.

31. Youngjohn JR, Lees–Haley PR, Binder LM. Comment: Warning Malingerers Produces More Sophisticated Malingering. Archives of Clinical Neuropsychology 1999; 14(6): 511–515.

32. Youngjohn JR. Confirmed attorney coaching prior to neuropsychological evaluation. Assessment 1995; 2: 279–283.

33. Bernard LC. The detection of faked deficits on the Rey Auditory Verbal Learning Test: the effect of serial position. Archives of Clinical Neuropsychology 1991; 6(1–2):81–8.

34. Gerardi RJ, Blanchard EB, Kolb LC. Ability of Vietnam veterans to dissimulate a psychophysiological assessment for posttraumatic stress disorder. Behavior Therapy 1989; 20: 229–243.

35. Tucker PM, Pfefferbaum B, North CS et al. Physiologic reactivity despite emotional resilience several years after direct exposure to terrorism. American Journal of Psychiatry 2007; 164(2):230–5.

15 | Future directions

Joseph Zohar, Murray B Stein, and David Nutt

This second volume of our posttraumatic stress disorder (PTSD) book allows us to see how far we have come over the past 7 years. It is clear that some aspects of knowledge regarding PTSD have progressed significantly, whereas others have moved on only a little. In this chapter we pick up some of the critical issues relating to knowledge gaps and future research needs.

THE BRAIN MECHANISMS OF PTSD

One of the major advances in research in PTSD has been in identifying the brain circuits that underpin the disorder. The Liberzon chapter pulls together a significant body of work that has defined a circuitry of emotion and its dysregulation in PTSD, showing relevant overlaps with brain regions involved in other anxiety disorders and in emotional regulation. The emerging evidence for some dysregulation of cortical function in the medial PFC is potentially very exciting. What is now needed is to know to what extent this region directs the full panoply of symptom expression in PTSD, that is, is it linked to the three symptom clusters or preferentially to one such as memory? Moreover, we need to know the origins of the fMRI abnormalities. One exciting possibility is that they might reflect alterations in GABA-A receptor function as suggested by the PET imaging data detailed in the chapter also.

A deficiency of GABA-A benzodiazepine receptors could lead to local PFC regulation as reported in the PET scans. How can we reconcile this with the fact that drugs that might be predicted to rectify this binding deficit, the benzodiazepines, seem to be ineffective in preventing PTSD development or in its treatment (see chapter 10). One reason for this might be that the benzodiazepines tend to produce adaptive changes in their binding sites that lead to a reduction in their function over time, thus undermining any therapeutic actions (see 1). If this is the case then there are potential ways to investigate such possibilities; in particular, one would predict that in animals that had been given a course of a benzodiazepine, with the course suspended after a specific period, the receptors would be in a state that could predispose to PTSD. An effective rat model of PTSD has now been developed (see chapter 10) so testing this theory is now possible. Of course, a GABA-A benzodiazepine deficit might be amenable to treatment with other new agents that do not suffer from the long-term problems that the traditional benzodiazepines cause. Such new drugs include subtype-selective agonists such for the a2 and a3 subtypes of the receptor.(2) These drugs are being trialed in the treatment of GAD and panic disorder, so exploring their action in PTSD is a possibility. Moreover, as these two specific subtypes have rather specific distribution in brain, being particularly located in circuits that regulate emotion and sleep, abnormalities of them might well be candidates for the pathogenesis of symptom generation in PTSD; such studies would again be amenable to investigation in animal models where both whole brain imaging and localized receptor mapping could be carried out.

The other main neurotransmitter in the cortex is glutamate, which is almost certainly involved in the learning of traumatic memories. Although imaging glutamate is currently not possible in humans, there are new tracers in development that may allow this in future years. Again animal studies might point to the best direction—would a marker of the ion-channel–linked (ionotropic) receptors be more informative than one for the metabotropic ones? One can make credible cases for either ionotropic or metabotropic receptors, or indeed both, being involved in PTSD, and there is some research underway, manipulating each of these in anxiety as well as other brain disorders. In particular, the work to augment ionotropic glutamate function with drugs that mimic the cotransmitter glycine (e.g., D-cycloserine) is well established in both animal and human models of stress learning. It is now established that learning to overcome stress-related anxiety in animals, for example, extinction of fear-based behavior, requires new learning, and this can be enhanced by D-cycloserine (see chapter by 9). Early human studies in phobic humans found similar results and so there are ongoing studies now in patients with PTSD who are engaging in psychotherapy treatment. Results should be available in a year or two, so watch this space!

HOW DO CURRENT TREATMENTS WORK?

It is now generally agreed (see 3) that SSRIs are the preferred first-line treatment of PTSD. However, they do not work immediately; usually it takes 3 or more weeks for a clear therapeutic action to emerge. The usual explanation for this is that the immediate action of SSRIs is to increase 5HT levels; this increase in 5HT then stimulates the 5HT1A autoreceptors on the raphe cell bodies and dendrites. As these are inhibitory receptors, the firing rate of the 5HT neurones is slowed down, limiting the potential increase of 5HT in the synaptic cleft that reuptake blockade can produce. However, over time the 5HT1A autoreceptors desensitize; thus the firing rate returns to normal and the 5HT released from cell firing cannot be taken up due to the SSRI effects, which leads to increased postsynaptic 5HT function. Subsequently, there may be adaptive changes in postsynaptic processes such as receptors, second messengers, gene products, and even new neurones (neurogenesis) that may produce the final therapeutic outcome.

In the treatment of depression with SSRIs there is considerable discussion about the role of synaptic versus postsynaptic mechanisms in the action of antidepressants. Although postsynaptic changes are well described in rodent models, they are harder to demonstrate in humans, possibly for technical reasons. One exception is the paroxetine study reported in chapter 5, which found that long-term treatment of PTSD with paroxetine increased hippocampal volume, suggesting some neurogenerating actions of 5HT. This increase in size was also associated with improved memory function. In another anxiety disorder, that is, panic disorder, clinical recovery on SSRI treatment has been found to restore the deficit in 5HT1A receptors found on PET scanning in untreated patients.(4) Again this suggests some role for 5HT in restoring normal neuronal function.

However, it may be that persistent elevations of 5HT are necessary for the therapeutic effects of SSRIs, for if brain 5HT is depleted using the tryptophan depletion paradigm then the antidepressant efficacy of SSRIs is undermined (5–7), although the same effect was not seen in OCD. (8) Recently we have shown that in panic (9) social anxiety disorder (10) tryptophan depletion produces relapse in patients who recovered using SSRIs suggesting that tonic 5HT function is necessary to maintain wellness in recovery. Since then we have been able to conduct a similar study in PTSD.(11) A total 10 patients who had made a good recovery on SSRIs (so they were rated fully or very markedly recovered on the CGI) underwent tryptophan depletion or sham depletion in a randomized crossover design. At the time of peak depletion (5 hours), patients were exposed to their traumas using autobiographical scripts. These provoked the full range of PTSD anxiety symptoms with physiological changes in blood pressure and heart rate despite the patients all being recovered. However, on the tryptophan depletion day, all measures of symptoms and physiology were significantly enhanced compared with the control day. This suggests that 5HT is critical to restraining the expression of anxiety in PTSD when treated with SSRIs and that there may be commonalities of action of the SSRIs across the range of anxiety disorders. It would be very interesting to see whether similar reductions in 5HT1A receptors are found in untreated PTSD as found in panic (4) and social anxiety (12) and whether they recover on successful treatment.

ANTISTRESS TREATMENTS?

One of the great goals of PTSD medicine is to find preventative mechanisms. Of course, such agents would be challenging to develop due to the relatively small percentage of exposed individuals going on to develop PTSD (though in incidents like rape this is the majority) and the need to ensure that other sequelae of trauma, especially depression, were also remedied or at least prevented from getting worse than the existing state.

Therefore, what are the processes that underlie the development of PTSD that could be amenable to early intervention? In essence, they are those relating to memory formation, that

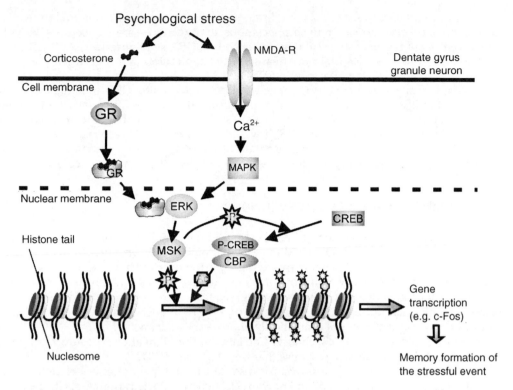

Figure 15.1 The necessary confluence of cortisol [through GR receptors] and glutamate [through NMDA receptors] in the production of memory.(15)

is, glutamate and GABA, and those related to emotional processing (noradrenaline 5HT) and those related to stress (cortisol plus related central regulators of this axis, for example, CRF and ACTH). The potential role of glutamate drugs in "unlearning" PTSD has been discussed briefly in the chapter on treatment (chapter 9), but even if this is successful, there is still the question of whether antiglutamate drugs could prevent the acquisition of the traumatic memories in the first place.(13)

As we have seen in Bisson et al.'s (chapter 10), GABA-A drugs, in particular the benzodiazepines, are not effective as prophylaxis; however, so far only nonselective benzodiazepines have been used. Given the multiple subtypes of the GABA-A/benzodiazepine receptor and new selective agents that are now being studied in humans, at some stage, it would be sensible to see whether these might have utility in PTSD prevention; certainly they seem to have less disadvantages in terms of tolerance abuse liability and withdrawal than the nonselective benzodiazepines.(2)

As Bisson et al mentioned in chapter 10, antinoradrenaline drugs, especially beta blockers and the a1 antagonist prazosin, have already been considered. A very recent paper extends the studies on b-blockers, describing the finding that a dose of 40 mg propranolol has been shown to "erase the expression of the fear memory" when given prior to the fear memory being reactivated.(14) If such an effect could be demonstrated in patients with PTSD then it could have significant clinical utility.

Another approach is to use established treatments but earlier in the course of the illness. The potential prophylactic role of the SSRI escitalopram is under investigation in a major Israeli study led by Shalev that will soon report its findings. But what of anticortisol agents? The central regulation and actions of cortisol are well understood and provide new treatment targets. Cortisol release is controlled by CRF (corticotrophin-releasing factor), a peptide found in a number of brain regions that regulates aspects of behavior such as grooming, eating, sexual drive, and sleep as well as stimulating ACTH release from the hypothalamus. ACTH then stimulates cortisol production and release from the adrenal glands, sending feedback onto the brain, to the inhibition of both CRF and ACTH release through two receptors, namely, the mineralocorticoid (MR) and glucocorticoid (GR) receptors. These receptors are highly expressed in limbic brain regions and regulate emotional as well as endocrine responses to cortisol. In the hippocampus, they are necessary coreceptors with glutamate receptors to regulate stressful memory encoding.(15 – see figure 15.1) Anti-GR drugs have been developed as potential new treatments of depression (16) that, therefore, could potentially be explored in the treatment of PTSD.

A complementary approach is to reduce CRF activation using CRF antagonists, several of which exist and which are being tested in depression also.(17) We have shown that a new CRF 1 receptor antagonist reduces anxiety in a stress model in normal volunteers involved in a 20-minute CO2 inhalation procedure.(18) It would be of great interest to test these agents in PTSD as soon as possible. Given the proviso that the cortisol system in chronic PTSD may be subfunctioning, the primary target would need to be prophylactic rather than curative.

AN OPPORTUNITY FOR EARLY INTERVENTION?

Following a cerebrovascular accident (CVA), there is a 3-hour "window" from the onset in which "clot-busting" drugs can be administered to relieve thrombosis. After a myocardial infarction ("heart attack"), reperfusion of the infarct-related artery in the very first hour significantly reduces mortality rates. The common denominator is that immediate intervention is given in order to prevent/decrease the impending (usually devastating) sequelae of those events, which often trigger a chain of pathological processes. The concept is that if the right intervention is given during the "window of opportunity," it might dramatically improve the outcome.

Is there a "golden hour" in psychiatry? Can intervention right after exposure to traumatic events attenuate the pathological response that we refer to as PTSD?

PTSD is unique among other psychiatric disorders in that the trigger is well defined, not only with regard to time (we can often know exactly when it started) but also with regard to cause (a "Criterion A" traumatic event). Hence, it would be quite straightforward to develop an animal model, as one can induce PTSD, for example, by exposure of animal to the predator (19), and carefully monitoring behavior afterwards. What is unique for PTSD is that most of the individuals who are exposed to traumatic events eventually recover from it, and only a minority (10–20%; 20) develop PTSD. An animal model has been developed that involves exposing the rat to its natural predator (a cat) and also mimics PTSD by setting apart the minority of those affected (via cutoff behavioral criteria; 21–23 and chapter 7 of this book). This animal model of PTSD may be unique among animal models of psychiatric disorders because in PTSD it is feasible to create a situation that might eventually lead to the disorder (this is certainly not the case for any other psychiatric disorder, in which neither the precipitating event, nor the timing of the disorder is defined).

The authors submit that use of translational research, in which a valid animal model will be used, might be able to provide better insight with regard to beneficial versus harmful interventions in this narrow (albeit as yet poorly defined as to whether it is hours or days) window of opportunity. We anticipate that the pendulum in PTSD research will shift from treatment of established (and often very chronic) PTSD to innovative approaches aiming at limiting the development of PTSD (and other related forms of psychopathology, such as depression) following trauma exposure. Such approaches will focus at administering preventive interventions during these golden hours.

Actually, there are some initial encouraging data pertaining to administration of pharmacological agents early in the aftermath of traumatic stress, such as cortisol (22), galanin (24), and oxytocin.(24) There are also some hints regarding the potential benefit of early administration of SSRIs (25), opiate agonists such as morphine (26), and possibly betaadrenergic blocking agents such as propranolol (27); the list will probably be expanded. It might be that, ultimately, PTSD will be the first psychiatric disorder in which the focus could be on prevention as opposed to treatment. This of course will depend on whether the field will be able to develop effective interventions in the golden hours— the first few hours immediately after the traumatic event. Animal models suggest that targeting the consolidation or reconsolidation of the traumatic event will be instrumental for such treatments. If we can manage to interfere with the consolidation or maintenance of the traumatic memory during the golden hours (28, 29), it may be possible to prevent the development of PTSD.

Along these lines, sophisticated psychotherapeutic approaches aimed at altering or reducing the impact of the traumatic memories could be another potential approach to be followed. There are, in fact, strong data supporting the use of cognitive–behavioral approaches in the aftermath of trauma to prevent the development (or reduce the progression into chronicity) of PTSD.(30) It may someday be possible to use pharmacotherapy to augment the effects of exposure on extinction of fear.(14) For those individuals whose minds are trapped in traumatic pasts, the future is bright!

REFERENCES

1. Nutt DJ. Death and dependence: current controversies over the selective serotonin reuptake inhibitors. J Psychopharmacol 2003; 17: 355–64.
2. Nutt DJ. GABA-A receptors: subtypes, regional distribution and function. In J Clin Sleep Med 2006; 2(2): 5–11.
3. Stein D, Cloitre M, Nemeroff CB et al. Cape Town Consensus on Posttraumatic Stress Disorder. CNS Spectr 2008; 13: 12 (Suppl 19).
4. Nash JR, Sargent PA, Rabiner EA et al. A positron emission tomography study of serotonin 5-HT$_{1A}$ receptor availability in untreated and recovered patients with panic disorder. Br J Psychiatry 2008; 193: 1–6.
5. Delgado PL, Charney DS, Price LH et al. Serotonin function and the mechanism of antidepressant action. Reversal of antidepressant-induced remission by rapid depletion of plasma tryptophan. Arch Gen Psychiatry 1990; 47: 411–8.
6. Hood SD, Bell CJ, Nutt DJ. Acute tryptophan depletion part 1: rationale and methodology: Australia and New Zealand. J of Psychiatry 2005; 39: 558–64.
7. Bell CJ, Hood SD, Nutt DJ. Acute tryptophan depletion part 2: Australia and New Zealand. J of Psychiatry 2005; 39: 565–74.
8. Barr LC, Goodman WK, McDougle. Tryptophan depletion in patients with obsessive compulsive disorder who respond to SSRIs. Arch Gen Psychiatry 2004; 51: 309–17.
9. Bell C, Forshall S, Adrover M et al. Does 5-HT restrain panic? A tryptophan depletion study in panic disorder patients recovered on paroxetine. J Psychopharmacol 2002; 16: 5–14.
10. Argyropoulos S, Hood SD, Adrover M et al. Tryptophan depletion reverses the therapeutic effect of selective serotonin reuptake inhibitors in social anxiety disorder. Biological psychiatr 2004; 56: 503–9.
11. Corchs F, Nutt DJ, Hood S, Bernik M. 5HT and sensitivity to trauma-related exposure in SSRI-recovered PTSD. Biol Psychiatry 2009; Biol Psychiatry 2009; 66(1):17–24.
12. Lanzenberger RR, Mitterhauser M, Spindelegger C et al. Reduced serotonin-1A receptor binding in social anxiety disorder. Biol Psychiatry 2007; 61: 1081–9.
13. O'Brien M, Nutt D. Loss of consciousness and post-traumatic stress disorder. A clue to aetiology and treatment. Br J Psychiatry 1998; 173: 102–4.
14. Kindt M, Soeter M, Vervliet B. Beyond extinction: erasing human fear responses and preventing the return of fear. Nat. Neurosci 2009; 12(3): 256-8.
15. Reul H and Nutt DJ. Cortisol and glutamate—a critical confluence in PTSD? J Psychopharmacol 2008; 22:469–72.
16. Schatzberg AF, Lindley S. Glucocorticoid antagonists in neuropsychotic disorders. Eur J Pharmacol 2008; 583: 358–64.
17. Ising M, Holsboer F. CRH1 receptor antagonists for the treatment of depression and anxiety. Exp Clin Psychopharmacol 2007; 15(6): 519–28.
18. Bailey JE, Papadopoulos A, Diaper A et al. Preliminary Evidence of Efficacy of a CRF1 Receptor Antagonist in the7.5% CO2 Model of Anxiety. Journal of Psychopharmacology Summer meeting supplement 2008.
19. Adamec RE, Shallow T. Lasting effects on rodent anxiety of a single exposure to a cat. Physiol Behav 1993; 54: 101–9.
20. Yehuda R, McFarlane AC. Conflict between current knowledge about posttraumatic stress disorder and its original conceptual basis. Am J Psychiatry 1995; 152(12): 1705–13.
21. Cohen H, Zohar J, Matar M. The Relevance of differential response to trauma in an animal model of post-traumatic stress disorder. Biological Psychiatry 2003; 53: 463–73.
22. Cohen H, Matar MA, Buskila D, Kaplan Z, Zohar J. Early post-stressor intervention with high-dose corticosterone attenuates posttraumatic stress response in an animal model of posttraumatic stress disorder. Biol Psychiatry 2008; 64(8): 708–17.
23. Cohen H, Matar M, Zohar J. Animal models of posttraumatic stress disorder. In: P.M. Conn (Ed) Sourcebook of Models for Biomedical Research. Humana Press 2008; 591–602.

24. Kozlovsky N, Matar MA, Kaplan Z, Zohar J, Cohen H. The role of the galaninergic system in modulating stress-related responses in an animal model of posttraumatic stress disorder. Biol Psychiatry 2009; 65(5): 383–91.

25. Matar MA, Cohen H, Kaplan Z, Zohar J. The effect of early poststressor intervention with sertraline on behavioral responses in an animal model of posttraumatic stress disorder. Neuropsychopharmacology 2006; 31(12):2610–8.

26. Bryant RA, Creamer M, O'Donnell M, Silove D, McFarlane AC. A study of the protective function of acute morphine administration on subsequent posttraumatic stress disorder. Biol Psychiatry 2009; 65(5): 438–40.

27. Brunet A, Orr SP, Tremblay J et al. Effect of post-retrieval propranolol on psychophysiologic responding during subsequent script-driven traumatic imagery in post-traumatic stress disorder. J Psychiatr Res 2008; 42(6): 503–6.

28. Kozlovsky N, Kaplan Z, Zohar J et al. Protein synthesis inhibition before or after stress exposure results in divergent endocrine and BDNF responses disassociated from behavioral responses. Depress Anxiety 2008; 25(5): E24–34.

29. Cohen H, Kozlovsky N, Matar MA, Kaplan Z, Zohar J. Mapping the brain pathways of traumatic memory: inactivation of protein kinase M zeta in different brain regions disrupts traumatic memory processes and attenuates traumatic stress responses; submitted.

30. Bryant RA, Moulds ML, Nixon RVD. Cognitive behaviour therapy of acute stress disorder: a four-year follow-up. Behav Res Ther 2003; 41(4): 489–94.

Index

Page numbers in *italics* refer to tables; those in **bold** to figures.

[123I]iomazenil 46
99mTc hexamethylpropyleneamineoxime (HMPAO) SPECT 37

acute PTSD 7–8
acute stress disorder 7
  and pediatric PTSD 148–9
  symptoms 7
adrenergic agents 122
afferent sensory input 52
Alprazolam 95
amnesia 52
amygdala 40, 52, 59–60
  aversive conditioning 43
animal genetic studies 80–1
  knockout models 80
animal model 88
  behavioral assessments 89
  cutoff behavioral criteria
    classifications 89–91
    selective study 91–5
Anisomycin 95
anterior cingulate gyrus 52
anticonvulsants 120–1
antidepressants 116–20
  selective serotonin reuptake
    inhibitors 116–18
  dual reuptake inhibitors 118
  tricyclic antidepressants 118–19
  Bupropion 119
  monoamine oxidase inhibitors 119
  Mirtazapine 119–20
antipsychotics 121–2
antistress treatments 196–8
anxiety disorders 105, 109
anxiety 56
anxiogenic' memories 55
apolipoprotein E gene 76
avoidance symptoms 30–1

behavior therapy
  anxiety disorders 109

behavioral sensitization 54
  see enhanced stress sensitivity
benzodiazepine 95, 121
blood oxygen level–dependent method
    (BOLD) signal 37
brain circuits
  cognitive appraisal 52
  default network 62
  finding
  memory function 52–3
  neuroimaging
    functional study 58
    activity 58–9
  neurological working model 51–2
    fear behavior 52
  performance 57–8
  traumatic memory
    formation of 54–7
brain mechanisms 195
brain-derived neurotrophic
    factor gene 76
Brodmann Area 32 52
Bupropion 119

catecholamines 55
childhood
  abuse in 28
  see also pediatric PTSD
Chromatin 54
chronic PTSD 7–8
Clinician-Administered PTSD
    Scale (CAPS) 103
Cochrane Database review 101
cognitive activation studies 39
cognitive appraisal 44–5
cognitive reappraisal 45
cognitive–behavioral therapy (CBT)
  anxiety management techniques (AMT)
    105
  exposure therapy 101–4
  eye movement desensitization and
    reprocessing 106–7

pediatric PTSD 155–6
  systematic desensitization 105–6
  virtual reality exposure
      therapy 104–5
cognitive–emotional interactions 44–6
comorbid disorders
  and genetics 79–80
  pediatric PTSD 149–50
  postdisasters 180
comorbidity 6
  mental health 20–1
  physical health conditions 21–2
  suicidal behavior 21
  and trauma spectrum 33
corticosteroid 94
cross-cultural study 167–9
  ethnoculture 167–9
  trauma-related disorder 170–2
culture 163
  trauma on 169
  see also ethnoculture
cutoff behavioral criteria (CBC), *90, 91*
  classification 89–90
    minimal behavioral response 89
    extreme behavioral response 89
  time factor 91
  physiological data 91–2
  strain/genetic studies 92
  molecular neurobiology,
      correlation 93
  drug study 93–5

D-cycloserine (DCS) 109
delayed-onset PTSD 8
*Diagnostic and Statistical Manual of Mental
    Disorders* 12
diagnostic dilemmas, in assessment
  of trauma 26–9
  symptoms 29–32
  structured instrument 33
dissociative symptoms 32
Dopamine-related genes 72, 75
dual reuptake inhibitors
duloxetine 118
dynamic psychotherapy 100–1

early interventions 198–9
  theoretical models 128
  social models 128
  psychological models 128–9
  biological models 129–30
  types of 130–1

efficacy of 131
    multiple session interventions *132–40*
earthquake imagery 38
emotion regulation 44
emotions 28–9
enhanced stress sensitivity 54
ethnoculture
  cross-cultural study 167–9
  culture, definition 163–4
  individual and social
      conflicts 165–6
  meaning of 165
  symptoms, presentation of 169
  trauma, impact on 169–70
  traumatic memory 166–7
exposure
  characterization of 179
  postdisasters 180
exposure therapy 101–4
extreme behavioral response 89
extreme fear 52
eye movement desensitization and
    reprocessing (EMDR) 106
  pediatric PTSD 156

fear conditioning
  inhibition of 109
  extinction 56–7
FK506 binding protein 5 (FKBP5)
    gene 77–8
frontal cortical areas 53
functional imaging techniques 58
functional magnetic resonance imaging
    (fMRI) 36–7
  and receptor imaging 46

gamma-aminobutyric acid gene (GABA)
    46, 76–7, 195
gene expression 78–9
General Health Questionnaire 103
general population studies
  on PTSD 12, 13
    lifetime and prevalence of *14*
  on traumatic events 12
genes 54
genetic mechanism 70
  animal genetic studies 80
  apolipoprotein E gene 76
  brain-derived neurotrophic factor
      gene 76
  comorbidity 79–80
  Dopamine-related genes 72, 75

familial aggregation studies 70–1
FK506 binding protein 5 (FKBP5)
    gene 77–8
gamma-aminobutyric acid
    gene 76–7
gene expression 78–9
glucocorticoid receptor gene 77
molecular studies 71–2
monoamine oxidase gene 75–6
neuropeptide Y gene 78
serotonin transporter gene 75
twin studies 71
glucocorticoid dysregulation
    mechanisms 123
glucocorticoid receptor gene 77
glucocorticoids 55

hippocampus 43, 52, 60
horror 28
human-made disaster 176–7
hyperarousal symptoms 31–2
hypnosis 99
hypnotherapy 99
hypnotics 121

Impact of Event Scale (IES) 99
incident disorders
    postdisaster, assessment of 179–80
Institute of Medicine 101
interventional studies
    postdisasters 181

longitudinal study
    postdisasters 181

malingering 187
medial prefrontal cortex (MPF) 53
memories 54
    see also traumatic memories
mental health comorbidities 20–1
Miller Forensic Assessment of Symptoms
    (M-FAST) 191
minimal behavioral response 89
Minnesota Multiphasic Personality
    Inventory 190–1
Mirtazapine 119–20
molecular genetic studies 71–2
monoamine oxidase gene 75–6
monoamine oxidase inhibitors 119
motor cortex 53
MPFC 59–60
multiple traumatic events 15

N methyl D aspartase (NMDA) 54
natural disasters 168, 177–8
Nefazodone 120
neural activation 38
neural circuitry 51–2
    fear behavior 52
    sensitization 54
neuroimaging 36
    of brain 58–9
    cognitive activation study 39–41
    cross-sectional symptom
        severity 38–9
    functional connectivity
        analyses 41
    functional magnetic resonance imaging
        (fMRI) 36–7
    functions 41–2
    symptom provocation study 37–8
    threat-related process 43–4
neuropeptide Y gene 78
neurotrophins 93
novel agent 122–3

olfactory sensory input 52
orbitofrontal cortex (OFC) 52

parahippocampus 61
parietal cortex 53
pediatric PTSD
    community surveys 147–8
    and acute stress disorder 148–9
    comorbidity 149–50
    neurobiology 150–1
    risk and resilience 151–2
    assessment 152–4
    treatment 154
        psychotherapies 155–7
        pharmacotherapies 157–8
    selective serotonin reuptake inhibitors
        157–8
pharmacotherapy
    adrenergic agents 122
    anticonvulsants 120–1
    antidepressants 116–20
    antipsychotics 121–2
    benzodiazepines 121
    hypnotics 121
    novel agent 122–3
    pediatric PTSD 157–8
physical health comorbidities 21–2
Positive Feedback Cycle 130
positron emission tomography (PET) 36

postdisasters
  human-made and technological disasters 176–7
  interventional studies 181
  longitudinal studies 181
  methodological changes 178–80
  natural disasters 177–8
  research directions 180–1
posterior cingulate cortex 53
posttraumatic stress disorder (PTSD)
  association studies 73–4
  course of 181
  definition 1
  diagnosis 2
  heterogeneity 62
  mental and physical comorbidities 20–2
  neuroanatomical impairments 39
  neuroimaging studies 36
  population studies 12
  prevalence of 17–18
    sex difference 18–19
  process implicated 43–4
  risk factors for 20
  time course 6, 43
    habituation and extinction 43–4
  and traumatic events 12
  types 7–8
precuneus 61
predator-scent stress paradigm 88–9
  PSS 89
prolonged exposure 102
psychosocial treatments
  anxiety management techniques (AMT) 105
  combined treatment approaches 107–10
  exposure therapy 101–4
  psychotherapy 108–10
  virtual reality exposure therapy 104–5
psychotherapy 108–10, 155
  pediatric PTSD 155–7
PTSD symptoms 5

rape 28, 102
  anxiety management techniques 105
  conditions, in PTSD 102
receptor imaging 46
  on inhibitory systems 46
reexperience symptoms 29–30
regional cerebral blood flow (rCBF) 37

Screening Tool for Early Predictors 156–7
  early identification 156–7
secondary traumatization 28
selective serotonin reuptake inhibitors (SSRI) 196
  pediatric PTSD 157–8
  treatment, duration 117–18
  Sertraline 93
sensitization
serotonin transporter gene 75
serotonin/norepinephrine reuptake inhibitors 118
severity 187
  exacerbation 6
sex differences
  in prevalence of PTSD 18–19
  traumatic events 15–16
single-photon emission tomography (SPECT) 36
spider phobia 110
Sertraline 93
startle reflex 56
stress inoculation training (SIT) 102, 105
striatum 53
Structured Interview of Reported Symptoms 191
suicidal behavior 21
symptom exaggeration
  classical basic approach 189
  clinical and social implications 187–8
  cognitive testing 191–2
  financial loss 188–9
  identify 189–90
    scales 190–1
  obstacles 189
  physiological measures 192
  vs. malingering 187
symptom severity
  correlation with 38–9
symptoms assessment 29
  for acute stress disorder 7
  avoidance symptoms 30–1
  dissociative symptoms 32
  hyperarousal symptoms 31–2
  reexperience symptoms 29–30
systematic desensitization 105–6

technological disaster 177
thalamus 61
threat-related neurocircuitry 43

time course 6
trauma
  childhood abuse 28
  DSM-IV
    diagnostic criteria 26
    definition 27
trauma-focused cognitive–behavior therapy
  pediatric PTSD 155–6
trauma-induced personality
    changes 8
trauma-related disorder 170–2
  cross-cultural study 167–9
trauma spectrum
  and comorbidity 33
Trauma Symptom Inventory (TSI) 191
traumatic cues 55
traumatic events
  amnesia 52
  definition 12
  dilemmas, in assessment 26–27
  exposures 19–20
  methods of assessing 12
  multiple traumatic events 15
  population studies 13
  prevalence of 13–15, 17–18

risk factors 16
sex difference 15–16
traumatic memories 52
  extinction, failure of 56–7
  fear conditioning 55–6
traumatic memory
  ethnoculture
    problem and nature 166–7
  grasping 167
  in children 148
  neurological working model
    features 51–2
traumatic stress–induced disorders
  time factor 91
tricyclic antidepressants 118–19

U.S. National Comorbidity Study 6

Venlafaxine 118
vicarious traumatization 28
Vietnam veterans 104
virtual reality exposure therapy 104–5

World War I 169
World War II 169